Medical Radiology

Diagnostic Imaging

For further volumes:
http://www.springer.com/series/4354

Stefan Hähnel
Editor

Inflammatory Diseases of the Brain

Second Edition

Springer

Editor
Prof. Dr. Stefan Hähnel
Neurologische Klinik
Abt. Neuroradiologie
Universitätsklinikum Heidelberg
Heidelberg
Germany

ISSN 0942-5373
ISBN 978-3-642-30519-1 ISBN 978-3-642-30520-7 (eBook)
DOI 10.1007/978-3-642-30520-7
Springer Heidelberg New York Dordrecht London

Library of Congress Control Number: 2013932336

Printed on acid-free paper

Springer is part of Springer Science+Business Media (www.springer.com)

Für Claudia, Theresa, Paulina und Felizia

Preface

Inflammatory diseases of the central nervous system (CNS) play an increasingly important role in the clinical practice of neuroradiology: Infections of the CNS frequently involve immunocompromised patients and come more and more along with the employment of innovative and aggressive immunosuppressive and immunomodulatory therapies. Noninfectious inflammations such as multiple sclerosis account for about 10 % of all neurological diseases.

In the second edition of this textbook special attendance was again credited to advanced MR techniques such as diffusion-weighted imaging, perfusion imaging, susceptibility weighted imaging as well as MR spectroscopy. These techniques provide important information for the differentiation between inflammatory brain diseases and other entities, such as neoplastic, metabolic, or ischemic diseases which have to be considered in the differential diagnosis.

Chapters with special topics are dealing with brain inflammation in childhood, with granulomatous diseases, and with MR imaging and spectroscopic specifics in the context of recommendations for imaging protocols.

The uniform structure of the particular chapters should help the reader to find one's way in the complexity of the diseases and to understand the coherence of clinical, epidemiological, pathological, and radiological specifics of brain inflammation.

We are aware that there are some repetitions between the chapters and themes: They should support learning and memorizing certain topics from different points of view.

Special importance was attached to furnish the book with many instructive figures—a neuroradiological book is living from abundant picturing. For those who are in hurry, therefore it might be worth to flick through the book while only looking at the images. In this second edition several images have been supplemented.

We hope that also the second edition will be of value not only for neuroradiologists but also for neurologists, pediatricians, and general radiologists. The co-authors and I would be thankful for constructive criticism from the reader: Please let us know if something can be improved in the next edition.

A lot of people contributed substantially to this book beside the actively involved authorship. First, I would like to thank my former chief Klaus Sartor (Heidelberg/Heppenheim), who had woken my interest for diagnostic neuroradiology as academic teacher more than 20 years ago, and who had inspired me to publish this book. Michael Knauth (Göttingen) accompanied me not only during publishing this book but also during my professional career, and as friend and companion. Further, I thank my current chief, Martin Bendszus, for giving me ample space to be myself for creating and editing this book. Last but not least, I thank Corinna Schäfer and Martina Wiese from Springer-Verlag who patiently assisted me during editing the manuscript book and advised me excellently regarding the structure of this book.

Heidelberg, November 2012 Stefan Hähnel

Contents

Contributors

Martin Bendszus Division of Neuroradiology, University of Heidelberg Medical Center, Im Neuenheimer Feld 400, 69120 Heidelberg, Germany

Birgit Ertl-Wagner Institute of Clinical Radiology, Ludwig Maximilians University Munich, Grosshadern Campus, Marchioninistrasse 15, 81377 Munich, Germany

Jens Fiehler Department of Diagnostic and Interventional Neuroradiology, Clinic and Policlinic of Neuroradiology, University of Hamburg-Eppendorf Medical Center, Martinistrasse 52, 20246 Hamburg, Germany

Stefan Hähnel Division of Neuroradiology, University of Heidelberg Medical Center, Im Neuenheimer Feld 400, 69120 Heidelberg, Germany

Christian Jacobi Department of Neurology, Krankenhaus Nordwest GmbH, Steinbacher Hohl 2-26, 60488 Frankfurt am Main, Germany

Thilo Kollmann Department of Psychiatry, University Hospital Basel, Wilhelm Kleinstrasse 27, 4012 Basel, Switzerland

Bodo Kress Department Neuroradiology, Central Institute of Radiology and Neuroradiology, Steinbacher Hohl 2-26, 60488 Frankfurt, Germany

Michael Lettau Division of Neuroradiology, Department of Neurosurgery, University of Freiburg Medical Center, Breisacher Strasse 64, 79106 Freiburg, Germany

Markus Möhlenbruch Division of Neuroradiology, University of Heidelberg Medical Center, Im Neuenheimer Feld 400, 69120 Heidelberg, Germany

Stefan Rohde Division of Neuroradiology, University of Heidelberg Medical Center, Im Neuenheimer Feld 400, 69120 Heidelberg, Germany

Angelika Seitz Department of Neuroradiology, Kopfklinik, University of Heidelberg, Im Neuenheimer Feld 400, 69120 Heidelberg, Germany

Joachim Spreer Department Neuroradiology, Cologne Medical Center, Ostmerheimer Strasse 200, 51109 Köln, Germany

Christoph Stippich Universitätsspital Basel, Klinik für Radiologie, Neuroradiologie und Nuklearmedizin, Petersgraben 4, 4031 Basel, Switzerland

Brigitte Storch-Hagenlocher Division of Neuroradiology, University of Heidelberg Medical Center, Im Neuenheimer Feld 400, 69120 Heidelberg, Germany

Henriette Tschampa Department of Radiology/Neuroradiology, Sigmund Freud-Strasse 25, 53105 Bonn, Germany

Horst Urbach Department of Radiology/Neuroradiology, Sigmund Freud-Strasse 25, 53105 Bonn, Germany

Martina Wengenroth Department of Radiology, Marchioninistrasse 15, 81377 Munich, Germany

Axel Wetter Institute of Diagnostic and Interventional Radiology and Neuroradiology, University Hospital Essen, Hufelandstrasse 55, 45147 Essen, Germany

Stephan G. Wetzel Department of Diagnostic and Interventional Neuroradiology, University Hospital Basel, Petersgraben 4, 4031 Basel, Switzerland

Brigitte Wildemann Division of Molecular Neuroimmunology, Department of Neurology, University of Heidelberg Medical Center, Im Neuenheimer Feld 400, 69120 Heidelberg, Germany

Part I

Brain Parenchyma

Multiple Sclerosis and Other Demyelinating Diseases

Martin Bendszus and Brigitte Storch-Hagenlocher

Contents

M. Bendszus (✉) · B. Storch-Hagenlocher
Division of Neuroradiology,
University of Heidelberg Medical Center,
Im Neuenheimer Feld 400,
69120 Heidelberg, Germany
e-mail: martin.bendszus@med.uni-heidelberg.de

Abstract

Multiple sclerosis (MS) is the most frequent idiopathic inflammatory demyelinating disease of the central nervous system. Magnetic resonance imaging is the most important paraclinical parameter in the diagnosis of MS. If the MR criteria for dissemination in time and space are positive, the early diagnosis of MS may be established already after one clinical event; thus, MRI has an important impact on the initiation of early therapy in MS. Moreover, MRI is essential in monitoring disease activity and therapy effects. Atypical inflammatory demyelinating diseases include ADEM, neuromyelitis optica (Devic disease), Baló's concentric sclerosis, Schilder's disease, Marburg's disease, tumefactive demyelinating lesions, and acute transverse myelitis. These entities may be separated from MS by a different clinical course and a particular appearance on MRI. Occasionally, these variants merge with MS.

1 Multiple Sclerosis

Brigitte Storch-Hagenlocher
and Martin Bendszus

1.1 Introduction

Multiple sclerosis is a chronic autoimmune condition of the central nervous system (CNS) characterized by blood–brain barrier breakdown, inflammation, myelin damage, and axonal loss. The pathogenesis of MS is unknown; apart from a genetic predisposition, previous virus infections are thought to be relevant. Multiple sclerosis is estimated to affect 2.5 million individuals worldwide. Multiple sclerosis typically presents in young Caucasian adults, with a peak between 20 and 40 years. There is increasing evidence for first manifestations of MS at childhood and older ages as well. Multiple

S. Hähnel (ed.), *Inflammatory Diseases of the Brain*, Medical Radiology. Diagnostic Imaging,
DOI: 10.1007/174_2012_787, © Springer-Verlag Berlin Heidelberg 2013
Published Online: 01 February 2013

sclerosis is twice as common in women than in men. The first manifestation of MS may be a clinically isolated syndrome (CIS) occurring with typical clinical symptoms indicating demyelination, but without evidence of dissemination in time. The clinical courses include relapsing-remitting (RRMS), secondary progressive (SPMS), and primary progressive (PPMS) MS. Patients with RRMS exhibit neurological symptoms that remit over a period of weeks to months with or without complete recovery. A large proportion of patients with RRMS evolve after 10–15 years the SPMS form of the disease, in which neurological deficits become fixed and cumulative. In contrast, patients with PPMS exhibit a continuous steady progression of neurological symptoms from the onset of the disease without periods of relapse or remission. Patients with PRMS also experience steady disease progression from the outset with or without superimposed relapses and remissions.

The clinical diagnosis of MS requires evidence for at least two anatomically distinct lesions consistent with (CNS) white matter damage in an individual with a history of at least two distinct episodes of focal neurological dysfunction (so-called symptom dissemination in time and space). These criteria are not difficult to demonstrate in well-established MS, but considerable problems can arise early in the course of the disease presenting with a clinically isolated symptom typical of MS (e.g., unilateral optic neuritis, internuclear ophthalmoplegia, or partial myelopathy). In recent years, new drugs have been introduced in the treatment of MS proven to especially treat early stages of the disease. In order to establish an early diagnosis of MS and therefore initiate early treatment, new diagnostic criteria, including paraclinical parameters, have been introduced. According to 2010 revisions of the McDonald diagnostic criteria MS can be assumed after the first manifestation if there is evidence of clinical abnormalities in at least one functional system in the presence of additional two or more typical lesions in the initial MRI. Magnetic resonance imaging has become the most important of these paraclinical parameters. Already after one clinical event and positive MRI criteria, the diagnosis of MS may be established and treatment initiated; thereby, MRI has immediate impact on early treatment of MS.

1.2 Epidemiology, Clinical Presentation, and Therapy

Brigitte Storch-Hagenlocher

1.2.1 Epidemiology

Multiple sclerosis (MS) is a chronic inflammatory demyelinating disease of the central nervous system (CNS) that affects mainly young adults and is yet the most frequent cause of invalidity at an early stage. The proportion of women to men affected is about 2–3:1, and disease most frequently occurs between the ages of 20–40 years but also with increasing incidence during childhood and after the age of 50 years. PPMS is affecting men and women to about the same degree typically during the fourth or fifth decade of life.

The prevalence of MS varies considerably around the world, increasing with the distance from the equator. It is highest in northern Europe, southern Australia, and the middle part of North America, with 80–150 per 100,000 persons. Germany also belongs to high prevalence regions with about 120,000–150,000 MS patients. There has been a trend toward an increasing prevalence and incidence, particularly in southern Europe. It is uncertain to which extent the observed increases are explained by an enhanced awareness of the disease and improved diagnostic techniques. There is also a remarkable increase of contracted women documented in Scandinavian database. The reasons for the variation in the prevalence and incidence of MS worldwide are not well understood. Environmental and genetic factors probably play a role. People who migrate from high- to low-prevalence areas during childhood only take on the risk of the host country, and vice versa; however, the nature of putative environmental factors remains unclear in numerous case–control studies. The immunoregulatory role of Vitamin D has been focused as a cofactor for MS manifestation. This hypothesis is supported by evidence of low Vitamin D levels in children with MS and during the first manifestation in adults as well as by the geographic distribution of the disease.

1.2.2 Genetics

Evidence that genetic factors have a substantial effect on susceptibility to MS is unequivocal. The concordance rate is highest among monozygotic twins (about 30 %) and only about 2–5 % among dizygotic twins; however, the risk of disease in a first-degree relative of a patient with MS is 20–40 times higher than the risk in the general population. In 1972 the association between MS and the HLA region of the genome was established since narrowed down to the HLA-DRB1 gene on chromosome 6p21. Populations with a high frequency of the allele have the highest risk of MS. Furthermore, there is evidence of the involvement of two other interesting genes: IL2RA, which encodes the alpha subunit of the interleukin-2 receptor (synonym CD25) on chromosome 10p15; and IL7RA, which encodes the alpha chain of the interleukin-7 receptor on chromosome 5p13. These two interleukin-receptor genes are important in T cell-mediated immunity regulating T cell responses and homeostasis of the memory T cell pool and may be important in the generation of autoreactive T cells in MS. In addition within the last few years, genome-wide association studies have led to the identification of nearly 60 additional genetic risk loci.

1.2.3 Clinical Presentation

The heterogeneity of clinical symptoms and the temporal evolution of clinical findings may suggest the diagnosis of MS. In relapsing–remitting MS (RRMS), the type present in about 80 % of cases, symptoms and signs evolve over a period of some days, stabilize, and often improve spontaneously or in response to corticosteroids, within several weeks. A relapse is defined by symptoms lasting more than 24 h, not associated with an increase of body temperature (Uhthoff phenomenon) or infection and occurring at least $\geq$ 30 days after the beginning of a precedent relapse. Relapsing–remitting MS generally begins in the second or third decade of life with a female predominance. With the first treatment, symptoms usually respond very well to corticosteroids with fast and frequently complete recovery, but this effect often decreases over the years. The "benign" type of relapsing–remitting MS defined by only mild symptoms being present 30 years after disease onset is found only in about 10 % of cases. In the majority of cases disease passes into secondary progressive MS (SPMS) within 20–30 years.

Twenty percent of affected patients suffer from primary progressive MS (PPMS), which is characterized by a gradually progressive clinical course and a similar incidence among men and women.

Relapsing–remitting MS frequently starts with sensory disturbances and Lhermitte's sign (trunk and limb paresthesias evoked by neck flexion). Further initial signs are unilateral optic neuritis or diplopia (internuclear ophthalmoplegia). Limb weakness, clumsiness, gait ataxia, and neurogenic bladder and bowel symptoms at the beginning of disease more often indicate a less favorable course. The onset of symptoms post-partum and symptomatic worsening with increases in body temperature (Uhthoff's symptom), as well as pseudoexacerbations with fever, are suggestive of MS. Recurring, brief, stereotypical phenomena (paroxysmal pain or paresthesias, trigeminal neuralgia, episodic clumsiness or dysarthria, tonic limb posturing) also suggest the diagnosis of MS. Even at the beginning of the disease cognitive impairment, depression, emotional lability, dysarthria, dysphagia, vertigo, spasticity, progressive quadriparesis and sensory loss, pain, ataxic tremor, sexual dysfunction, and other manifestations of central nervous system dysfunction may impair affected patients; however, cortical signs (aphasia, apraxia, recurrent seizures, visual-field loss) as well as extrapyramidal symptoms generally only rarely occur.

Patients with primary progressive MS often develop a "chronic progressive myelopathy" with gradually evolving upper motor-neuron symptoms of the legs. Over time this variant worsens with quadriparesis, cognitive decline, visual impairment, brain-stem syndromes, and cerebellar, bowel, bladder, and sexual dysfunction.

There are several standardized clinical parameters and scales to evaluate disease progression. Relapse rates are important for determining disease severity in the short term. Neurological disability is most directly measured with the Expanded Disability Status Scale (EDSS), an ordinal rating scale that defines transitions between different disability states ranging from 0 = normal neurological examination, to 10 = death from MS. The cognitive decline can be assessed by several neuropsychological tests, such as the Paced Auditory Serial Addition Test (PASAT), which measure speed of information processing. The nine-hole peg test (9HPT) is a specific measure of upper limb function, whereas ambulation tasks, such as the 25-ft. walk, measure lower limb function. The combination of these function-specific measures is more sensitive for following clinical outcome than the individual measures alone and is provided by the Multiple Sclerosis Functional Composite (MSFC).

1.2.4 Clinical Diagnosis

To increase specificity of diagnosis, the use of both clinical and paraclinical criteria must be obtained including information MRI, evoked potentials (EP), and cerebrospinal fluid (CSF), all being only supportive and not diagnostic itself. In 2001, the "International Panel on the Diagnosis of Multiple Sclerosis" presented new diagnostic criteria for MS with particular emphasis on determining dissemination of lesions in time and space. Recent revision of the Diagnostic criteria in 2010 allows the diagnosis of MS even in the first manifestation of disease (CIS) in the presence of asymptomatic Gadolinium enhancing and non-enhancing lesions on MRI. Detection of new demyelinating lesions in control MRIs also confirms the diagnosis of MS in the course of time.

The value of CSF analysis is stressed in primary progressive MS but the importance of CSF analysis has declined in RRMS in favor to MRI criteria. However, for differential diagnosis CSF analysis remains essential. In addition, electrophysiological tests (visual and somatosensory evoked potentials, transcranial magnetic stimulation) can detect clinically asymptomatic dysfunctions and thus confirm dissemination and objectify described symptoms. When the results of these paraclinical tests are normal, this strongly suggests an alternative diagnosis, whereas when they are abnormal, they would support the diagnosis of MS. In addition, diagnostic criteria also demand that "there be no better explanation other than MS to account for the historical and objective evidence of neurological dysfunction"; therefore, other differential diagnoses must be ruled out very carefully (Table 1).

On MRI, findings of multifocal lesions of various ages, especially those involving the periventricular and

Table 1 Clinical differential diagnosis of multiple sclerosis

Variants of MS	Optic neuritis, neuromyelitis optica, acute disseminated encephalomyelitis
Autoimmune diseases	Sjögren's syndrome, systemic lupus erythematosus, Behçet's disease, sarcoidosis, antiphospholipid-antibody syndrome, paraneoplastic disorders
Infections	HIV-associated myelopathy, HTLV-1-associated myelopathy, neuroborreliosis, meningovascular syphilis
Metabolic disorders	Disorders of B12 and folate metabolism, leukodystrophies
Vascular disorders	Central nervous system vasculitis inclusive variants (e.g., Susac's syndrome, Cogan's disease), cerebral autosomal–dominant arteriopathy with subcortical infarcts and leukoencephalopathy
Genetic syndromes	Hereditary ataxias and hereditary paraplegias, Leber's atrophy, other mitochondrial cytopathies
Lesions of the posterior fossa and spinal cord	Arnold–Chiari malformation, nonhereditary ataxias, spondylotic, or other myelopathies
Psychiatric disorders	Conversion reaction

subcortical white matter, brain stem, cerebellum, and spinal cord white matter, support the clinical impression of MS. The presence of gadolinium-enhancing lesions on MRI indicates current active lesions. In the past few years numerous studies have also demonstrated brain atrophy due to early axonal loss resulting in progression of neurological deficits and development of cognitive impairment.

The CSF examinations include white blood cell (WBC) count, quantitative and qualitative protein analysis, as well as glucose and/or lactate level measurement. Higher than normal (N $<5 \times 10^6$/l) WBC counts are found in approximately 35 % of MS cases, but very high ($>50 \times 10^6$/l) CSF WBC counts are unusual. Plasma cells can be detected in about 70–80 % of cases, even in normal cell counts. CSF glucose and lactate levels usually are in normal ranges. Total protein and albumin quotient to indicate the blood–brain barrier function usually are normal. In MS the most important CSF findings are the detection of intrathecally produced IgG ("raised IgG index") in about 70–90 % of MS patients and oligoclonal bands different from those in serum in about 98 % of MS. Intrathecally produced IgM can also be detected in about 30–40 % of cases. In case of ambiguous results antibody-synthesis-indices of neurotropic viruses (measles, rubella, varicella zoster) may confirm the diagnosis. Although revised McDonald criteria do not require CSF analysis in either case for diagnosis of MS, in Europe CSF analysis is still recommended to eliminate alternative conditions that might "mimic" the disease.

1.2.5 Pathology and Pathogenesis

Multiple sclerosis is an immune-mediated disease with a complex pathogenesis involving both inflammatory and neurodegenerative components. The basic pathology is characterized by perivascular infiltration of lymphocytes and lipid-containing macrophages, as well as axonal transsection even in an early stage of disease. The destroying process not only involves white matter areas, but also thinly myelinated areas of gray matter and basal ganglia. The margins of the acute lesions can be indistinct due to ongoing demyelination and the lesion center may be edematous.

Even though exact details of MS pathogenesis remain elusive, it is assumed that activated autoreactive T-cells from the periphery pass the blood–brain barrier and initiate a cascade of inflammatory immune reactions within the CNS. This includes activation of macrophages and B-cells, production of antibodies, and release of proinflammatory cytokines. Initially, the generation of autoimmune T-cells may be promoted by an impaired suppressive function of CD4 + CD25 high-regulatory T-cells (Treg), a phenotype that may be relevant in controlling autoimmune diseases. In MS lesions CD4 + and CD8 + T-cells are present, with CD4 + T-cells being predominantly in the perivascular cuff, and CD8 + T-cells being more prevalent in the center and border zone of the lesion. Axonal damage may be promoted by activated CD8 + T-cells that directly target neurons, by destructive macrophages, inflammatory mediators, and toxic molecules, as well as binding of antibodies to neuronal surface antigens, followed by complement activation and antibody-mediated phagocytosis of axons. In addition, indirect mechanisms, such as loss of protective myelin, mitochondrial dysfunction, or release of glutamate nitric oxide, might contribute to axonal damage. Clinical course and histopathological findings suggest that in MS patients these multiple mechanisms of disease are present to a different extent. According to Lucchinetti and colleagues (2000), four different immunopathogenic patterns in acute MS lesions can be observed histopathologically. Two patterns (I and II) display T cells as the predominant cell population. Additional deposits of immunoglobulins and complement characterize pattern-II lesions. Patterns III and IV show primary oligodendrocyte dystrophy and pattern III also shows apoptotic oligodendrocytes. Patients with patterns I and II often show remyelinated plaques, but remyelination is absent in pattern-III and pattern-IV lesions.

1.2.6 Therapy

1.2.6.1 Relapse Treatment

Glucocorticoids are the standard treatment for acute relapses. They restore the blood–brain barrier, induce T-cell apoptosis, and decrease the release of proinflammatory cytokines; therefore, they have beneficial effects on inflammation, apoptosis, and demyelination. Although these drugs may shorten the duration of a relapse, they have no effect on the exacerbation rate or on the development of long-term disability. A relevant MS relapse should be treated with high-dose pulse therapy of methylprednisolone IV optionally followed by oral tapering. In case improvement is not satisfactory, treatment should be escalated either by solely repeating high-dose methylprednisolone or administering it in combination with a cytotoxic immunosuppressive agent (cyclophosphamide, mitoxantrone).

Plasma exchange (PE) or immunoadsorption is also an alternative escalating immunotherapy in patients with severe steroid-resistant relapses. In small trials the mean time point of improvement was after the third plasmapheresis session, and early initiation of plasma exchange therapy (within 1 month after start of relapse) was associated with better outcome.

1.2.6.2 Immunotherapy in Relapsing–Remitting MS

The therapy escalation and de-escalation scheme is illustrated in Fig. 1. In relapsing–remitting MS (RRMS), on the basis of the inflammatory nature of the disease, targeting at the immune response has thus far been the most widely used and only successful treatment. Strategies have been developed that range from nonselective immunosuppression to highly specific immune intervention. Such treatments bring undoubted benefits in reducing the risk of relapse and, potentially, the risk of acquiring irreversible neurological disability. Evidence from research suggests that many patients with clinically isolated syndromes or early MS should be treated with disease-modifying drugs at an early stage, since disease experience during the first few years is likely to have significant impact on the long-term evolution of disease. Natural-history studies have also shown that the number of relapses occurring during the first few years of disease is related to the amount of accrued disability.

Immunomodulation and Global Immunosuppression

Most people with immunotherapy in relapsing–remitting MS (RRMS) are currently treated with the immunomodulatory substances betainterferon (INF-β) or glatiramer acetate (GA). INF-β has multiple immunomodulatory effects: it curtails T-cell trafficking, redresses a Th1–Th2 imbalance that is in favor of proinflammatory Th1 responses in MS patients, and exhibits antiviral properties. Glatiramer acetate, a synthetic polypeptide composed of the most prevalent amino acids inmyelin basic protein (MBP), is a main target antigen in MS-related immune response. Glatiramer acetate is believed to modulate autoreactive T-cells, inhibit monocyte activity, and induce bystander immune suppression at lesion sites in the CNS. As GA-reactive T-cells have been reported to release neurotrophic factors, GA might theoretically also promote neuroregeneration. These drugs have shown a reduction of relapse rates at about 30–35 % and reduction of inflammatory activity and lesion load at about 60 % as measured by MRI.

Other immunomodulating substances (fumaric acid, teriflunomide, laquinimod, phosphodiesterase inhibitors) are being tested for therapeutic properties in phase-II or phase-III trials. But these drugs are not licensed until now.

Alternatively, global immunosuppression can be applied with immunosuppressant drugs, most frequently with azathioprine or cyclosporine, both well-known drugs in other autoimmune diseases. Mycophenolate mofetil, another member of the antimetabolite group of immunosuppressants, has also shown positive effects on relapsing rates in a small number of patients. Additional immunosuppressant drugs (e.g., cladribine, treosulfan, temsirolimus) are also being investigated in clinical trials at this time.

In addition, combination therapies with azathioprine and INF-β or azathioprine and GA are being explored.

Intravenous immunoglobulin G (IVIG) can modify the balance between Th1 and Th2 subtypes and produce a downregulation of proinflammatory cytokines. It is applied to several autoimmune diseases and has also shown reduced relapse rates and gadolinium-enhancing lesions in RRMS but failed to show a benefit in secondary progressive MS (SPMS). Presently, IVIG is only a therapeutic option in pregnancy and post-partum to prevent new relapses.

Selective Immune Intervention

With the introduction of humanized monoclonal antibodies and small specific molecules (e.g., receptor agonists or antagonists), specific ablation of distinct immune populations or selective blockade or activation of immune molecules has become possible. Antibodies that bind cell-specific surface molecules allow depletion of T cells, B cells, and other immune-cell subsets via antibody binding and complement-mediated cell lysis.

Modulation of Immune-Cell Migration

If first-step immunomodulation fails in controlling disease activity, an escalating therapy should be adopted. Natalizumab, a humanized monoclonal antibody against the adhesion molecule α-4 integrin, blocks this epitope on leukocytes and therefore prevents leukocyte binding to the vessel wall and thereby hampers leukocyte passage across the

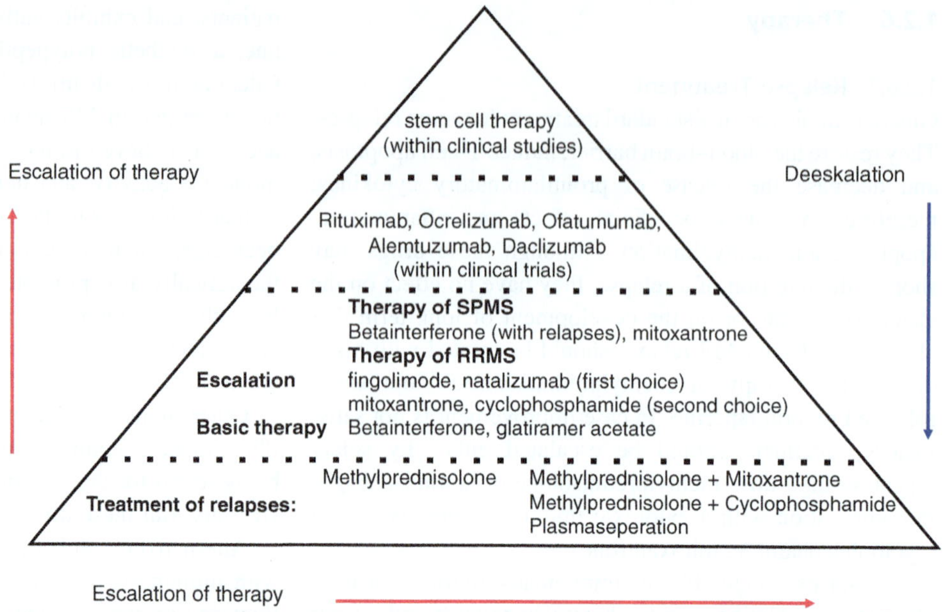

Fig. 1 Escalation scheme for therapy of multiple sclerosis

blood–brain barrier. This drug effectively reduces disease activity and has already been approved for very active RRMS. Side effects may be severe and patients must be controlled very carefully. The application of natalizumab is associated with a certain risk of developing progressive multifocal leukoencephalitis (PML) caused by JC-virus. The risk of PML increases with a positive serological JCV status and duration of natalizumab therapy. Therefore it is recommended to test for JCV and to stop therapy after 2 years of treatment. FTY20 (fingolimode), a fungal metabolite with sphingosine-1-phosphate-receptor agonist activity, induces homing of lymphocytes to the lymph nodes and traps them at this site, thereby preventing their migration to inflamed organ departments. Clinical trials in patients with MS revealed positive results, and the drug is now available and licensed for highly active RRMS in case of failure of basic therapy with betainterferons or glatiramer acetate.

Depletion of Immune Cells

The monoclonal antibodies mentioned below have already demonstrated effectiveness in reducing contrast-enhancing lesions and improving clinical scores in patients with RRMS in phase-II or small open-label trials. Further studies are intended or have already been started.

Alemtuzumab (Campath1H) is a humanized anti-leukocyte (CD52) monoclonal antibody that is cytolytic and produces prolonged lymphocyte depletion. Positive effects in RRMS have been shown, and a study in SPMS has generated not unequivocal results; thus, there is a need for more data. Results of recently presented or ongoing studies are encouraging but side effects may be severe.

Daclizumab is a humanized monoclonal antibody specific for the IL-2-receptor alpha chain that inhibits activation of lymphocytes. Further clinical trials and more data about long-term efficacy and safety are required. Phase-II studies of daclizumab as monotherapy or combined with other treatments are now underway.

Rituximab, a human-murine chimeric monoclonal antibody that binds specifically to the CD20 antigen, causes rapid depletion of CD20-positive B-cells in the peripheral blood. In small studies treating patients with RRMS rituximab was able to reduce disease activity and frequency of relapses significantly. Rituximab may be an alternative escalating therapy in highly active RRMS.

Other antibodies against CD20-positive B-lymphocytes are Ocrelizumab and Ofatumumab, which were effective in RRMS in very small phase-II studies.

Stem Cell Transplantation

Experimental and clinical observations suggest that high-dose immunosuppression followed by autologous stem cell transplantation can induce remissions in severe, refractory autoimmune diseases, including MS. Stem cells have the capacity to enter the CNS and trans-differentiate into microglia and possibly neurons, and therefore might be of significant importance in producing remyelination and neuron repair. Initial studies were associated with significant morbidity and mortality but were promising in terms of clinical stability and impact on disease activity at MRI. Patients with severe, rapidly worsening MS who are unresponsive to approved therapies could be candidates for this treatment, but only within clinical trials.

1.2.6.3 Therapy of Secondary Progressive Multiple Sclerosis

In secondary progressive multiple sclerosis (SPMS) treatment options are limited. Interferon-β might ameliorate disease progression slightly, although this effect could not be demonstrated in all studies. Nevertheless, interferon-β (Betaferon, Bayer Schering Pharma, Berlin, Germany) is approved for this indication, especially in the presence of relapses. In MS patients with rapidly progressive disease activity (e.g., deterioration in the EDSS of $\geq$1 point within 1 year) mitoxantrone, an antineoplastic agent, has shown efficacy on disability progression. Due to restricted cumulative life dose, mitoxantrone can be given for about 2 years (cumulative dose rate about 100 mg/qm), and thus far there is ambiguity as to which immunotherapy should be applied after mitoxantrone treatment.

1.2.6.4 Therapy of Primary Progressive MS

In primary progressive multiple sclerosis (PPMS) treatment only limited data are available from small studies. Beneficial effects in reducing progression of disability could be achieved by combined low-dose mitoxantrone and methylprednisolone therapy. Also, repeated IV methylprednisolone administration has the ability to decelerate disease progression. An alternative therapy option is the treatment with low-dose oral methotrexate resulting in a slowed deterioration of motor function.

1.2.6.5 Symptomatic Therapy

A large panel of various symptomatic therapies to treat MS patients is necessary and available. Physiotherapy and occupational therapy are essential as well as antispastic, anticholinergic, or analgetic drugs. Therapeutically, problems in coping with the disease should be considered as well as fatigue or depression, which are the main problems in about half of all MS patients.

1.3 Imaging

Martin Bendszus

1.3.1 Technical Aspects

Magnetic resonance imaging is the imaging modality of choice in MS. Lesion conspicuity is related to the field strength of the MR scanner; therefore, high-magnetic-field scanners ($\geq$1 T) should be preferred. Lower field-strength magnets with an open configuration, however, may be the only option for examining extremely claustrophobic or obese patients. With the advance of 3-T scanners in clinical routine detection and delineation of MS, lesions have once again increased (Wattjes 2006). Most MS patients undergo serial MR examinations. In order to assure interindividual comparability, exact and reproducible slice positioning is essential; therefore, a scout sequence in three directions should be performed initially. Axial slices should be aligned with the subcallosal line on the mid-sagittal scout image (Simon et al. 2006). Another approach to assure exact slice repositioning is the acquisition of 3D data sets with secondary image reconstruction with isotropic voxel. Sequence parameters, angulation, and the amount of contrast medium should be kept identical for every patient. For clinical routine, a concentration of 0.1 mmol Gd-DTPA per kilogram body weight is well established (Simon 2006); however, higher concentrations (e.g., 0.2 or 0.3 mmol) reveal more contrast-enhancing lesions (Fillipi 1998). Another factor that directly influences the number and extent of contrast-enhancing lesions is the time between application of contrast medium and the beginning and duration of the MR sequence. This time should be at least 5 min and should always be kept constant (Simon 2006). Magnetization transfer sequences may increase sensitivity in detecting contrast-enhancing lesions (Fillipi 1998). Lesion number and volume are directly related to slice thickness. For MR studies in MS a slice thickness of 3 mm for the axial slices is recommended (Polman 2005). In clinical practice, a slice thickness of 3–5 mm has been suggested (Simon 2006). For routine imaging of the brain in MS, the following sequence protocol has been suggested: sagittal FLAIR images, axial fast spin-echo (FSE) PD- and T2-weighted images, and axial T1-weighted images spin-echo (SE) images before and administration of Gd-DTPA (Simon 2006). For MRI of the spine sagittal T1-weighted and T2-weighted FSE sequences have been proposed, supplemented by axial T1-weighted and T2-weighted sequences (see also Neurotuberculosis).

1.3.2 Imaging Findings in Typical MS

Magnetic resonance imaging is the most relevant paraclinical diagnostic criterion for MS as well as a surrogate parameter for monitoring disease activity. Unenhanced T2-weighted images are highly sensitive for the detection of hyperintense MS lesions and therefore useful for diagnosing MS, monitoring short-term disease activity, and assessing the overall disease burden; however, these lesions are nonspecific for the underlying pathologic findings, and correlations with clinical status seem to be weak. Hypointense lesions on T1-weighted images (so-called black holes) may represent areas with severe tissue damage as demyelination and axonal loss. Hyperintense lesions on unenhanced T1-weighted images are possibly related to a local deposition of free radicals, and recent studies indicate an association between the presence of hyperintense T1-lesions and disability; therefore, post-gadolinium T1-weighted sequences should always be preceded by unenhanced T1-weighted images. Enhancement of gadolinium on T1-weighted images scans allows discrimination between active and inactive MS lesions, since Gd-DTPA enhancement is a consequence of a disruption of the blood–brain barrier and corresponds to areas with acute inflammation. Typical localizations for MS lesions include the posterior fossa (in particular, pons, pedunculus cerebelli, and cerebellar white matter), the optic radiatio, the internal and external capsule, the corpus callosum, and the periventricular and subcortical region. Subcortical lesions typically include the subcortical U-fibers and are also referred to as "juxtacortical" lesions. Spinal cord imaging can be extremely helpful in excluding other differential diagnoses. Whereas lesions in the brain can develop in healthy aging people, this is not typical in the spinal cord. Lesions on spinal MRI may contribute to the dissemination in space. Spinal cord lesions should be focal (i.e., clearly delineated and circumscribed as seen on heavily T2-weighted images) in nature for consideration in MS diagnosis. Moreover, they should be at least 3 mm in size, but less than two vertebral segments in length and occupying only part of the cord cross section.

In 2001, an international panel suggested diagnostic MR criteria for MS (so-called McDonald criteria; McDonald 2001). These criteria were revised and simplified in 2005 and most recently 2011 (Polman 2005, 2011). According to these criteria, the early diagnosis of MS may be established after one clinical event. The clinical concept of dissemination in space and time was adapted to MRI. Similar to the clinical diagnosis of MS, the MR diagnosis of MS requires a dissemination of lesions in space and time. ***Dissemination in space*** requires at least one lesion on T2-w images in at least two of the four following localizations: periventricular, subcortical, fossa posterior, spinal cord. (Fig. 2, 3, 4 and 5, Table 2); *Dissemination in time* is fulfilled by any new T2 lesion compared to a baseline scan irrespective of the timing of the baseline scan. Alternatively, dissemination in time can be fulfilled on one MR examination only by the coexistence of a nonenhancing (considered as old lesion) and an enhancing lesion (considered as acute lesion) on contrast-enhanced T1-w images (Fig. 6, 7, Table 2). The most recent modification of the original McDonald criteria has increased sensitivity in the diagnosis of early MS without losing specificity (Swanton et al. 2007) (Table 3).

In the most recent revision of the McDonald Criteria (Polman et al. 2011) neuromyelitis optica (NMO) has been recognized as a separate entity which should be considered if (a) myelopathy is associated with MRI-detected spinal cord lesions longer than three spinal segments and primarily involving the central part of the spinal cord on axial sections, (b) optic neuritis is bilateral and severe or associated with a swollen optic nerve or chiasm, and (c) intractable hiccough or nausea/vomiting is present for >2 days with evidence of a periaqueductal medullary lesion on MRI. In these patients aquaporin-4 autoantibodies should be tested to make a differential diagnosis between NMO and MS.

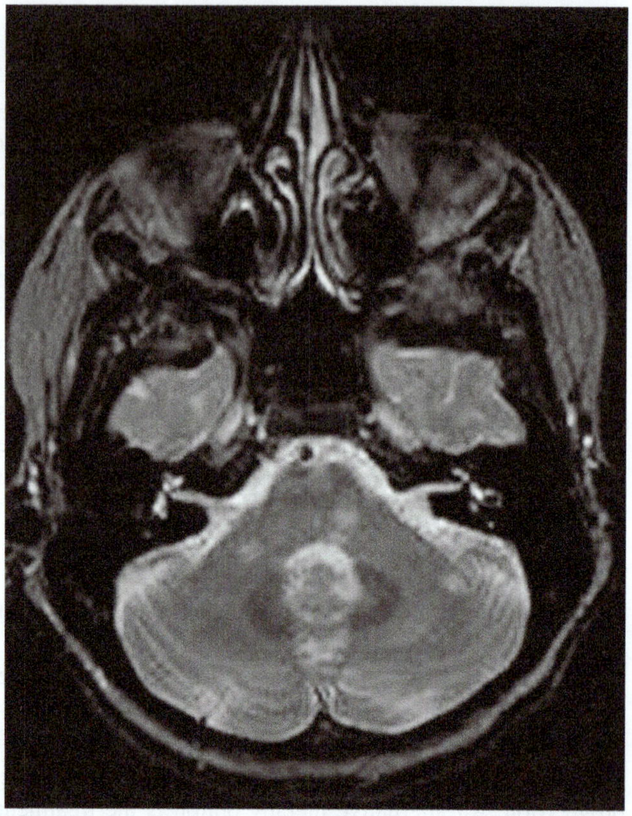

Fig. 2 Infratentorial MS plaques. Axial T2-weighted image. Hyperintense lesions in the pons, pedunculus cerebelli medius, and the white matter of the left cerebellar hemisphere. These are typical localizations for inflammatory lesions. One criterion for dissemination in space is fulfilled if at least one infratentorial lesion is present

1.3.3 Imaging Findings in PPMS

Beside acute relapsing–remitting, the beginning of MS onset may be primarily chronic in 10–15 % of patients. Clinically, the diagnosis of primarily chronic MS represents a challenge. Compared with a relapsing–remitting course of disease, patients with PPMS are older at onset and a higher proportion is male. Inflammatory white matter lesions are less evident, but diffuse axonal loss is seen in normal-appearing white matter, in addition to cortical demyelination. Spinal cord atrophy corresponds to the frequent clinical presentation of progressive spastic paraplegia. In 2011 (Polman et al. 2011), new diagnostic criteria were introduced by an international panel to diagnose primarily chronic MS. Apart from 1 year of disease progression (retrospectively or prospectively assessed) the diagnosis of PPMS requires at least two out of the following three criteria: (1) cerebral involvement with at least one T2 lesion in at least one area characteristic for MS (periventricular,

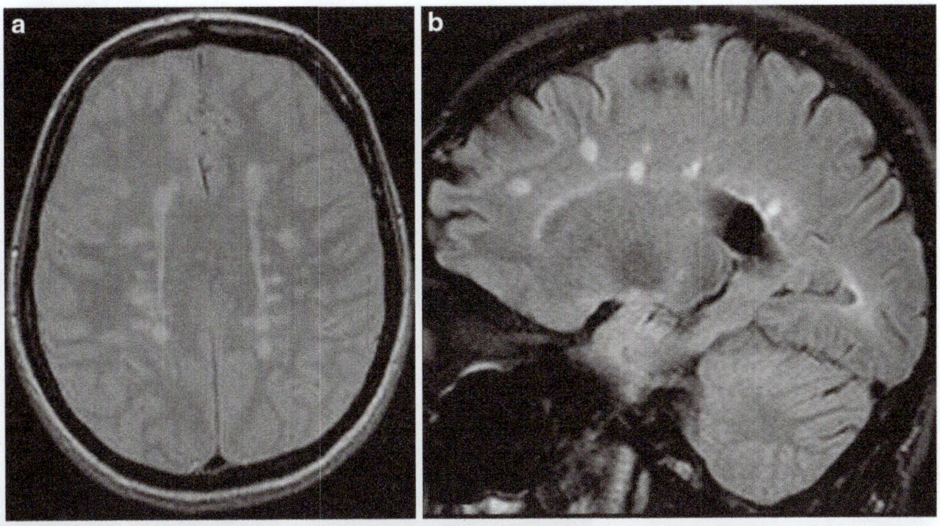

Fig. 3 Multiple periventricular lesions. **a** Axial PD-weighted image. **b** Sagittal FLAIR image. These lesions typically have an ovoid shape with immediate contact to the lateral ventricles ("Dawson finger"). The immediate contact to the lateral ventricles is demonstrated best on sagittal FLAIR images (**b**)

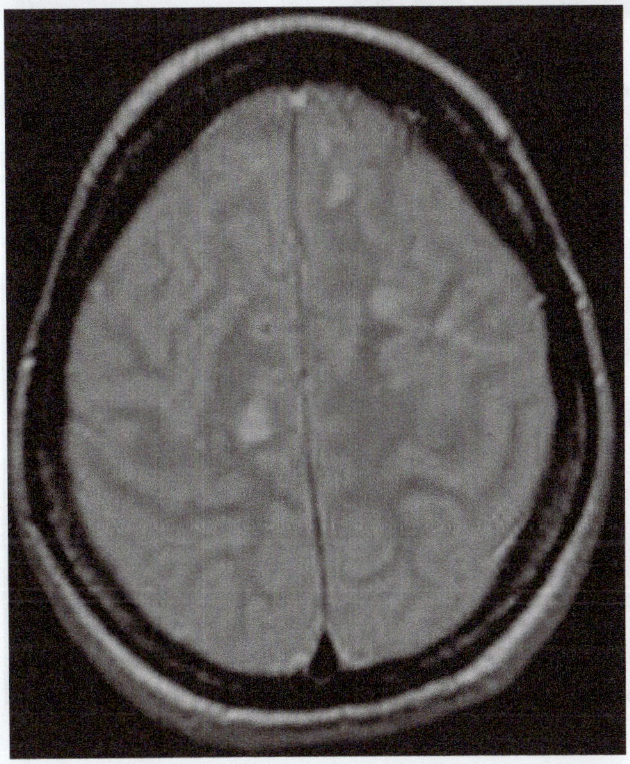

Fig. 4 Subcortical lesions. Axial PD-weighted image. Hyperintense subcortical lesions. In contrast to microangiopathic lesions, MS lesions involve the subcortical U-fibers (so-called juxtacortical lesions)

subcortical, infratentorial), (2) spinal lesions with at lease two focal T2 lesions, (3) positive CSF (defined as oligoclonal IgG bands and/or increased IgG index).

1.3.4 Differential Diagnosis

The differential diagnosis of MS includes other white matter lesions such as unspecific or microangiopathic white matter changes, acute disseminated encephalomyelitis (ADEM), cerebral autosomal-dominant arteriopathy with

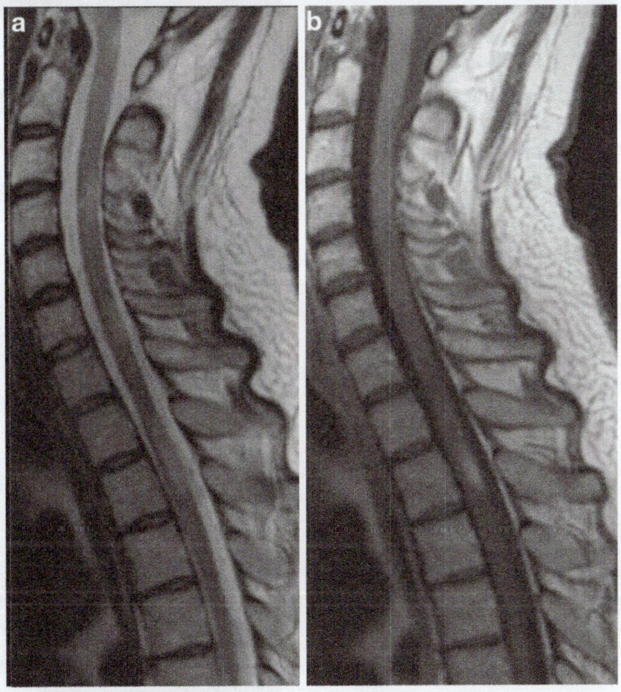

Fig. 5 Spinal lesions. **a** Sagittal T2-weighted image. **b** Sagittal T1-weighted image after contrast administration. Hyperintense lesions in the cervico-thoracic spine on sagittal T2-weighted images (**a**) extending over one to two segments. One of these lesions reveals enhancement of Gd-DTPA on sagittal T1-weighted images (**b**)

Table 2 2010 Criteria for demonstration of dissemination in space (DIS) in MS. DIS can be demonstrated by ≥ 1 T2 lesion (1) in at least 2 of 4 areas of the CNS

– Periventricular
– Juxtacortical
– Infratentorial
– Spinal cord (2)

(1) Gadolinium enhancement of lesions is not required for DIS

(2) If a subject has a brain-stem or spinal cord syndrome, the symptomatic lesions are excluded from the Criteria and do not contribute to lesion count

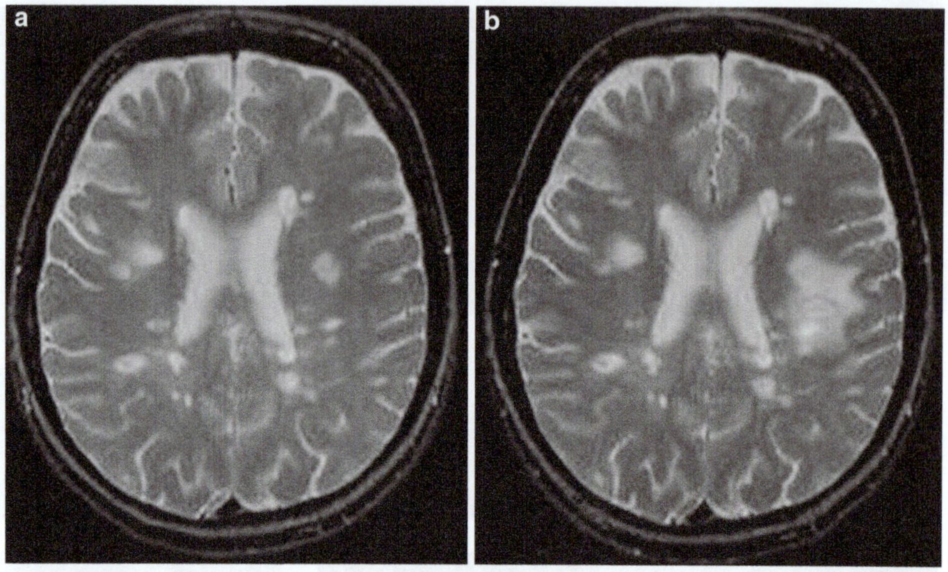

Fig. 6 Dissemination in time (I). **a** Axial T2-weighted image in a patient with optical neuritis shows T2-lesions fulfilling the criteria for a dissemination in space for MS. **b** Follow-up axial T2-weighted image shows a new large T2 lesion with perifocal edema; thereby, dissemination in time is fulfilled. Dissemination in time on the basis of T2 lesions requires two MRI examinations

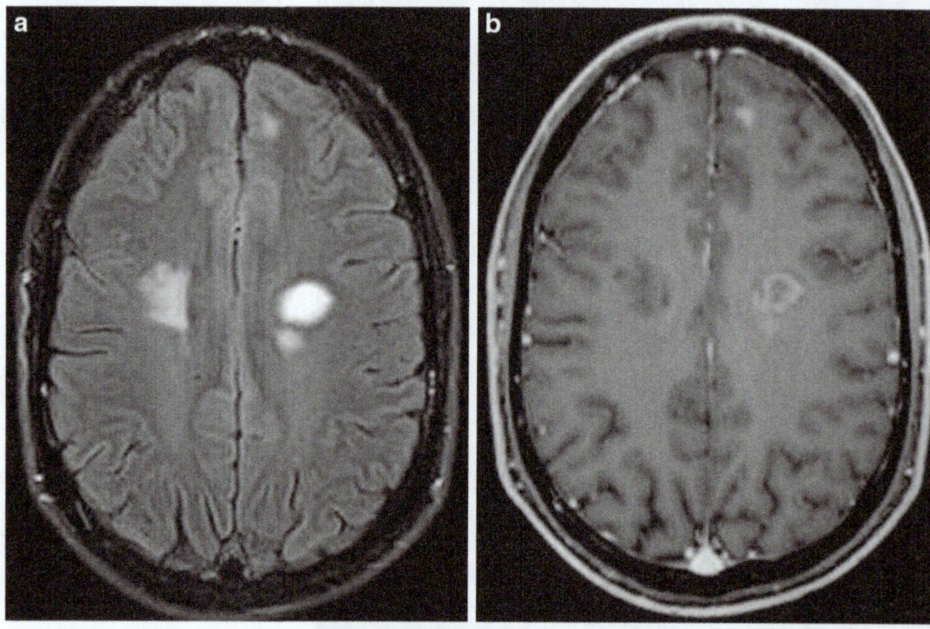

Fig. 7 Dissemination in time (II). Axial FLAIR and contrast-enhanced T1-w images in a patient with an clinically isolated syndrome shows multiple lesions on FLAIR images fulfilling dissemination in space. On contrast-enhanced images the majority of the lesions appear hypointense ("black holes"), whereas some of the lesions are hyperintense due to uptake of contrast medium. The coexistence of old lesions (hypointense) and acute lesions (uptake of contrast medium) demonstrate the dissemination in time of the inflammatory lesions

subcortical infarcts and leukoencephalopathy (CADASIL), neurosarcoidosis, viral encephalitis, cerebral vasculitis, and metastasis. Microangiopathic white matter lesions have a more bandlike configuration and have no preferential manifestation in the corpus callosum, as is true for MS. In contrast to cerebral microangiopathy, MS only rarely manifests in the central gray matter (basal ganglia, thalamus). Moreover, posterior fossa and spinal cord lesions are very rare in microangiopathy. Lesions from ADEM are often more asymmetric than MS plaques, may also be manifested in the central gray matter, and have no predilection for the corpus callosum, as is the case with MS. Furthermore, ADEM lesions are mostly in the same stage regarding contrast enhancement. The CADASIL lesion typically involves the subcortical white matter of the frontal and temporal lobes, and the inner capsule. Neurosarcoidosis often involves the cranial nerves, the pituitary gland, the hypothalamus, and the leptomeninges, and the signal of granulomas on T2-weighted images is mostly iso- to hypointense (see also Pyogenic Cerebritis and Brain Abscess). The most common viral encephalitis which may mimic MS in imaging is neuroborreliosis (Lyme disease). In neuroborreliosis cranial nerves are often involved (see also Other Bacterial Infections of the Brain). The imaging pattern in CNS vasculitis depends on the number, the site, and the size of the involved vessels; therefore, in contrast to MS,

Table 3 2010 McDonald Criteria for demonstration of dissemination in time (DIT) DIT can be demonstrated by

A new T2 and/or gadolinium-enhancing lesion(s) on follow-up MRI, with reference to a baseline scan, irrespective of the timing of the baseline MRI
Simultaneous presence of asymptomatic gadolinium-enhancing and nonenhancing lesions at any time

cerebral vasculitis may also involve cerebral gray matter. In some patients with vasculitis vessel stenoses or occlusions may be detected using MRA or DSA (see also Cerebral Vasculitis). Cerebral metastases are typically located at the gray–white matter interface (corticomedullary junction), are space occupying, sometimes reveal hemorrhage, and show contrast enhancement throughout.

2 Other Demyelinating Diseases

Brigitte Storch-Hagenlocher
and Martin Bendszus

2.1 Summary

In addition to MS there are several other idiopathic inflammatory demyelinating diseases (IIDDs) which differ in clinical course, severity, and lesion distribution as well as in imaging, laboratory, and pathological findings. Some IIDDs have a restricted topographical distribution such as optic neuritis, transverse myelitis, and neuromyelitis optica (Devic). Acute disseminated encephalomyelitis (ADEM) is a clinical monophasic inflammatory disease with a broad spectrum of clinical and radiologic features. The differentiation of tumor-like lesions sometimes may be challenging. Fulminant variants of IIDDs are Marburg's disease, Baló's concentric sclerosis, and Schilder's disease characterized by acute and severe attacks, and lesions seen as typical on MRI.

2.2 Introduction

Demyelinating lesions of the brain most frequently present with a typical clinical and morphological pattern of MS; however, atypical findings also exist and may represent differential diagnostic problems. Herein the most frequent types of idiopathic inflammatory demyelinating lesions of the brain are outlined.

2.3 Clinically Isolated Symptoms

Patients with monofocal inflammatory demyelinating symptoms, such as transverse myelitis, optic neuritis, or isolated brain-stem manifestation, not always but frequently develop MS especially in the presence of positive MRI and cerebral spinal fluid (CSF) findings. Patients with isolated symptoms who present with disseminated demyelinating lesions on MRI and oligoclonal bands present in the CSF have an 88 % chance of developing clinically definite MS within 10–15 years, as compared with about 20 % of such patients with normal MRI and CSF findings.

2.4 Acute Disseminated Encephalomyelitis

Acute disseminated encephalomyelitis (ADEM) is an immune-mediated acute inflammatory disorder of the central nervous system characterized by extensive demyelination predominantly involving the white matter of the brain and spinal cord. Most frequently, the disease is precipitated by a vaccination or viral infection. Patients commonly present with nonspecific symptoms, including headache, vomiting, drowsiness, fever, and lethargy, all of which are relatively uncommon in MS. Gender ratio of the disease is equal, but children and young adults are more affected than the elderly. The CSF findings usually differ from those of MS patients. The CSF cell count is frequently elevated (>50/µl) but may also be normal, and the presence of oligoclonal bands is variable. Thus far, however, the diagnosis of ADEM is still based on the clinical and radiological features, since no other typical biological markers are available. Lesions in ADEM are typically large, multiple, and symmetric (Fig. 8). In most cases, lesions involve the subcortical and central white matter as well as the cortical gray–white matter junction of cerebral and cerebellar hemispheres, brain stem, and spinal cord. Moreover, the deep gray matter of the thalami and basal ganglia are commonly involved. A symmetrical pattern of lesion distribution is common. The corpus callosum is not typically involved but may be affected in large lesions. Four patterns of cerebral involvement have been proposed to describe the MRI findings in ADEM: (1) ADEM with small lesions (<5 mm); (2) ADEM with large, confluent, or tumefactive lesions, with frequent extensive perilesional edema and mass effect; (3) ADEM with additional symmetric bithalamic involvement; and (4) acute hemorrhagic encephalomyelitis (AHEM, Hurst), when hemorrhage can be identified in large demyelinating lesions. The MRI pattern was not introduced to provide information about outcome or disability, since the clinical course usually is monophasic and "black holes" should not exist. Most lesions resolve on follow-up imaging studies, but frequently new lesions emerge within the first 3 months after the beginning of the disease and

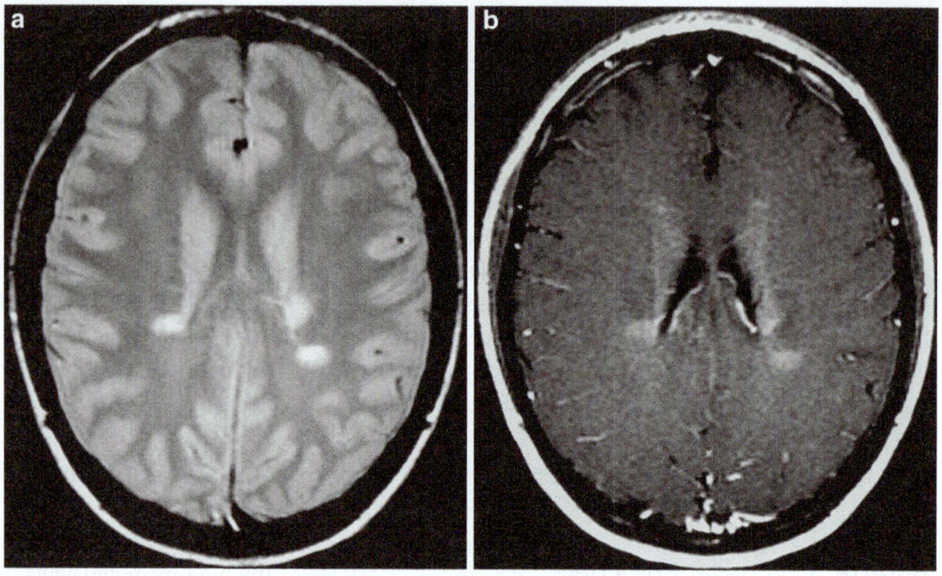

Fig. 8 Acute disseminated encephalomyelitis. **a** Axial FLAIR image. **b** Axial T1-weighted image after contrast administration. Bilateral symmetric and subcortical lesions on FLAIR images, one of which reveals contrast enhancement

even then are defined only as "one attack." In "recurrent" ADEM a second attack is required more than 3 months after the first event but involving the same anatomic area. "Multiphasic" ADEM is defined by a second attack with new areas of involvement. In these cases transition to MS is ambiguous; however, this classification may be useful when considering the differential diagnosis of ADEM and may identify patients for whom the initial ADEM phenotype is really the first manifestation of MS (Fig. 9).

2.5 Neuromyelitis Optica

Neuromyelitis optica (NMO, Devic syndrome) is a rare inflammatory demyelinating disease that typically affects optic nerves and spinal cord. Optic neuritis with a sudden complete or partial uni- or bilateral vision loss and myelitis, paresthesias, and rapidly developing paresis or quadriparesis and bowel and bladder disturbances, may occur weeks or even years apart. Symptoms implicating other CNS regions usually exclude the diagnosis. The CSF reveals $\geq$50 WBC/μl or $\geq$5 neutrophils/μl, especially in an acute phase of disease. Oligoclonal bands are usually not detected in the CSF or are only temporary. In addition, in patients presenting with an optic–spinal syndrome, a highly specific serum autoantibody (NMO-IgG) has been detected that targets aquaporin 4, the most abundant water channel in the CNS, which is highly concentrated in astrocytic foot processes. NMO-IgG is found in the serum of about 80 % of patients with typical clinical and radiological findings of NMO. Histopathologically, NMO lesions resemble the MS pattern II described by Lucchinetti et al. (2000), but are different from them. Lesions are characterized by deposits of IgG and IgM co-localizing with products of complement activation in a vasculocentric pattern around thickened hyalinized blood vessels, suggesting a pathogenic role of humoral immunity targeting an antigen in the perivascular space pointing to the importance of humoral immunity.

Myelitis usually involves several spinal segments but can also cause complete transverse myelitis at a single segment. Also, enhancement of the affected optic nerves or lesions involving the optic nerve can be observed. The brain stem, cerebellum, and the cerebral hemispheres are typically not involved initially but may be affected in the later course of disease. In 2011, differential diagnostic criteria of NMO versus MS have been proposed (Polman et al. 2011). NMO should be considered if (a) myelopathy is associated with MRI-detected spinal cord lesions longer than three spinal segments and primarily involving the central part of the spinal cord on axial sections, (b) optic neuritis is bilateral and severe or associated with a swollen optic nerve or chiasm, and (c) intractable hiccough or nausea/vomiting is present for >2 days with evidence of a periaqueductal medullary lesion on MRI. In these patients aquaporin-4 autoantibodies should be tested to make a differential diagnosis between NMO and MS.

Treatment strategies are preferentially focused on humoral immunity. Patients are treated with high-dose glucocorticosteroids, plasma exchange, or immunoadsorption, and in some cases also with intravenous immunoglobulins. For preventing relapses immunosuppressants (e.g., azathioprine, mitoxantrone, cyclophosphamide) are applied. Interferon-β may deteriorate the clinical course. The first results from preliminary studies with rituximab have been positive. Rituximab is a monoclonal antibody targeting CD20 that induces B-cell depletion for many months. A controlled multicenter study has been started.

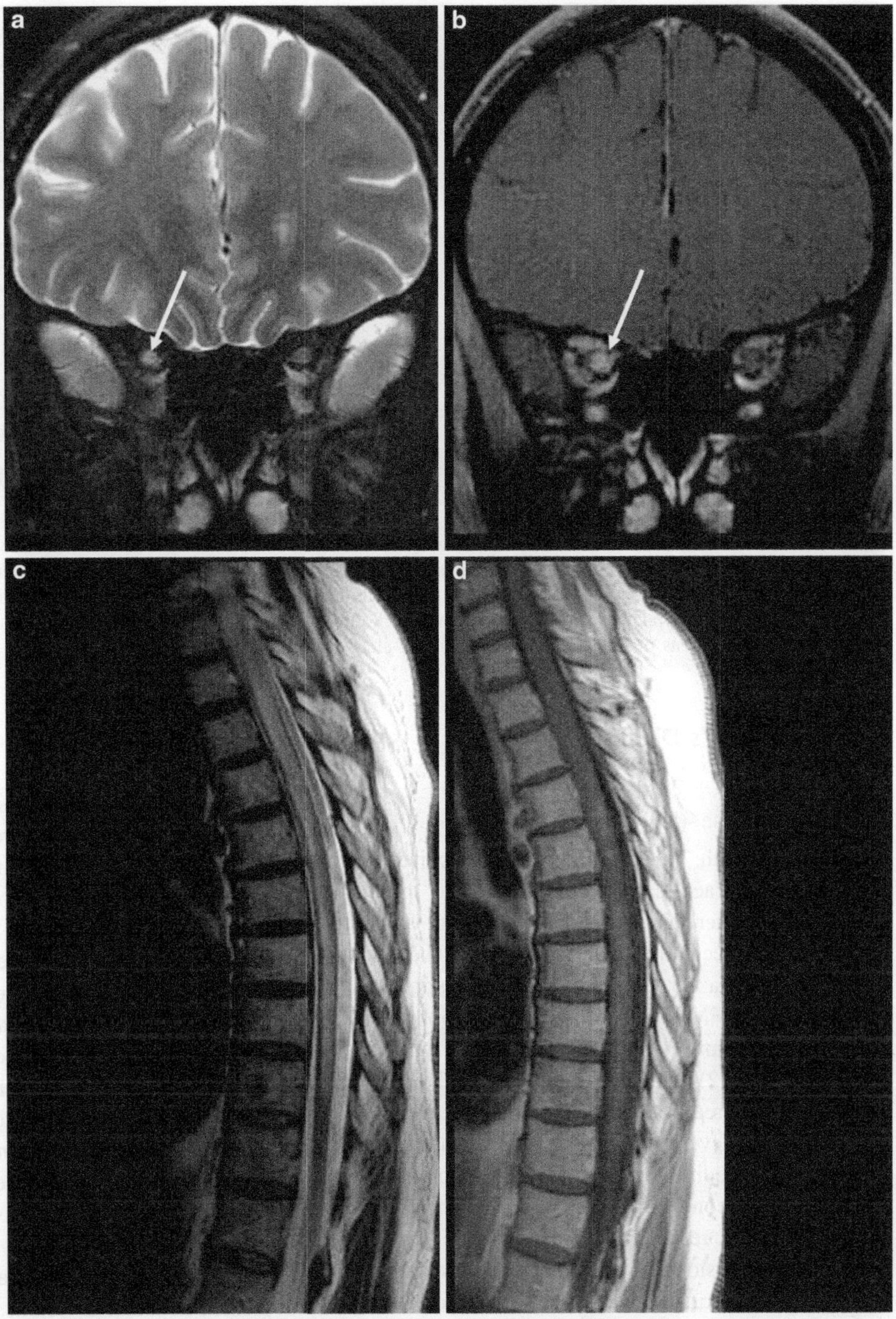

Fig. 9 Neuromyelitis optica (Devic's disease). **a** Coronal fat-suppressed T2-weighted image. **b** T1-weighted image with fat saturation after contrast administration. **c** Sagittal T2-weighted image. **d** Sagittal T2-weighted image after contrast administration. Swelling and hyperintense signal of the right optic nerve (**a**, *arrow*) with contrast enhancement (**b**, *arrow*). Spinal MRI shows multisegmental extensive hyperintensity (**c**) and swelling of the thoracic spinal cord with contrast enhancement (**d**)

2.6 Marburg's Disease

Marburg's disease is a variant of MS clinically characterized by relatively acute onset of headache, vomiting, mental confusion, and focal neurological symptoms. This rare relapsing subtype of MS has a dramatically progressive clinical course with frequent, severe relapses leading to severe disability or death within weeks to months. Most of the survivors develop a relapsing form of MS subsequently.

On MRI Marburg's disease typically presents with multifocal lesions of variable size on T2-weighted images that may join together with large white matter lesions throughout the periventricular white matter and brain stem. These lesions may show enhancement and perifocal edema.

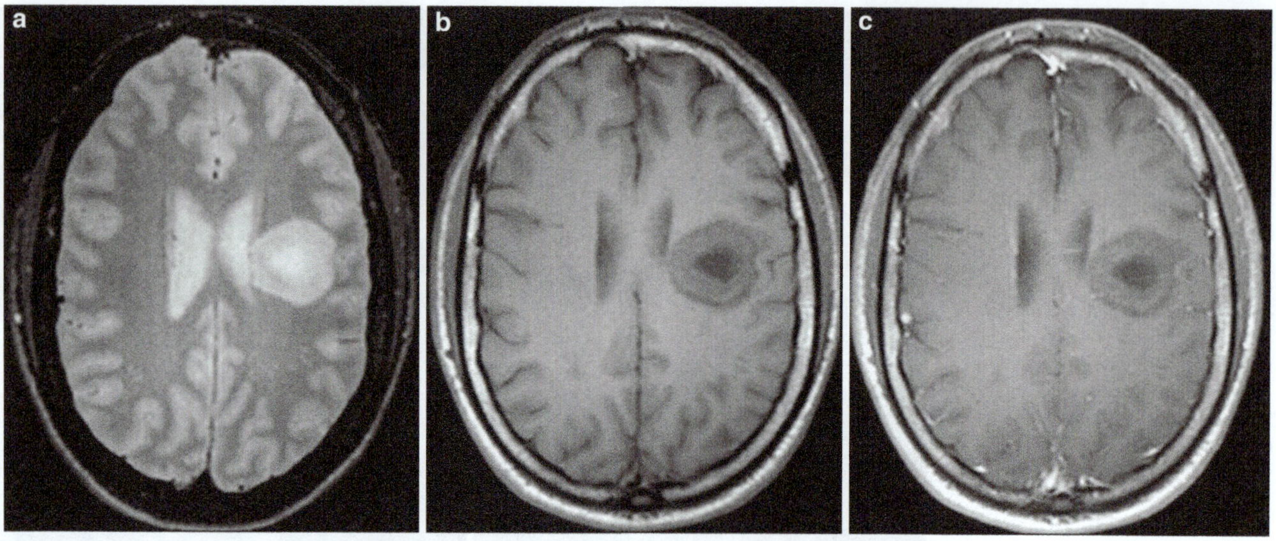

Fig. 10 Baló's concentric sclerosis. **a** Axial T2-weighted image. **b** Axial T1-weighted image before contrast administration. **c** Axial T1-weighted image after contrast administration. Periventricular lesion with concentric hypointense bands on T2-weighted images (**a**) corresponding to areas of demyelination and gliosis, alternating with isointense bands on T2-weighted images (**a**) corresponding to normal myelinated white matter (onion-like pattern). The lesion center reveals a homogeneous hyperintensity on T2-weighted images (**a**) due to extensive demyelination. There is only little contrast enhancement (**c**)

2.7 Schilder's Disease

Schilder's disease (SD) commonly affects children and young adults with an acute onset of psychiatric symptoms, acute intracranial hypertension, and progressive deterioration. There is no association with proceeding infections or vaccinations, and no fever. The following diagnostic criteria for SD emphasize its distinction from typical MS, ADEM, and adrenoleukodystrophy: (1) clinical symptoms and signs often atypical for the early course of MS; (2) CSF normal or atypical for MS; (3) bilateral large areas of demyelination of cerebral white matter; (4) no fever, viral, or mycoplasma infection, or vaccination preceding the neurological symptoms; and (5) normal serum concentrations of very long-chain fatty acids. Magnetic resonance imaging demonstrates large ring-enhancing lesions involving both hemispheres, which may be symmetrical. Frequently, there is little mass effect, incomplete ring enhancement, and the brain stem is spared. Lesions are most commonly located in the white matter of the parieto-occipital lobes and may mimic a brain tumor, an abscess, or even adrenoleukodystrophy. Histopathologically, SD shows well-demarcated demyelination and reactive gliosis, but no involvement of the axons. Clinical and imaging features usually show a dramatic response to steroids. In some cases treatment with immunosuppressants (cyclophosphamide, azathioprine) is necessary.

2.8 Baló's Disease

Baló's concentric sclerosis has a fulminant clinical course and is thought to be a rare and aggressive variant of MS. Clinically, Baló's concentric sclerosis leads to death in weeks to months. The histopathological characteristic of the lesions is a distinct pattern of alternating layers of preserved and destroyed myelin. These alternating layers also represent the characteristic pattern that can be identified on MR images. T2-weighted images typically show concentric hypointense bands corresponding to areas of demyelination and gliosis, alternating with isointense bands corresponding to normal myelinated white matter (Fig. 10) with an onion-like pattern. The lesion center usually does not reveal these layers due to extensive demyelination. Contrast enhancement and decreased diffusivity are frequent in the outer rings (acute inflammation at the outer edge) of the lesion. This imaging pattern of Baló's concentric sclerosis may be present in isolated lesions, multiple or mixed with typical MS-like lesions. Usually symptoms are severe and monophasic. Treatment includes glucocorticosteroids and other immunosuppressant substances.

2.9 Tumefactive or Pseudotumoral Demyelinating Disease

Occasionally, idiopathic inflammatory lesions may present as single or multifocal mass lesions that may be clinically

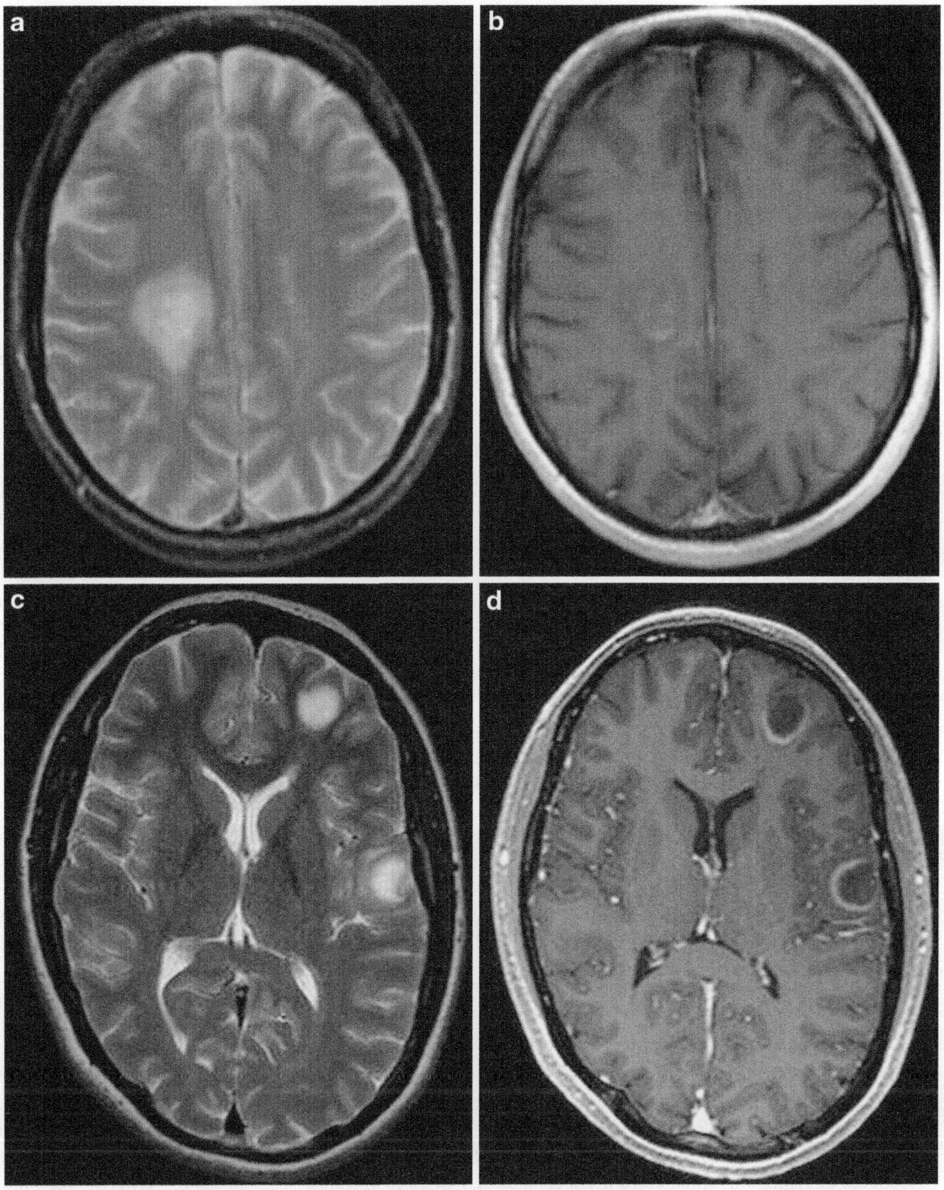

Fig. 11 Tumefactive lesions. **a, c** Axial T2-weighted image. **b, d** Axial T1-weighted image after contrast administration. All images have the same slice positions and are from the same patients. Singular, predominantly solid mass lesion in the periventricular white matter with perifocal edema (**a**) and contrast enhancement (**b**). These lesions are hardly distinguishable from intrinsic brain tumors on the basis on MRI and may require biopsy. Two subcortical cystic lesions with incomplete ring enhancement (**c**) and perifocal edema (**a**; biopsy proven inflammatory lesions). The differential diagnosis includes metastases, cystic gliomas, and abscesses

and radiographically indistinguishable from brain neoplasms. This represents a differential-diagnostic challenge, frequently requiring brain biopsy despite the clinical suspicion of demyelination; however, even the histological specimen may imitate a brain tumor in view of the hypercellularity of the lesions.

Occasionally, tumefactive demyelinating lesions may also represent the first clinical and radiological manifestation of MS. More commonly, though, these lesions affect patients with already established diagnosis of MS. In these cases, the pseudotumoral lesions do not usually represent a diagnostic problem; however, cystic or solid lesions presenting initially as idiopathic inflammatory demyelinating lesions may hardly be distinguished from neoplasms on MRI (Fig. 11). Single large lesions mostly resolve without relapse. Only in rare cases do pseudotumoral lesions have a relapsing course, with single or multiple pseudotumoral lesions appearing over time in different locations.

2.10 Acute Transverse Myelitis

Acute transverse myelitis (ATM) may be a monophasic disease, but it may also be the first manifestation of MS or Devic's neuromyelitis optica. Occasionally, there may be recurrence exclusively at the spinal cord (recurrent acute transverse myelitis). Acute ATM is defined by bilateral, and not necessarily symmetric, sensory, motor, or autonomous dysfunction attributable to the spinal cord, a sensory level, and the proof of inflammation within the spinal cord by MRI or CSF examination. An extra-axial compressive lesion, a vascular (anterior spinal artery thrombosis, arteriovenous malformation), etiology and a history of radiation to the spine have to be excluded. Transverse myelitis can be idiopathic or develop subsequent to viral or bacterial infections, after vaccinations as well as in the course of systemic autoimmune diseases. Magnetic resonance imaging abnormalities of the spinal cord commonly include large lesions extending over several vertebral segments with swelling of the cord. Gadolinium enhancement is usually present at the acute stage. There is no linear correspondence between MR findings and neurological signs.

Further Reading

Hemmer B, Nessler S, Zhou D, Kieseier B, Hatung HP (2006) Immunopathogenesis and immunotherapy of multiple sclerosis. Nat Clin Pract Neurol 2(4):201–211

Lucchinetti CF, Brück W, Parisi J, Scheithauer B, Rodrigues M, Lassmann H (2000) Heterogeneity of multiple sclerosis lesions: implications for the pathogenesis of demyelination. Ann Neurol 47(6):707–717

McDonald WI, Compston A et al (International Panel on MS diagnosis) (2001) Recommended diagnostic criteria for multiple sclerosis: guidelines from the International Panel on the diagnosis of multiple sclerosis. Ann Neurol 50(1):121–127

Poser S, Luer W, Bruhn H, Frahm J, Bruck Y, Felgenhauer K (1992) Acute demyelinating disease. Classification and non-invasive diagnosis. Acta Neurol Scand 86:579–585

Silvia Tenembaum S, Chitnis T, Ness J, Hahn JS (2007) Acute disseminated encephalomyelitis. Neurology 68:23–36

Wingerchuk DM, Lennon VA, Pittock SJ, Lucchinetti CF, Weinshenker BG (2006) Revised diagnostic criteria for neuromyelitis optica. Neurology 66(10):1485–1489

Young NP, Weinshenker BG, Lucchinetti CF (2008) Acute disseminated encephalomyelitis: current understanding and controversies. Semin Neurol 28(1):84–94

References

Filippi M, Rovaris M, Capra R, Gasperini C, Yousry TA, Sormani MP, Prandini F, Horsfield MA, Martinelli V, Bastianello S, Kuhne I, Pozzilli C, Comi G (1998) A multi-centre longitudinal study comparing the sensitivity of monthly MRI after standard and triple dose gadolinium-DTPA for monitoring disease activity in multiple sclerosis. Implications for phase II clinical trials. Brain 121:2011–2020

McDonald WI, Compston A, Edan G, Goodkin D, Hartung HP, Lublin FD, McFarland HF, Paty DW, Polman CH, Reingold SC, Sandberg-Wollheim M, Sibley W, Thompson A, van den Noort S, Weinshenker BY, Wolinsky JS (2001) Recommended diagnostic criteria for multiple sclerosis: guidelines from the international panel on the diagnosis of multiple sclerosis. Ann Neurol 50:121–127

Polman CH, Reingold SC, Edan G, Filippi M, Hartung HP, Kappos L, Lublin FD, Metz LM, McFarland HF, O'Connor PW, Sandberg-Wollheim M, Thompson AJ, Weinshenker BG, Wolinsky JS (2005) Diagnostic criteria for multiple sclerosis: 2005 revisions to the "McDonald Criteria". Ann Neurol 58:840–846

Polman CH, Reingold SC, Banwell B, Clanet M, Cohen JA, Filippi M, Fujihara K, Havrdova E, Hutchinson M, Kappos L, Lublin FD, Montalban X, O' Connor P, Sandberg-Wollheim M, Thompson AJ, Waubant E, WEinshenker B, Wolinsky JS (2011) Diagnostic criteria for multiple sclerosis: 2010 revisions to the McDonald criteria. Ann Neurol 69:292–302

Simon JH, Li D, Traboulsee A, Coyle PK, Arnold DL, Barkhof F, Frank JA, Grossman R, Paty DW, Radue EW, Wolinsky JS (2006) Standardized MR imaging protocol for multiple sclerosis: consortium of MS centers consensus guidelines. Am J Neuroradiol 27(2):455–461

Swanton JK, Rovira A, Tintore M, Altmann DR, Barkhof F, Filippi M, Huerga E, Miszkiel KA, Plant GT, Polman C, Rovaris M, Thompson AJ, Montalban X, Miller DH (2007) MRI criteria for multiple sclerosis in patients presenting with clinically isolated syndromes: a multicentre retrospective study. Lancet Neurol 6:677–686

Wattjes MP, Harzheim M, Kuhl CK, Gieseke J, Schmidt S, Klotz L, Klockgether T, Schild HH, Lutterbey GG (2006) Does high-field MR imaging have an influence on the classification of patients with clinically isolated syndromes according to current diagnostic MR imaging criteria for multiple sclerosis? Am J Neuroradiol 27(8):1794–1798

Cerebral Vasculitis

Martina Wengenroth, Christian Jacobi and Brigitte Wildemann

Contents

M. Wengenroth (✉)
Department of Radiology, Marchioninistrasse 15,
81377 Munich, Germany
e-mail: martina.wengenroth@med.uni-muenchen.de

C. Jacobi
Department of Neurology,
Krankenhaus Nordwest GmbH, Steinbacher Hohl 2-26,
60488 Frankfurt am Main, Germany

B. Wildemann
Division of Molecular Neuroimmunology,
Department of Neurology,
University of Heidelberg Medical Center,
Im Neuenheimer Feld 400, 69120 Heidelberg, Germany

Abstract

Vasculitis is an inflammation of blood vessels due to various origins. Vessels of the peripheral and/or central nervous systems may be involved. Clinical and radiological diagnosis of cerebral vasculitis is challenging as there is no vasculitis-specific symptom or imaging sign. Furthermore, it may mimic other neurological diseases, which would require different treatment approaches. Neuroimaging of cerebral vasculitis should begin with initial MRI to assess the degree of parenchymal damage and to detect vessel wall changes. If the results are indefinite DSA should be pursued in order to detect potential changes of medium-sized vessels. Vasculitides of small vessels cannot be detected by vascular imaging and require brain or leptomeningeal biopsy.

1 Epidemiology, Clinical Presentation and Therapy

Christian Jacobi and Brigitte Wildemann

Summary

Vasculitis is defined as inflammation of blood vessels with or without necrosis of the vessel wall. Vasculitis can be further classified based on the origin of vessel pathology into immunoallergic, infectious and neoplastic forms, and divided into primary and secondary subtypes. To confirm the diagnosis, histology is usually required. Vasculitis may involve vessels of both the peripheral and central nervous systems (CNS). Vasculitis of the CNS is rare and occurs in the context of systemic diseases or as primary angiitis of the CNS. The clinical diagnosis of CNS vasculitis is difficult, as there is a wide spectrum of neurological signs and symptoms, and specific technical examinations to confirm the CNS manifestation do not exist.

S. Hähnel (ed.), *Inflammatory Diseases of the Brain*, Medical Radiology. Diagnostic Imaging,
DOI: 10.1007/174_2012_661, © Springer-Verlag Berlin Heidelberg 2012
Published Online: 07 December 2012

Table 1 Examples for primary and secondary vasculitis affecting the nervous system

Primary vasculitis
Churg–Strauss syndrome
Polyarteritis nodosa
Microscopic polyangiitis
Wegener's granulomatosis
Takayasu arteritis
Hypersensitivity vasculitis
Cryoglobulin-associated vasculitis
Primary vasculitis of the central nervous system
Secondary vasculitis
Connective tissue diseases and other systemic autoimmune diseases
Sjögren syndrome
Rheumatoid arthritis
Systemic lupus erythematosus
Mixed connective tissue disease
Behçet's disease
Infections (e.g. HIV, CMV, spirochetes)
Neoplastic diseases (e.g. lymphoma, solid tumours)
Drug exposure (e.g. morphine, cocaine)

1.1 Classification

Cerebral vasculitis can be classified in different ways. One classification is based on the differentiation between primary and secondary subtypes (Table 1).

Primary vasculitis can be further classified depending on the size of the affected vessels (small, medium, large). The international consensus classification (Chapel Hill classification from 1994) defines the vessel size depending on the smallest affected vessel. Other classifications include histological (e.g. granulomas) and immunological markers (e.g. the association with antineutrophil cytoplasm antibodies, ANCAs).

1.2 Epidemiology

The overall incidence of primary vasculitis is about 40/1,000,000 persons [excluding giant cell (temporal) arteritis, GCA]. Its incidence increases with age. The incidence of GCA is much higher (around 200/1,000,000 persons in the age group >50 years).

The frequency of CNS manifestations in primary vasculitis is not well examined. Published data exist for polyarteritis nodosa (10–40 %), Wegener's granulomatosis (10 %) and Churg–Strauss syndrome (10 %). In all other primary vasculitides CNS manifestations seem to be rare.

In secondary vasculitis valid data as to the frequency of CNS involvement are not uniformly available. CNS vasculitis is reported in around 5 % of cases in Sjögren syndrome and in 10–30 % of patients diagnosed with mixed connective tissue diseases. In systemic lupus erythematosus CNS involvement affects 40–60 % of patients but is attributable to vasculitis in 7–13 % of cases only. The frequency of neuro-Behçet is around 10–40 %.

1.3 Clinical Presentation

Clinical and pathological presentation in CNS vasculitis represents a wide spectrum. Among others, headache, cranial nerve affections, encephalopathy, seizures, psychosis, myelitis, stroke, intracranial haemorrhage and aseptic meningoencephalitis are described.

Aside from clinical examination (comprehensive clinical history and clinical examination), the diagnosis of vasculitis requires multiple technical examinations: laboratory tests (blood cell count, erythrocyte sedimentation rate (ESR); clinical chemistry panel [including C-reactive protein (CRP), liver and renal functions], anti-double stranded (ds) DNA, antinuclear antibody (ANA) and, if positive, ANA fine specificities (anti-Sm, anti-SSB, anti-SSA, antihistone, anticentromere, anti-Scl70, anti-nRNP, anti-Jo-1, anti-PM-Sd), ANCA, complement (C3 and C4) and cryoglobulin levels, rheumatoid factor, immunofixation electrophoresis, quantitative immunoglobulins, lupus anticoagulant (LA), anticardiolipin antibody (aCL), serology for hepatitis B and C virus) as well as radiographic examinations (e.g. CT, MRI, PET and SPECT). In case of suspected CNS involvement, electrophysiological studies, such as electroencephalography and evoked potentials, may be helpful. CSF analysis is another powerful tool to detect CNS involvement. Pleocytosis and intrathecal immunogobulin synthesis are the most prominent abnormalities; however, these abnormalities are non-specific. The gold standard to diagnose CNS vasculitis remains the histopathological examination of affected organs.

In the following sections selected primary and secondary vasculitides leading more frequently to CNS manifestations are discussed in more detail.

1.3.1 Primary Vasculitides

1.3.1.1 Large-Vessel Vasculitis

Giant Cell (Temporal) Arteritis

Giant cell (temporal) arteritis (GCA) involves the ophthalmic, posterior ciliary, superficial temporal, occipital, internal maxillary and facial arteries. In around 20 % of cases it is associated with polymyalgia rheumatica. Initial symptoms are exhaustion, myalgia, fever and weight loss.

The patients complain of parietal headache and visual disturbances. The temporal artery is often tender to touch. During the course of disease the temporal artery gets thicker and loses its pulse. Ptosis and diplopia, due to ischaemia of the extraocular muscles and claudication of the jaw, are other possible symptoms. In some cases ischaemia of the tongue and scalp may arise. Diagnostic criteria of the American College of Rheumatology (ACR) are defined and include the following (positive if at least three are present):

1. Age at disease onset >50 years
2. Blood sedimentation reaction >50 mm/h (first hour)
3. New headache
4. Temporal artery tenderness to palpation or decreased pulsation, unrelated to arteriosclerosis of cervical arteries
5. Typical histology in temporal artery biopsy

Untreated GCA can lead to visual loss.

Rarely GCA affects intracranial vessels and may cause transient ischaemic attacks (TIA) and stroke.

Takayasu Arteritis

Takayasu arteritis is a granulomatous vasculitis of the great elastic branches (aorta and its major extracranial vessels, pulmonary arteries). It usually affects young patients <40 years and is more common in women. Japanese and Mexicans are more frequently affected compared with Caucasians. The ACR criteria are defined as follows (positive if at least three are present):

1. Age at disease onset <40 years
2. Claudication of extremities
3. Difference of >10 mm Hg in systolic blood pressure between arms
4. Decreased brachial artery pulse
5. Bruit over the subclavian arteries or aorta arteriogram abnormality
6. Syncope is the most frequent neurological symptom; less common are TIA or stroke

1.3.1.2 Medium-Sized Vessel Vasculitis

Polyarteritis Nodosa

Polyarteritis nodosa (PAN) is commonly associated with viral infections (e.g. hepatitis B and C, HIV). In this necrotizing vasculitis medium and small vessels are affected. The first systemic symptoms are malaise, fever and weight loss. Skin lesions and renal involvement occur in up to 70 % of the patients and 45 % suffer from gastrointestinal symptoms. Laboratory examinations reveal increased ESR, CRP, decreased complement (C3 and C4) and circulating immune complexes. The most common neurological manifestation is peripheral neuropathy. The CNS involvement in PAN leads to headache, retinopathy and encephalopathy with seizures and cognitive decline (small-sized vessels). In around 10 % of the patients with neurological manifestations stroke and intracerebral haemorrhage are the leading CNS disorders (medium-sized vessels). Other symptoms may arise from affection of the cranial nerves or the spinal cord.

1.3.1.3 Primary Angiitis of the CNS

Primary angiitis of the CNS (PACNS) is an isolated vasculitis of the central nervous system affecting small and medium-sized vessels in the brain and spinal cord. The most frequent clinical signs and symptoms (40–80 %) are chronic headache, encephalopathy and focal signs and symptoms (most frequently aphasia and hemiparesis). Stroke (ischaemia or intracerebral haemorrhage) is rare. The disease course is usually subacute (around 80 %) and may be relapsing or continuously progressive. Only in around 20 % of cases does the course fluctuate. CSF findings can be normal, but in most cases a pleocytosis can be detected during follow-up. The only possibility to confirm the diagnosis is a brain/leptomeningeal biopsy.

1.3.1.4 Small-Sized Vessel Vasculitis

Wegener's Granulomatosis

Wegener's granulomatosis affects the respiratory tract and the kidney with frequent glomerulonephritis. Usually anti-proteinase 3 (PR3, c-ANCA in around 90 % of the cases) can be measured in serum. The ACR defined the following diagnostic criteria for Wegener's granulomatosis (positive if at least two are present):

1. Development of painful or painless oral ulcers or purulent or bloody nasal discharge.
2. Urinary sediment showing microhaematuria or red cell casts.
3. Abnormal chest radiograph with the presence of nodules, fixed infiltrates or cavities.
4. Histological changes showing granulomatous inflammation within the wall of an artery or in the peri-vascular or extravascular area (artery or arteriole).

Stroke is a rare complication (4 %) of Wegener's granulomatosis. Intracranial granuloma following direct invasion from the nasal cavity may lead to an affection of the basal cranial nerves. Other possible neurological complications are aseptic meningitis, encephalopathy and sinus thrombosis.

1.3.2 Secondary Vasculitis in Connective Tissue Diseases

Connective tissue diseases, such as systemic lupus erythematosus (SLE), scleroderma, rheumatoid arthritis, mixed connective disease and Sjögren syndrome, are systemic immune-mediated diseases that lead to multiple organ affections. Diagnostic criteria for these diseases are defined by the rheumatological societies. A spectrum of antinuclear antibodies (ANA) is measurable in serum. In mixed connective disease, scleroderma, rheumatoid arthritis and Sjögren syndrome CNS manifestations are usually caused by vasculitis, while in SLE vasculitis of cerebral vessels is rather uncommon and occurs in around 10 % of cases. The CNS involvement may cause headache, stroke (intracranial haemorrhage and ischaemia), sinus thrombosis, encephalopathy, seizures and aseptic meningitis. The CSF examinations often reveal a pleocytosis and intrathecal antibody synthesis including positive CSF oligoclonal bands.

1.3.3 Behçet's Disease

Behçet's disease usually affects the small blood vessels including arteries and veins. The major clinical signs are oral ulcers, genital ulcers, ocular lesions (mainly uveitis) and cutaneous involvement. CNS involvement is present in 10–40 % of patients and can be subdivided into parenchymatous (inflammation of the CNS tissue) and vascular neuro-Behçet. The most common neurological symptom of neuro-Behçet is headache. The parenchymatous manifestation leads to encephalitis and meningoencephalitis often affecting the basal ganglia and the brain stem. Possible vascular manifestations of neuro-Behçet include pseudotumour cerebri, sinus thrombosis and stroke. The CSF shows pleocytosis and intrathecal immunoglobulin synthesis and is usually normal in patients with pure vascular disease (e.g. sinus thrombosis).

1.4 Therapy

Vasculitis is a serious disease that is potentially fatal or leads to permanent disability and requires rapid institution of immunosuppressive treatment. Possible therapeutic options include glucocorticoids, cyclophosphamide, azathioprine, intravenous immunoglobulins and mycophenolate mofetil.

Systemic vasculitis with CNS involvement is usually treated with a combined medication of oral glucocorticoids (1 mg/kg prednisone) and oral cyclophosphamide as recommended by the modified Fauci scheme (2 mg/kg/day). It may be initiated by i.v. therapy with 1,000 mg methylprednisolone for 3 days. In severe cases a dosage of up to 4 mg/kg day cyclophosphamide may be required. In some cases plasmapheresis may be helpful. Following remission, long-term treatment can be continued with other immunosuppressants such as azathioprine, cyclosporine A, methotrexate or mycophenolatmofetil.

In GCA rapid treatment with oral glucocorticoids (e.g. 100 mg methylprednisolone for 2 weeks) is mandatory to avoid visual loss. After 2 weeks, slow reduction of steroids may be considered and tapering should be adjusted over many weeks.

Primary vasculitis of the central nervous system is treated with combined oral glucocorticoids (1 mg/kg prednisone) and oral cyclophosphamide (2 mg/kg/day). The therapy may be initiated with i.v. glucocorticoids (3 days 1000 mg methylprednisolone) followed by cyclophosphamid pulse therapy before oral medication (Aksel S 2001; Berlit P 2004; Ferro JM 1998; Moore PM 1998).

2 Cerebral Vasculitis: Imaging and Differential Diagnosis

Martina Wengenroth

Summary

Vasculitides represent a heterogeneous group of inflammatory diseases that affect blood vessel walls of varying calibers (inflammatory vasculopathy). Cerebral vasculitis is defined as inflammation of leptomeningeal and/or parenchymal vessels of the brain. It is a rare but severe condition which can occur in all ages and often poses diagnostic challenges to clinicians and neuroradiologists alike. Clinically it can present with a panoply of manifestations such as headache, seizures, psychosis, and neurological deficits. In neuroimaging there is no vasculitis-specific sign and vasculitis may be mistaken for several other diseases such as multiple sclerosis, infections, or brain tumors, which all require different treatment approaches. Since the devastating symptoms of CNS vasculitis are at least partially reversible, early diagnosis and appropriate treatment are important. In order to establish a differential diagnosis clinical features, disease progression, age of onset, blood results, as well as CSF examinations have to be taken into consideration. Neuroimaging techniques, such as MRI and DSA, play a central role in the diagnosis and disease monitoring. The diagnostic protocol for cerebral vasculitis should include initial MRI to assess the degree of parenchymal damage and to detect vessel wall changes, in particular in large-vessel vasculitis. If the results are ambiguous or medium-sized arteries are affected (beyond the spatial resolution of MRI) DSA should follow. Small-vessel vasculitides entirely evade detection by vascular imaging and consequently require brain or leptomeningeal biopsy.

2.1 Neuroimaging of Cerebral Vasculitides

In cerebral vasculitis diverse causes may trigger leptomeningeal and/or parenchymal vessel wall inflammation of the brain. The term “arteritis” defines arterial inflammation, whereas “angiitis” is characterized by the inflammation of either arteries or veins. “Primary central nervous system vasculitis” (PCNSV) is restricted to the central nervous system. In contrast, secondary vasculitides may occur in the course of underlying systemic inflammation such as infections, neoplasias, drug abuse as well as connective tissue diseases and other systemic autoimmune disorders.

Table 2 Examples for the classification of primary vasculitides depending on the affected vessel size

	Large-sized vessels (ICA, A1, M1, P1, VA, BA)	Medium-sized vessels (M2, ACA, Pcom)	Small-sized vessels (arterioles, venules, capillaries)
Takayasu arteritis	X		
Giant cell (temporal) arteritis	X		
Polyarteritis nodosa		X	
Primary angiitis of the central nervous system	(X)	X	X
Wegener's granulomatosis			X
Vasculitis in connective tissue diseases			X
Behçet's disease			X
Vasculitis in connective tissue diseases (e.g. SLE)			X

Table 3 Imaging signs of cerebral vasculitides

	MRI	DSA
Vascular changes	T1-weighted: increased thickness of vessel wall	Abnormal straightening and/or kinking of arteries
	Postcontrast T1-weighted: mural enhancement	Multiple micro-aneurysms (rare, but highly specific)
	T2-weighted: vessel wall edema (may persist despite clinical remission)	Stenoses (one or multiple)
	Non-atherosclerotic arterial stenoses and occlusions	No prevalence of stenoses to vascular branching points
Parenchymal changes	Ischemic brain lesions (multiple infarcts of different ages; located in various vascular territories)	
	Intracerebral or subarachnoid hemorrhage	
	Cerebral perfusion deficits	
	Postcontrast T1-weighted: enhancement of leptomeningeal tissue adjacent to affected vessels	

Various inflammatory pathways induce endothelial cell activation. Subsequent changes of the intima may lead to accelerated atherosclerosis with occlusion, micro-aneurysms, and/or rupture of the respective vessel.

Since the caliber of the affected vessels may be indicative with regard to possible differential diagnoses, a classification of vasculitides according to the vessel size is helpful from the neuroradiological point of view. According to the traditional Chapel Hill nomenclature which was developed for systemic diseases, most intracranial vessels would fall into the category of either small- or medium-sized (Jennette et al. 1994); hence, this chapter categorizes intracranial vasculitides according to the vessel size as proposed by (Kueker 2007), whereby cerebral vessels with a diameter of more than 2 mm would be considered large (Table 2). They comprise the ICA, the M1 segment of the MCA, the A1 segment of the ACA, the P1 segment of the PCA, the intracranial VA, and the BA. Vasculitides that may target large vessels include giant cell (temporal) arteritis, Takayasu's arteritis, PCNSV as well as virus and bacterial-associated vasculitides. In patients who present solely with large-vessel involvement, tissue biopsies are not feasible; hence, neuroimaging becomes an indispensable diagnostic tool. Direct signs of vessel wall changes may be detected by DSA, MRA, and MRI (Table 3; Kueker et al. 2008). Thickened vessel walls may be visualized by advanced MR sequences, which help to distinguish between noninflammatory and inflammatory (edema, contrast enhancement of vessel wall) origin (Giannini et al. 2012). Indirect signs of vasculitis as deduced from the pattern of parenchymal damage can be assessed by MRI.

Medium-vessel vasculitides affect cerebral arteries distal to the bifurcation of the MCA as well as the anterior and posterior communicating arteries (ACA and Pcom). The prevalence appears to be higher in older patients. The prototypical medium-vessel vasculitis is panarteritis nodosa (PAN). Furthermore, medium-sized vessels may be involved in systemic lupus erythematosus (SLE) and Behçet's disease.

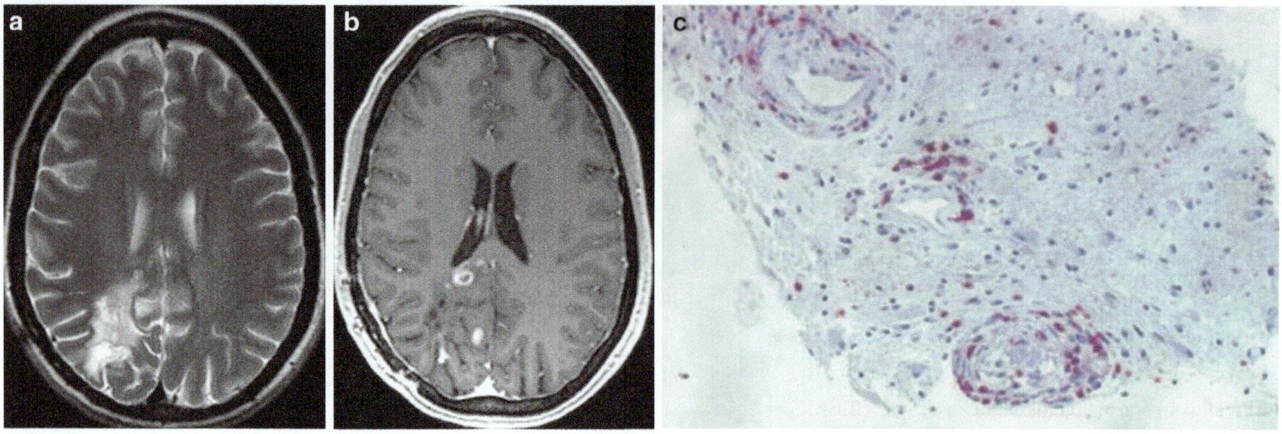

Fig. 1 Primary angiitis of the central nervous system (PACNS). A 27-year-old woman with headache and leg twitching. **a** Axial T2-weighted image. **b** Axial T1-weighted image after contrast administration. **c** Immunohistochemical preparation of stereotactic brain biopsy. Laminar hyperintensity of the right subcortical and cortical parietooccipital region on T2-weighted images (**a**). Multifocal patchy and circular contrast enhancement at the border between gray and white matter (**b**). Fibrinoid necrosis and CD8+ lymphocytic infiltration of cerebral vessels, consistent with the diagnosis of vasculitis (**c**; courtesy of M.D. Siegelin, Neuropathology Heidelberg)

Small-vessel vasculitides affect arterioles, venules, as well as capillaries. This rare type of vasculitis includes Wegener's granulomatosis, microscopic polyangiitis, Sjögren syndrome, and cryoglobulinemic vasculitis; however, often enough vasculitic syndromes, such as Wegener's granulomatosis, do not adhere to vessel-size boundaries. The inflammatory changes of small cerebral vessels are beyond the spatial resolution of currently routinely available vascular imaging techniques and consequently require brain or leptomeningeal biopsy. Nevertheless, that diagnostic pathway may possibly change with the introduction of ultra high field strength MRI in the clinical routine application.

MRI has a high sensitivity for cerebral vasculitides, particularly with respect to secondary tissue damage, but a low specificity. There is no imaging sign pathognomonic for vasculitis and the appearance can be similar irrespective of the underlying disease mechanism; however, multiple infarcts in various vascular territories and of different ages are suggestive of cerebral vasculitis, in particular in young patients.

Due to the higher spatial resolution of DSA (approximately 100–200 μm), conventional angiography should corroborate the presumed diagnosis when lab studies and clinical presentation are highly suspicious and if MRI or MRA results are negative or ambiguous.

In some cases biopsy may still be required to render a definitive diagnosis. Albeit still considered the gold standard in the diagnosis of vasculitis, with a sensitivity of approximately 75 %, even histopathology may yield inconclusive or false-negative results due to sampling error; thus, negative histopathology results do not forcibly exclude the diagnosis of vasculitis.

Taken together, large-vessel vasculitides may be diagnosed by MRI, medium-vessel vasculitides often require additional angiography, and small-vessel vasculitides may entirely evade detection by vascular imaging and therefore necessitate histological proof ("the smaller the affected vessel, the more invasive the required diagnostic procedure"). Despite the lack of specific signs, neuroimaging can be employed to assess the extent and type of lesions and to monitor the treatment response.

2.1.1 Primary Central Nervous System Vasculitis

Primary central nervous system vasculitis (PCNSV) is the most frequent vasculitis involving brain and spinal chord. Since it is limited to the nervous system it is being referred to as "primary angiitis of the CNS" (PACNS) or "primary central nervous system vasculitis" (PCNSV) (both terms are used synonymously).

Generally, patients of all age groups can be affected by this heterogeneous type of vasculitis, including children (cPCNSV or cPACNS = primary angiitis of the CNS in childhood). Most patients are between 40 and 60 years old at the time of diagnosis (Salvarani et al. 2007). In most cases the underlying pathophysiology is a noninfectious granulomatous angiitis affecting the nervous system; however, non-granulomatous histologies have been more and more reported recently (Giannini et al. 2012). Intracranial vessels of all sizes may be involved, predominantly leptomeningeal arteries and veins.

For clinicans and neuroradiologists alike, its diagnosis is challenging due to the absence of specific signs. Clinical symptoms include headache, non-focal and less frequently focal neurological signs. Imaging signs are typically multifocal caliber changes of the vessels; thus, multiple irregular-shaped stenoses or occlusions alternating with dilated segments. The most common MR imaging finding is multifocal infarctions in acute stages (in about 50 %), that typically involve the cortex and subcortical regions as well as deep

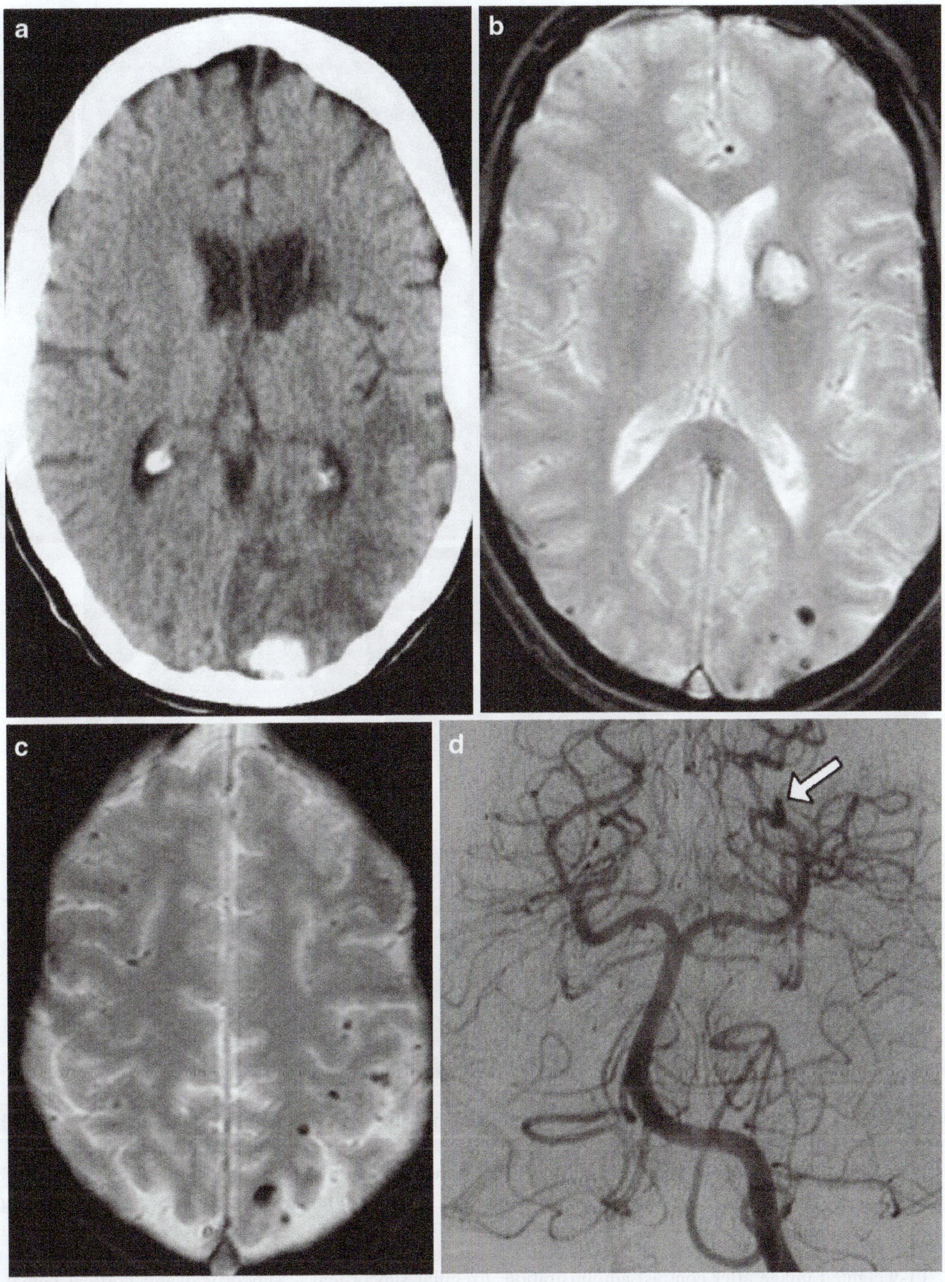

Fig. 2 Suspected primary angiitis of the central nervous system (PACNS). A 45-year-old woman with aphasia and right hemianopsia. Imaging signs are highly suggestive of cerebral vasculitis, despite negative CSF and histology results. Arguably, the posterior infarct might be a result of an embolus from an atrial myxoma which was found in this patient; however, this cannot sufficiently explain the multiple microaneurysms and petechial hemorrhages, which are typical findings in cerebral vasculitis. **a** Axial CT. **b**, **c** Axial T2*-weighted GRE image. **d** DSA of the left vertebral artery, frontal view. Old ischemic defect in the head of the left caudate nucleus, demarcated left posterior infarct and concomitant occipital parenchymal hemorrhage (**a**). Multifocal punctate areas of susceptibility low-signal intensity at the gray–white matter junction as a result of petechial hemorrhages, most prominently in the left parietal lobe (**b**, **c**). Classical appearance of vasculitis on DSA with multiple caliber changes including microaneurysms (**d**, *arrow*)

gray matter. Further MR signs include parenchymal and leptomeningeal enhancement, tumor-like masses, and signal-altered areas on FLAIR or T2-weighted images ((Birnbaum and Hellmann 2009, Zuccoli et al. 2011, Giannini et al. 2012). The SWI may present petechial hemorrhages with hemoglobin degradation products. MRA is relatively insensitive and may often be normal. (Figs. 1, 2).

2.1.2 Panarteritis Nodosa

Panarteritis Nodosa (PAN) is the most common systemic vasculitis that affects the CNS. The highest prevalence occurs in the fifth and sixth decades of life; young people are usually not affected. Characteristically, fibrinoid necrosis of the internal and external elastic lamina leads to the destruction of the vessel wall and consequent formation of microaneurysms and/or luminal obliteration (Fig. 3).

2.1.3 Giant Cell (Temporal) Arteritis

Giant cell arteritis results from granulomatous vessel wall infiltration of large arteries. Mainly the temporal arteries are affected (hence, the name), although occipital or other arteries may be involved additionally or alternatively. Temporal arteritis may be diagnosed by Doppler ultrasonography, which can depict both the vessel lumen and the vessel wall.

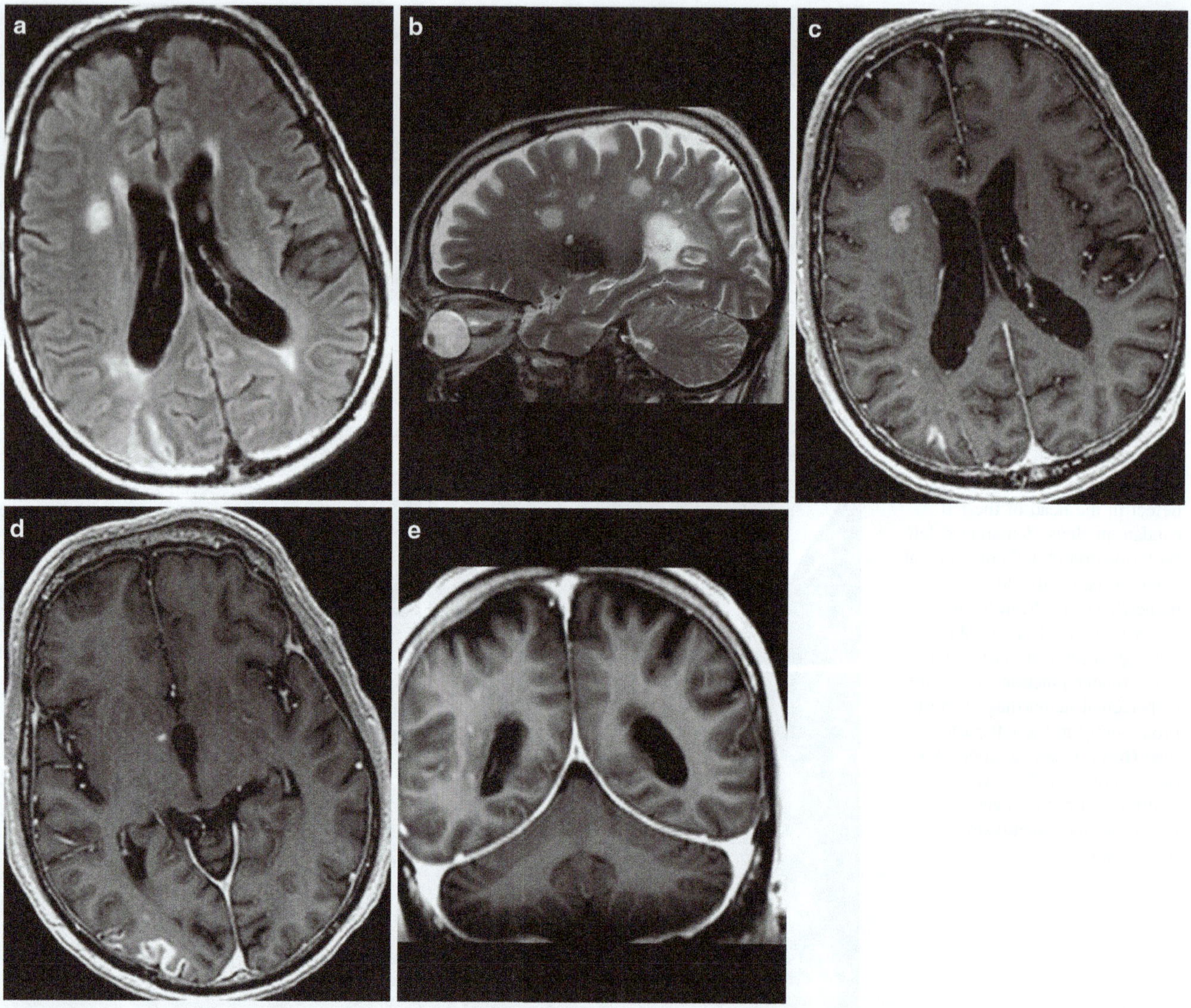

Fig. 3 Panarteritis nodosa (PAN). A 65-year-old man with loss of vigilance and intermittent hemiparesis of the left side. Biopsy of the cerebellum and meninges yielded pathological features compatible with those of cerebral vasculitis. He died 3 months after hospital admission. **a** Axial FLAIR image. **b** Sagittal T2-weighted image. **c**, **d** Axial T1-weighted images after contrast administration. **e** Coronal T1-weighted image after contrast administration. Irregular subcortical and cortical signal changes of the right hemisphere (**a**). Patchy hyperintense areas on T2-weighted images in the right cerebral hemisphere (**b**). Multiple right-hemispheric contrast-enhancing lesions, patchy in the periventricular white matter and garland-like in the cortex of the right occipital cortex (**c**, **d**). Punctate nodular contrast enhancement in the white matter of the right hemisphere (**e**). **e** Panarteritis nodosa (PAN). A 65-year-old man with loss of vigilance and intermittent hemiparesis of the left side. Biopsy of the cerebellum and meninges yielded pathological features compatible with those of cerebral vasculitis. He died 3 months after hospital admission. **e** Coronal T1-weighted image after contrast administration. Irregular subcortical and cortical signal changes of the right hemisphere (**a**). Patchy hyperintense areas on T2-weighted images in the right cerebral hemisphere (**b**). Multiple right-hemispheric contrast-enhancing lesions, patchy in the periventricular white matter and garland-like in the cortex of the right occipital cortex (**c**, **d**). Punctate nodular contrast enhancement in the white matter of the right hemisphere (**e**)

The vessel wall edema may be visualized by ultrasound as a characteristic and highly sensitive concentric hypoechogenic mural thickening ("halo sign"). Several studies have reported high sensitivity of MRI in giant cell arteritis (Bley et al. 2005). In particular, vessel wall changes, which are mural thickening and contrast enhancement of the temporal arteries and other large vessels, are sensitive signs. The higher the employed field strength of the MR scanner, the better is the sensitivity for vessel wall changes in MRI and MRA (Fig. 4; Pipitone et al. 2008).

2.1.4 Takayasu's Arteritis

Takayasu's arteritis ("pulseless disease") represents an idiopathic granulomatous giant cell arteritis, primarily affecting the aorta and its major branches. Characteristically marked thickening of the affected vessels with long, smooth

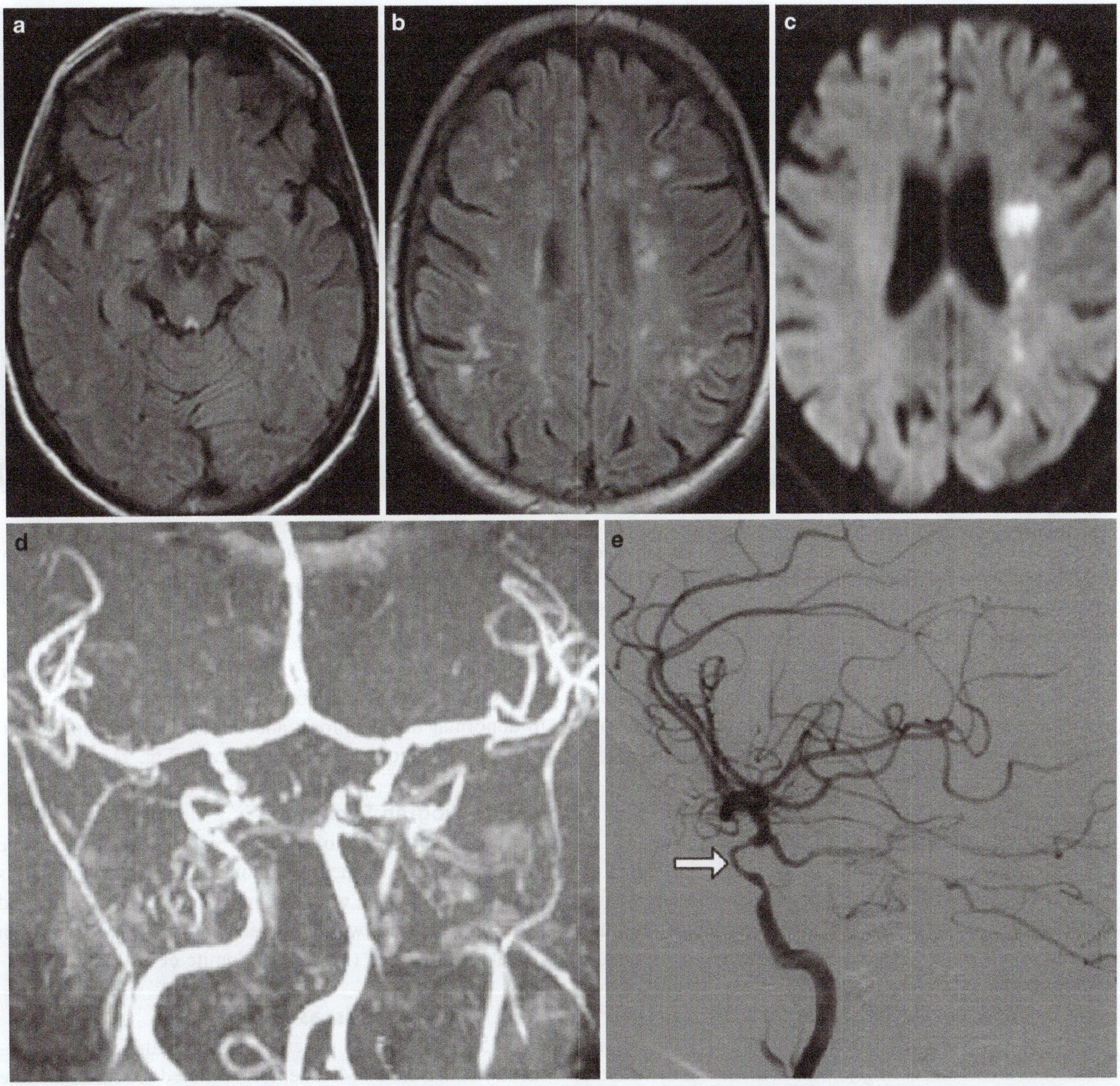

Fig. 4 Giant cell (temporal) arteritis. A 61-year-old woman presenting with hemiparesis of the right side and psychosis. The psychotic symptoms disappeared subsequent to the administration of high-dose steroids. **a, b** Axial FLAIR images. **c** Axial DWI. **d, e** Giant cell (temporal) arteritis. A 61-year-old woman presenting with hemiparesis of the right side and psychosis. The psychotic symptoms disappeared subsequent to the administration of high-dose steroids. **d** MIP of an arterial TOF MRA. **e** DSA of the right ICA, lateral view. Multifocal patchy signal changes in the subcortical and deep white matter of both hemispheres (**a**, **b**). Acute ischemic border zone infarction in the left corona radiata (**c**). Irregular and partially absent flow in the left ICA (**d**) and high-grade stenosis of the ophthalmic segment of the right ICA (**e**, *arrow*)

stenoses, and sometimes occlusions, becomes visible on DSA and MRA (Pipitone et al. 2008). Since large vessels are affected, vessel wall edema may be visualized using MR imaging. Diffuse dilations and aneurysms are not uncommon (Kelley 2004).

2.1.5 Wegener's Granulomatosis

This chronic systemic arteritis involves lungs, kidneys, and paranasal sinuses. The CNS is affected in less than 10 % of patients. In such cases, intracerebral and meningeal necrotizing granulomas or vasculitis may occur.

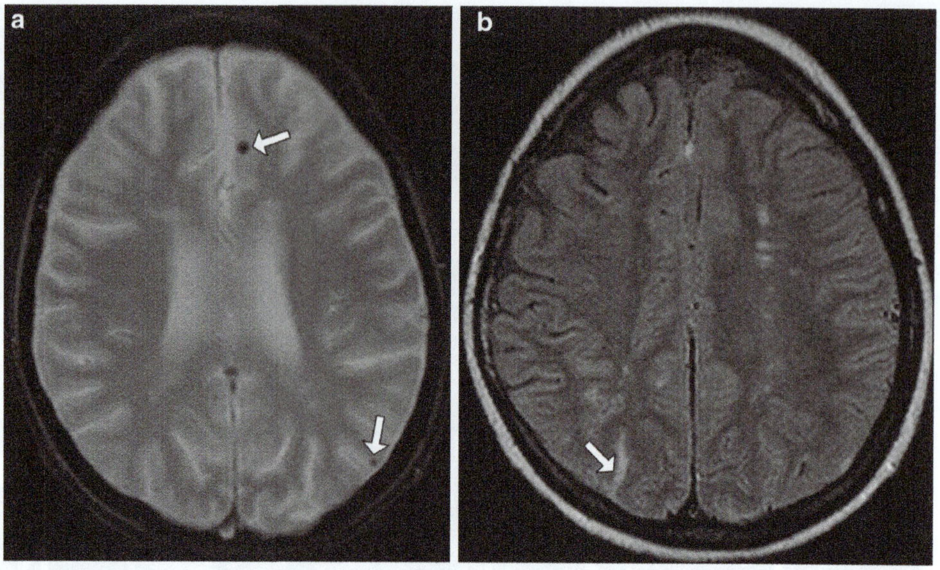

Fig. 5 Systemic lupus erythematosus (SLE) in a 21-year-old woman with renal and cerebral affection. **a** Axial T2* GRE-weighted image. **b** Axial FLAIR image. Petechial hemorrhages in the frontal and parietal cerebral cortex (**a**, *arrows*). Multifocal patchy white matter hyperintensities in the centrum semiovale as well as subarachnoid parietal hemorrhage (**b**, *arrows*)

Wegener's-associated vasculitis can lead to arterial or venous thrombosis as well as hemorrhage (Kelley 2004). Since the caliber of the affected vessels (50–300 μm in diameter) may be beyond the spatial resolution of DSA, and lesions of the brain parenchyma itself are rare, radiologically confirmed CNS vasculitis in Wegener's granulomatosis is exceptional; however, involvement of the dura with pachymeningitis may be detected on MR imaging after contrast administration (Chin and Latov 2005).

2.1.6 Systemic Lupus Erythematosus

Systemic lupus erythematosus is a chronic inflammatory connective tissue disorder that affects many organ systems. The CNS is involved in up to 75 % of cases and patients may present with a wide range of neurological and psychiatric manifestations (neuropsychiatric SLE). Cerebral SLE lesions occur as focal or multiple T2 hyperintensities, either as infarctions or as a correlate of symptomatic "migratory" edematous areas. Accordingly, water diffusion may be either restricted in early stages of ischemia (cytotoxic edema) or increased in vasculopathy (vasogenic edema).

The most common imaging findings in SLE are cortical atrophy, ventricular dilation, and fronto-parietal rounded or patchy lesions, which are not limited to the periventricular white matter. In fact, they can be localized in the gray–white junction, the cortex, or the basal ganglia. Contrast enhancement may be attributed to leakage in active lesions.

Venous MRA may show dural venous sinus thrombosis and should be performed particularly in antiphospholipid syndrome. Increased choline in proton MRS correlates with disease activity.

FDG-PET may be a useful tool in neuropsychiatric SLE if standard MRI appears to be normal: Active SLE with cerebral affection is correlated with decreased metabolism in parieto-occipital regions (Figs. 5, 6).

2.1.7 Scleroderma

In progressive systemic sclerosis, excessive collagen deposition in the skin, blood vessels, and other organs leads to abnormal tissue fibrosis and microvascular impairment. CNSmanifestations are extremely rare (Fig. 7).

2.1.8 Sjögren Syndrome

Approximately 20 % of patients with Sjögren syndrome present with neurological symptoms. The cerebral vasculitis resembles PAN with vessel stenoses and dilations. Enlarged ventricles due to white matter volume loss have been repeatedly reported (Fig. 8; Di Comite et al. 2005).

2.1.9 Behçet's Disease

Only 5 % of Behçet patients present with CNS involvement. In such cases, MRI depicts scattered subcortical white matter lesions which may show contrast enhancement in the acute phase. Characteristically, the lesions are preferentially located in the midbrain, whereas the cortex is usually spared (Fig. 9).

2.1.10 Viral Vasculitis

Varicella zoster virus is a frequent cause of cerebral vasculitis affecting mainly large cerebral vessels. Often the intracranial carotid bifurcation and the M1 segment of the MCA, but also the BA, are targeted. The clinical and neuroradiological characteristics of proven zoster vasculopathy and PACNS are so similar, that it may be speculated whether in a subgroup of PACNS the underlying cause is an undiagnosed zoster infection (Kueker 2007).

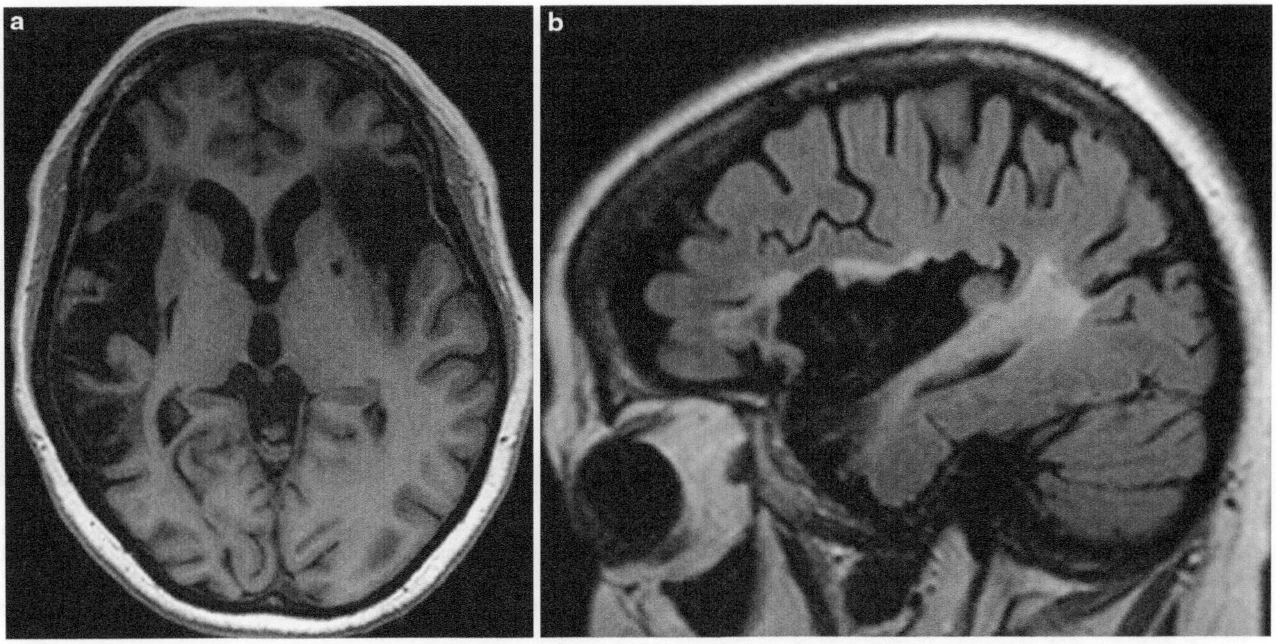

Fig. 6 Systemic lupus erythematosus (SLE). This 46-year-old woman has been diagnosed with SLE 26 years ago and has been suffering from cerebral affection for 24 years. **a** Axial T1-weighted image. **b** Sagittal FLAIR image. Chronic bilateral ischemic infarcts in the territory of the MCA (**a**) with reactive gliosis (perifocal hyperintensity on FLAIR images) (**b**). Note the enlarged ventricles as a result of white matter reduction

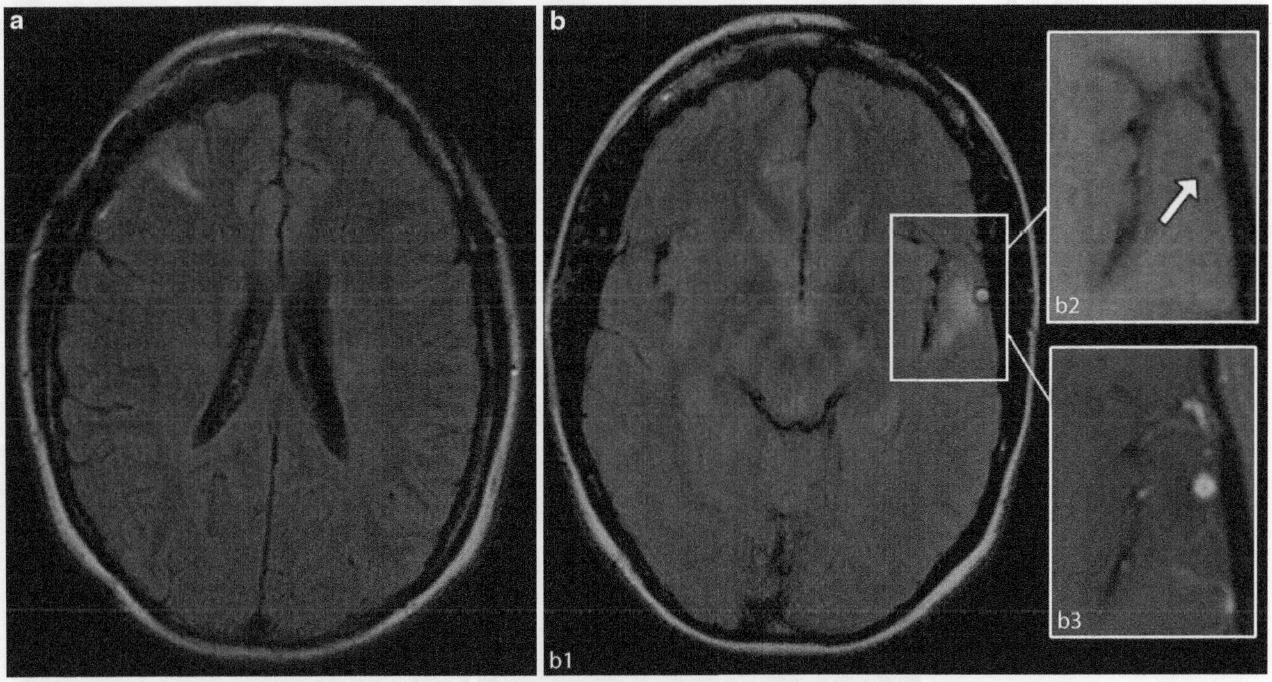

Fig. 7 Cerebral arteriopathy in scleroderma. A 32-year-old woman with linear scleroderma "en coup de sabre." Focal epilepsy starting five years ago was the first sign of cerebral affection. **a** Axial FLAIR-weighted image. **b** Axial FLAIR-weighted images (*b1*). Detail images of axial T1-weighted images of the left anterior temporal pole before (*b2*) and after contrast administration (*b3*). Right frontal (**a**) and left temporopolar (*b1*) cortical and subcortical white matter hyperintensities. Microaneurysm of a leptomeningeal vessel (*b1–b3*) with hyperintensity of the inner layer of the vessel wall on FLAIR image reflecting the intimal edema (*b1*). The vessel wall is thickened and therefore visible as a slightly hyperintense structure on non-enhanced T1-weighted images (*b2, arrow*). After gadolinium administration, all layers of the vessel wall exhibit severe contrast enhancement (*b3*)

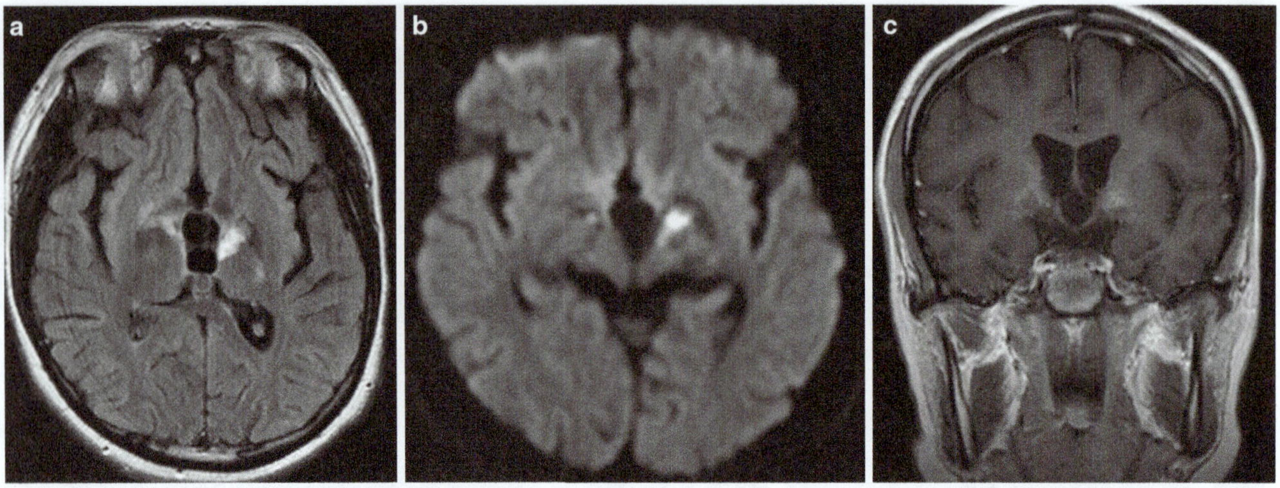

Fig. 8 A 20-year-old woman with Sjögren syndrome and associated CNS vasculitis. Since the age of 16 she has been suffering from sicca symptoms and hypothalamic dysfunction, the latter resulting in narcolepsy as well as postural and gait instability. **a** Axial FLAIR image. **b** Axial DWI. **c** Coronal T1-weighted MR image after contrast administration. Bilateral hyperintensities of the basal ganglia, predominantly of the left thalamus (**a**). Restricted diffusion in the left thalamus (**b**). Hemorrhagic transformation of bilateral thalamic infarctions with high signal on T1-weighted MR image (**c**). The basal ganglia hyperintensities were visible prior to contrast application as well (not shown). Note the enlarged ventricles due to loss of adjacent white matter

Fig. 9 Behçet's disease. A 56-year-old woman with dysarthria and labile affect due to brainstem encephalitis associated with neuro-Behçet syndrome. **a, b** Axial FLAIR images. **c** Axial T1-weighted image after contrast administration. **d** Sagittal T1-weighted image after contrast administration. Marked swelling and signal changes of the pons and cerebral peduncles (**a**, **b**). Lacunar pontine lesion (**c**) and abnormal contrast enhancement of the pons and mesencephalon (**c**, **d**)

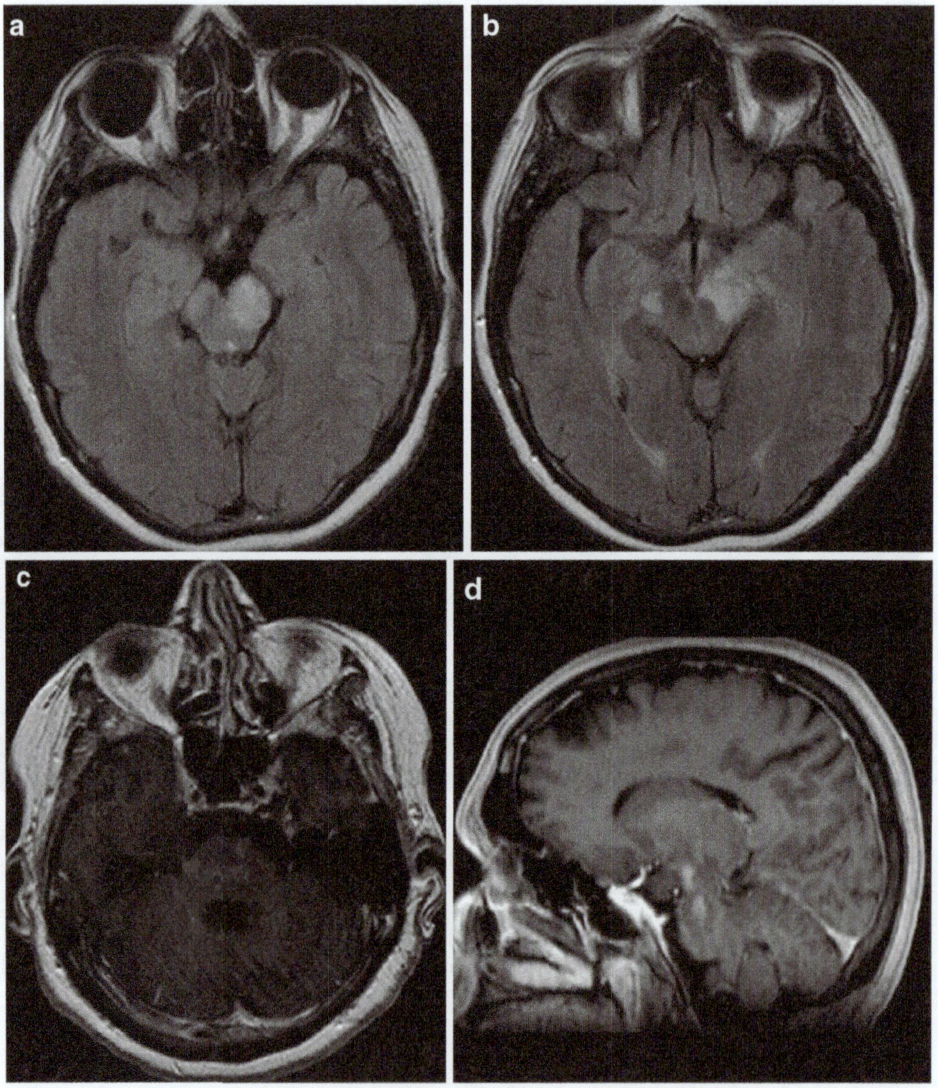

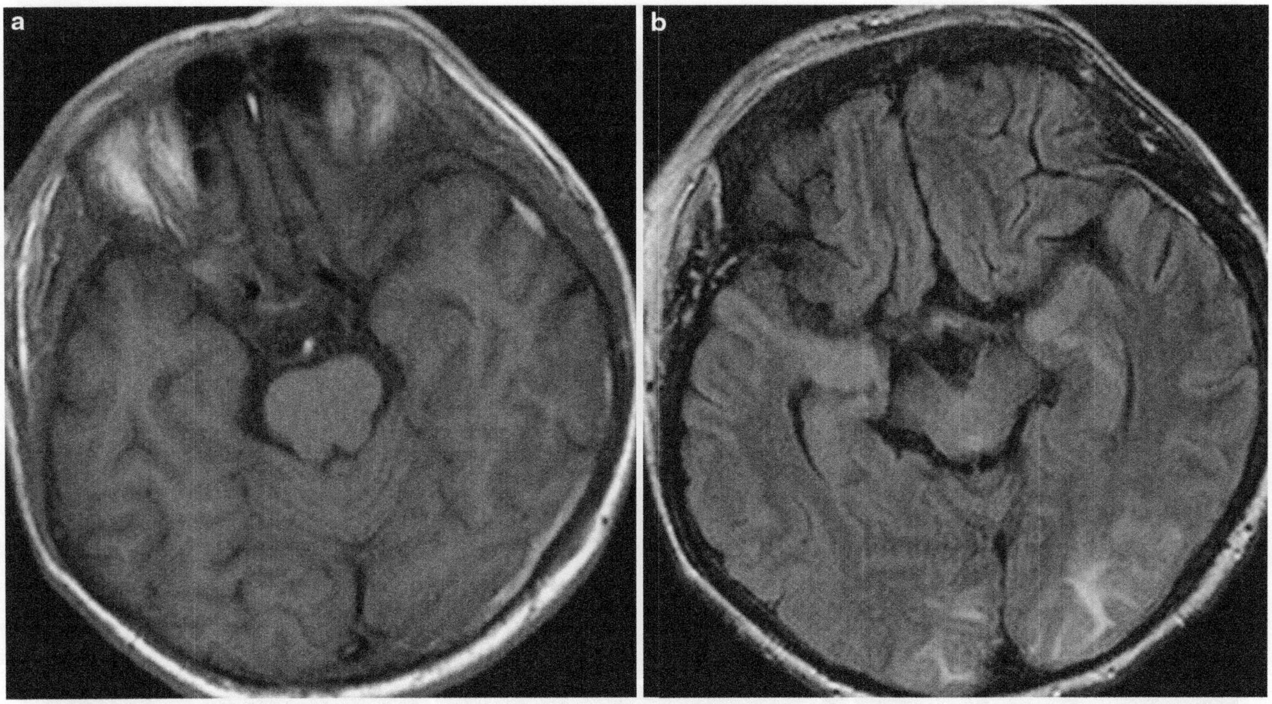

Fig. 10 Viral vasculitis (*Varicella zoster*). A 37-year-old immunocompromised man with ophthalmic zoster presenting with alternating phases of reduced vigilance and severe agitation. In the CSF *Varicella* viruses were found (as confirmed by PCR). **a** Axial T1-weighted image. **b** Axial FLAIR image. Left temporal acute, T1-hyperintense SDH. The traumatic SDH was acquired during an agitation phase in which the patient fell off the bed (**a**). Bioccipital hyperintense subcortical lesions resembling posterior reversible encephalopathy syndrome (PRES; **b**)

Other DNA viruses from the herpes family, such as herpes simplex virus type 1 and cytomegalovirus, may cause large-vessel vasculitis as well. Furthermore, RNA viruses, such as HIV, may be implicated. Indeed, the number of diagnosed HIV-associated vasculitides is increasing, especially in infants. The inflammatory response is particularly severe in AIDS patients (Fig 10; see also "Viral Encephalitis").

2.1.11 Bacterial Meningitis

A number of bacterial agents may cause acute septic meningitis and cerebral vasculitis. Firstly, purulent infection at the base of the brain may lead to inflammatory cell infiltration of vessel walls. Additionally, vessel wall damage may be aggravated by the activated immune response (such as cellular adhesion molecules, complement, reactive oxygen species, and proteolytic enzymes). Late complications might be septic thrombosis and thrombophlebitis (Younger 2004).

In tuberculosis, inflammation of the adventitia of small- and medium-sized arteries triggers proliferation of reactive subendothelial cells. This in turn, leads to stenosis of the vascular lumina; therefore, MRA and DSA demonstrate narrowing of the basal cerebral or cortical vessels. Typically, vessels at the skull base are most commonly involved, often leading to hemorrhages (Fig. 11; see "Neurotuberculosis").

2.1.12 Spirochetal Vasculitis

Treponema pallidum-associated cerebral vasculitis is caused by spirochetal invasion of the endothelial cells in the tertiary parenchymal syphilis syndrome. Diffuse vasculitis involves preferably cortical arteries and veins, whereas the gummatous vasculitis usually affects proximal MCA branches (see also "Neurolues").

Borrelia burgdorferi-associated cerebral vasculitis is believed to result from focal mononuclear inflammatory cell infiltration of blood vessels. The endothelial cell swelling may lead to stroke-like lesions as well as subarachnoid hemorrhage (Fig. 12; Younger 2004).

2.1.13 Drug-Induced Vasculitis

Currently it is well established that chronic drug abuse can damage vessels directly or indirectly (hypersensitivity to contaminants) and may therefore be associated with necrotizing arteritis. The severity of drug-induced cerebral vasculitis is influenced by the duration and degree of exposure, route of administration, immune status and, of course, the type of drug. In particular, drugs with sympathomimetic amine-type activity (amphetamines, cocaine, heroin etc.) have been repeatedly reported to induce cerebral vasculitis (Fig. 13).

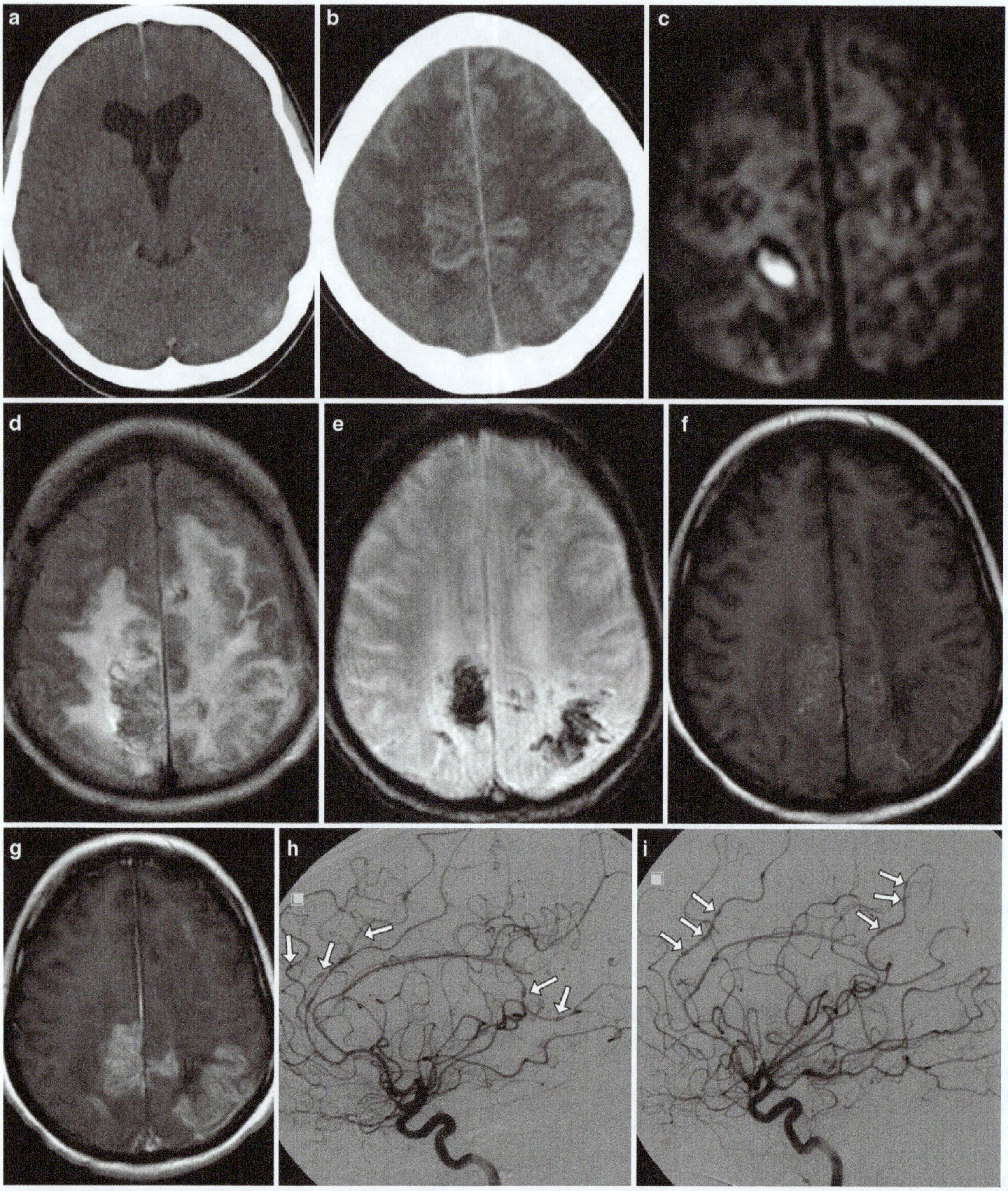

Fig. 11 Bacterial meningitis (*Mycobacterium* tuberculosis). A 40-year-old woman with tuberculosis for 15 years. She presented with acute pneumonia and reduced vigilance. **a, b** Axial CT. **c** Axial DWI. **d** Axial FLAIR image. **e–i** Bacterial meningitis (*Mycobacterium* tuberculosis). A 40-year-old woman with tuberculosis for 15 years. She presented with acute pneumonia and reduced vigilance. **e** Axial T2*-weighted image. **f** Axial T1-weighted image before contrast administration. **g** Axial T1-weighted image after contrast administration. **h, i** Bacterial meningitis (*Mycobacterium* tuberculosis). A 40-year-old woman with tuberculosis for 15 years. She presented with acute pneumonia and reduced vigilance. **h, i** DSA of the left ICA, lateral view. Initial CT demonstrated hydrocephalus (**a**) as well as cortical hyperdensities and white matter hypodensities (**b**). MR imaging revealed infarctions and hemorrhages (**c–g**). Focal area of restricted water diffusion in the subcortical white matter of the left hemisphere (**c**). Extensive laminar hyperintensities of bilateral gray and white matter (**d**) demonstrate severe parenchymal edema. Several large areas of signal loss on SWI due to hemoglobin degradation products (**e**). The cortex shows moderate hyperintensity (**f**) due to hemorrhagic transformation. Severe irregular cortical, subcortical, and even meningeal contrast enhancement (**g**). Alternating areas of vessel constriction and dilation of the anterior and middle cerebral artery, exhibiting "sausage-string" appearance (**h**, **i**, *arrows*: microaneurysms)

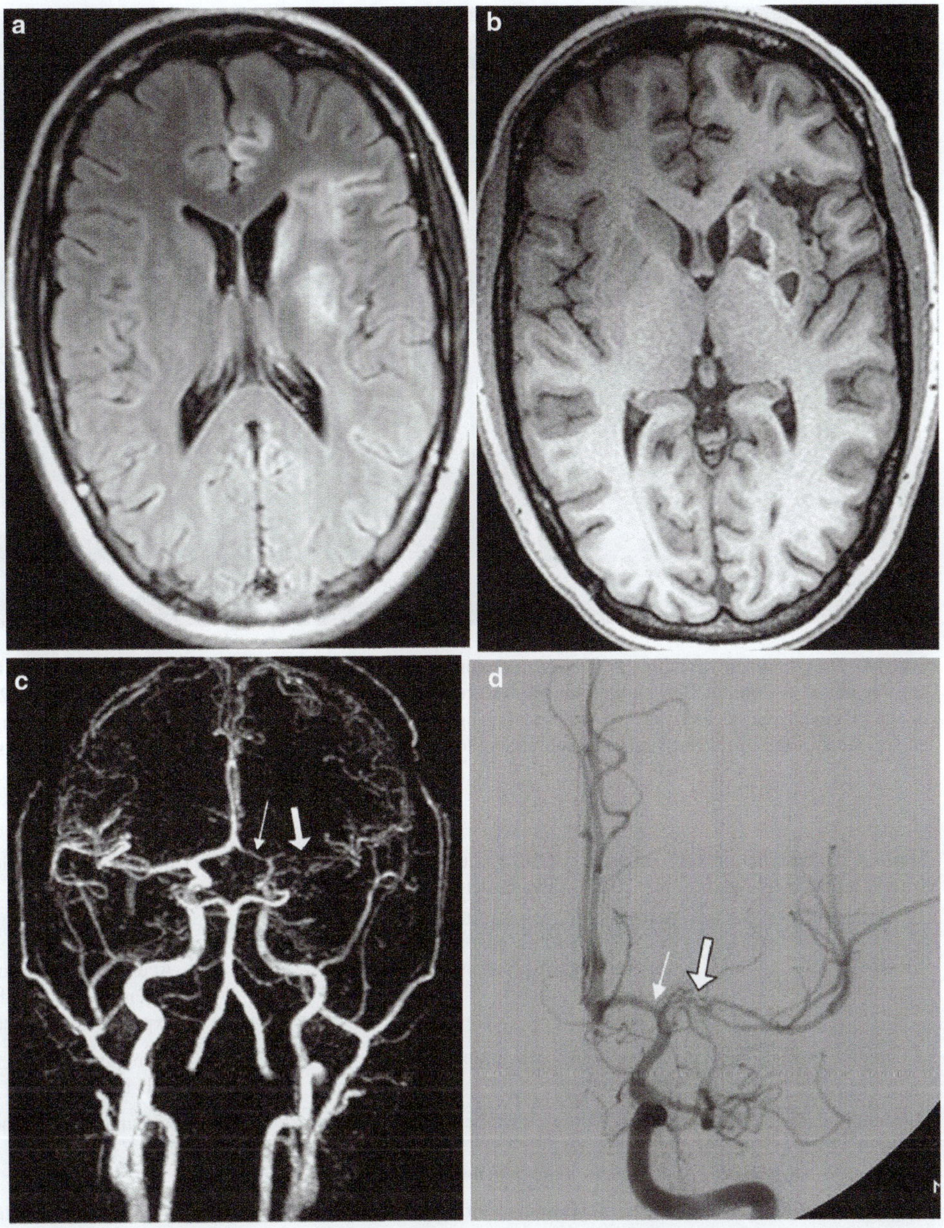

Fig. 12 Spirochetal vasculitis (*Borrelia burgdorferi*). A 20-year-old woman with erythema migrans, bilateral headaches, and recurring cramps in the right hand. **a** Axial FLAIR image. **b** Axial T1-weighted image. **c** MIP of a arterial TOF MRA. **d** DSA of the left ICA, frontal view. Left-hemispheric hyperintensities mainly affecting cortical and subcortical gray matter in the territory of the left anterior and medial cerebral arteries (**a**). Marked defect of the left lentiform nucleus with surrounding mild hemorrhages and focal brain atrophy (**b**). Distinct tapering of the left A1 segment (**c**, **d**, *thin arrows*) and severe stenosis of the proximal left MCA (**c**, **d**, *thick arrows*) with rarefaction in the periphery (**c**, **d**)

2.2 Differential Diagnoses of Cerebral Vasculitides

2.2.1 Intracranial Atherosclerotic Vascular Disease

In adults atherosclerosis is by far the most common cause of a vasculitis-mimicking angiographic pattern. ASVD affects mainly patients of advanced age and usually coincides with atherosclerosis of extracranial arteries such as coronaries. Atherosclerotic plaques preferentially affect the branching points of large vessels (which is unusual for vasculitis). In contrast, vasculitides usually involve smaller branches, and are more likely associated with haemorrhage.

2.2.2 Reversible Cerebral Vasoconstriction Syndrome

Reversible cerebral vasoconstriction syndrome (RCVS) is a rare disease, that can be easily mistaken for PCNSV. It presents with acute, very severe headaches ('thunderclap'), which may be recurrent over 1–3 weeks and might be associated with focal deficits and/or seizures. Although RCVS may occur spontaneously, in more than 50 % it follows "intracranial stress" such as exposure to vasoactive drugs (e.g. cocaine, amphetamine) or birth giving ("post-partum angiopathy") (Ducros et al. 2010).

Segmental multifocal arterial constriction and dilation leads to the characteristic "string of beads" or "sausage on

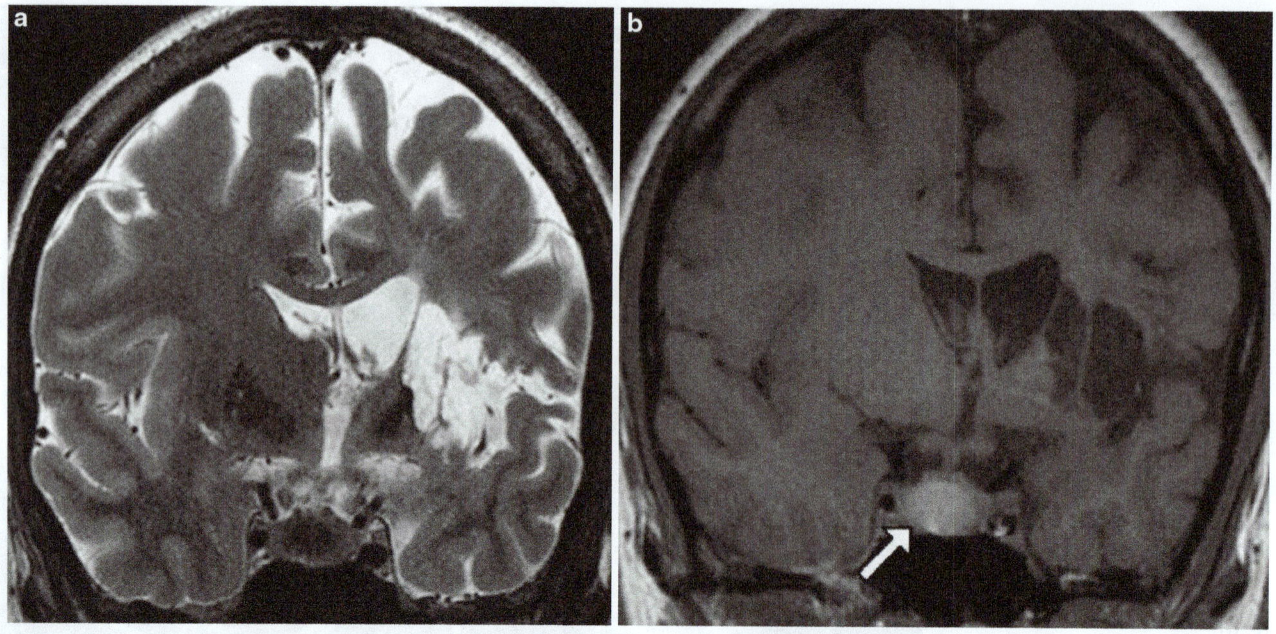

Fig. 13 Drug-induced vasculitis. A 22-year-old woman with chronic cocaine abuse. **a** Coronal T2-weighted image. **b** Coronal T1-weighted image. Parenchymal defects of the left basal ganglia and evacuo-enlargement of the ipsilateral ventricles subsequent to an infarct in the territory of the left MCA (**a**, **b**). Additionally, the pituitary gland is enlarged and demonstrates T2-hypointense (**a**) and T1-hyperintense signal changes (**b**) representing hemorrhage into the pituitary gland (*arrow*) possibly caused by vasculitis-associated hemorrhage

Table 4 Differentiation between primary CNS vasculitis (PCNSV) and Reversible Cerebral Vasoconstriction Syndrome (RCVS) [According to criteria reported by Sattar et al. (2010), Salvarani et al. (2012) and Giannini et al. (2012)]

	PCNSV	RCVS
Onset	Usually gradual and progressive	Acute, rapid development of symptoms Often precipitated in the postpartum or following exposure to vasoactive drugs
Course	Progressive with frequent appearance of cerebral infarcts	Monophasic Self-limited within 1–3 months
Commonest symptoms	Subacute and progressive headache, Altered cognition, Persistent neurologic deficit or stroke	"Thunderclap" headache (acute and severe)
Gender	Women are slightly more often affected than men	Women are more frequently affected than men (3:1)
CSF	Abnormal in 80–90 % of cases (white cell count and total protein concentration mildly increased)	Usually normal
MRI	Pathological in almost 100 %	Often normal during the first week MR angiography reveals diffuse segmental arterial constriction in up to 90 % after 1–2 weeks

a string" aspect on angiography. Since the initial vascular imaging may be normal in up to 90 %, a follow-up study 1–2 weeks after onset is usually required to demonstrate the characteristic segmental arterial constrictions. In the first week after onset, RCVS may be complicated by subarachnoid or intracerebral hemorrhage. In the second week, (additional) ischemic lesions may occur, typically in the arterial border zone regions (Sattar et al. 2010).

Distinguishing RCVS from PANCS is often a dilemma. In order to prevent RCVS patients from receiving cytotoxic medication, the following criteria may be helpful to differentiate these two disease entities (see Table 4).

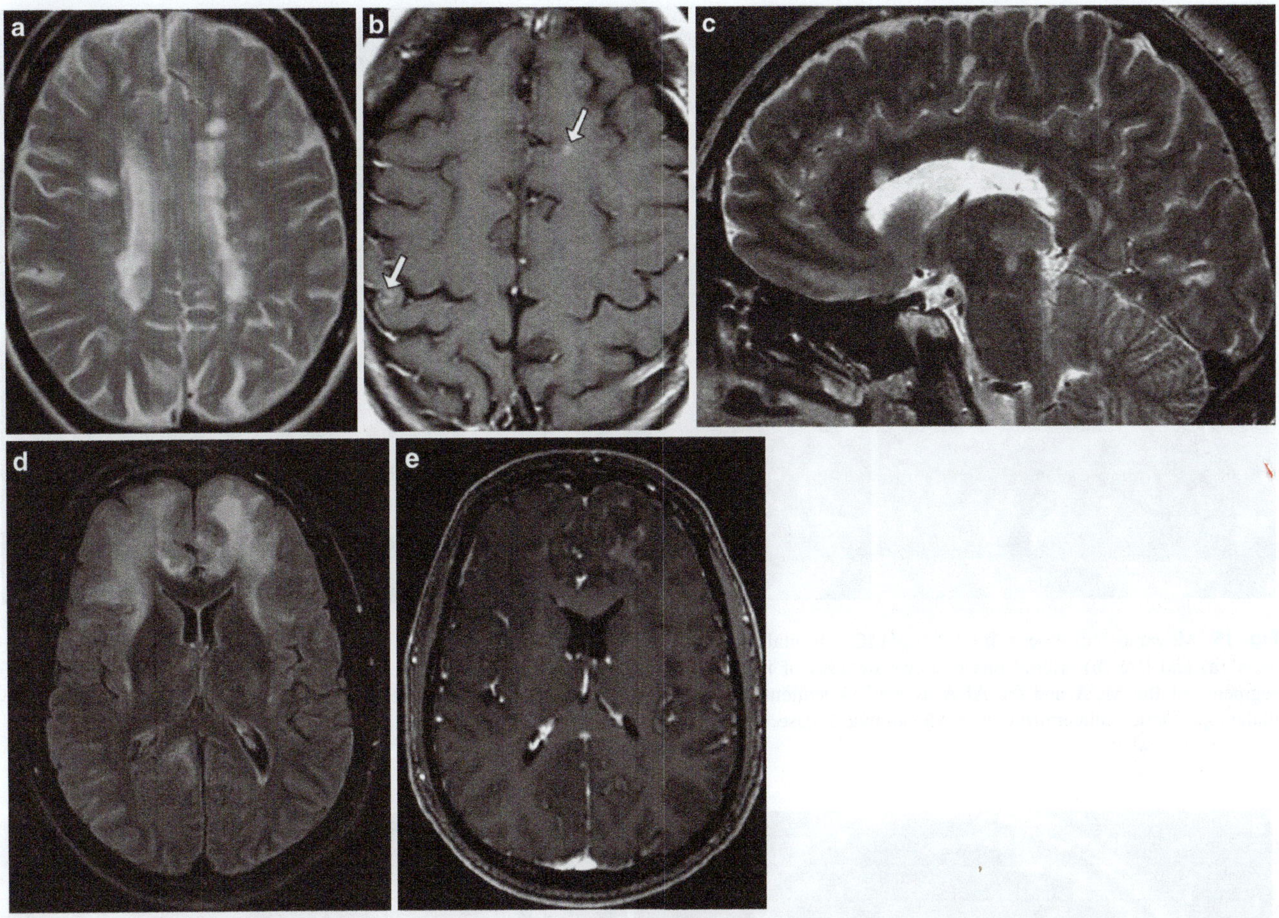

Fig. 14 Multiple sclerosis. **a** Axial T2-weighted image shows multiple bilateral periventricular round or ovoid hyperintensities. **b** Axial T1-weighted image after contrast administration depicts nodular enhancement as a correlate of active demyelination (*arrows*). **c** Multiple sclerosis. **c** The sagittal T2-weighted image through the midline demonstrates infra- and supratentorial MS plaques and the preferred affection of the corpus callosum. **d**, **e** PML in a patient with Multiple sclerosis under the treatment with natalizumab. **d** Axial FLAIR image. **e** Axial T1-weighted image after contrast administration. Bifrontal and right occipital slightly space occupying hyperintensities on the FLAIR images with involvement of the subcortical U-fibres. In contrast to classical PML the lesions reveal contrast enhancement

2.2.3 Multiple Sclerosis

Typical MS plaques appear as multiple round or ovoid T2-hyperintensities with temporal and spatial dissemination. Most lesions are located in the periventricular white matter. Pathognomonic for MS lesions is their perpendicular orientation at the calloseptal interface along penetrating venules ("Dawson fingers"). Transient contrast enhancement indicates acute breakdown of the blood–brain barrier as a correlate of active demyelisation. In vasculitis, however, lesions are usually less numerous and there is no preferred affection of the corpus callosum. Instead, gray matter is more often involved in vasculitis (Fig. 14; see Multiple Sclerosis).

A rare but important complication of the treatment with monoclonal antibodies is the development of atypical progressive multifocal leukoencephalopathy (PML), which might be difficult to differentiate from tumefactive MS (see "Viral Encephalitis"; Fig. 4).

2.2.4 Moyamoya Disease

Moyamoya disease is an angiographic pattern rather than a specific disease. It affects infants or young adults and is a frequent cause of stroke in Japanese children (idiopathic progressive arteriopathy of childhood). Probably triggered by various inflammatory causes, slow progressive (often bilateral) stenoses of the supraclinoid ICAs and later the BA lead to formation of abnormal lenticulostriate and thalamostriate collaterals which can be visualized on angiography as a cloudy net referred to as the "puff of smoke" sign (Japanese: "moyamoya"). The bright sulci on FLAIR and postcontrast T1-weighted MR images (leptomeningeal "ivy

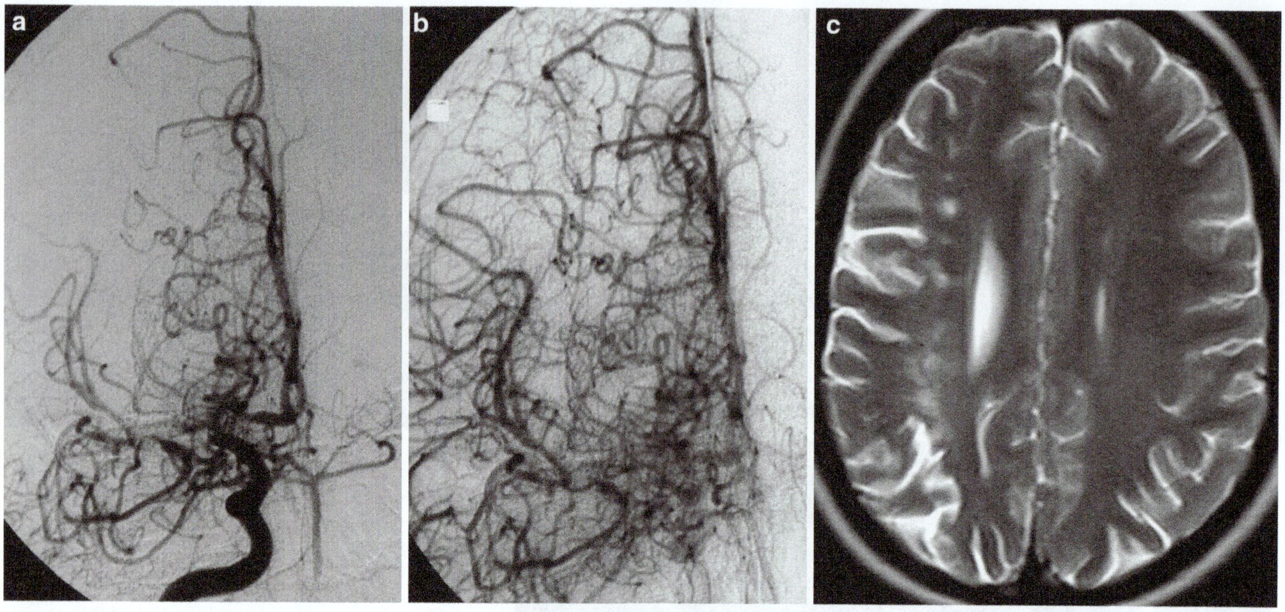

Fig. 15 Moyamoya disease. **a**, **b** DSA (right ICA; frontal view) at the early (**a**) and late (**b**) arterial phase shows stenoses of the proximal segments of the MCA and the ACA as well as lenticulostriate and thalamoperforate collateralization. **c** Moyamoya disease. **c** Axial T2-weighted image demonstrates increased signal in the right hemispheric border zone due to cortical and white matter ischemic infarcts. The prominent ipsilateral sulci are due to cortical atrophy. (From Ertl-Wagner 2007)

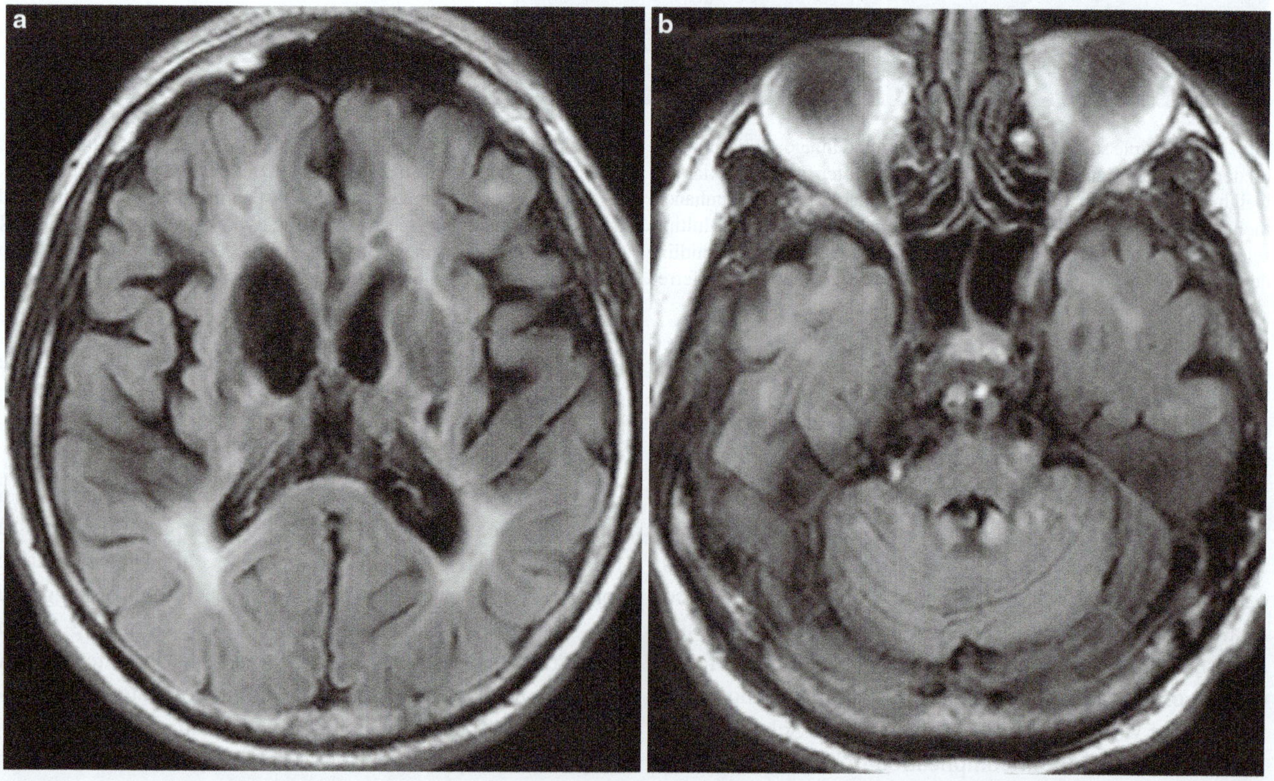

Fig. 16 Cerebral autosomal-dominant arteriopathy with subcortical infarcts and leukoencephalopathy (CADASIL). The axial FLAIR images (**a**, **b**) demonstrate bilateral subcortical hyperintensities of the anterior temporal poles. The periventricular white matter, including the external capsules, is involved as well

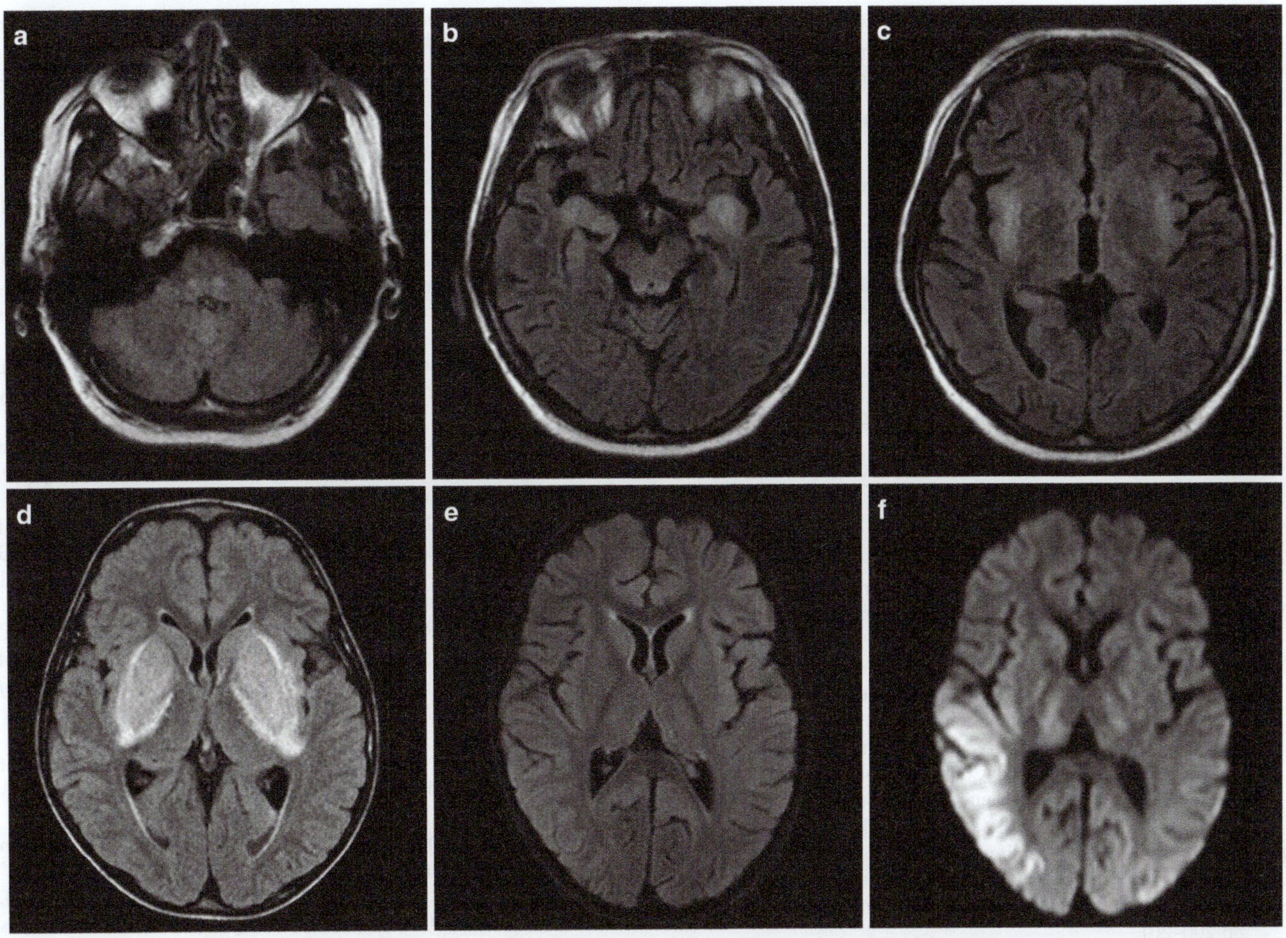

Fig. 17 HUS-associated encephalopathy. The axial FLAIR images (**a–e**) and the DWI image (**f**) show focal edematous signal changes in one adult patient (**a–c**) and two infants (**d–f**; Courtesy of A. Seitz, Pediatric Neuroradiology Heidelberg). In the pediatric population neuro-HUS typically affects bilateral basal ganglia (**d**) or the occiptotemporal cortex resembling PRES (**e**, **f**). The 61-year-old woman with epidemic HUS encephalopathy demonstrated transient symmetric signal changes of the pons (**a**) and persistently in mesolimbic structures and thalamus (**b**, **c**)

sign") are potentially reversible. To date, vessel wall changes on MR imaging have not been reported (Fig. 15).

2.2.5 Cerebral Autosomal-Dominant Arteriopathy with Subcortical Infarcts and Leukoencephalopathy

A hereditary point mutation in *Notch3* gene on chromosome 19 damages the vascular smooth muscle cells of small cerebral arteries manifesting in recurrent ischemic episodes in young adults (30–50 years). Bilateral subcortical lacunar infarcts of the anterior temporal poles are almost pathognomonic for CADASIL. Other affected regions are the superior frontal white matter and the external capsules leading to diffuse white matter hyperintensities in the course of the disease (leukoencephalopathy). As opposed to vasculitides, the cerebral cortex is mostly spared and the angiogram is usually normal (Fig. 16).

2.2.6 Radiation Vasculopathy

Radiochemotherapy can induce acute arteritis with associated transient white matter edema. Vessel wall changes due to edema and fibrosis may persist even beyond the acute stage. Chronic damage due to vasculopathy may be severe and include complete vessel obliteration, leukomalacia, calcifying microangiopathy, and brain atrophy.

2.2.7 Epidemic Hemolytic Uremic Syndrome

Hemolytic uremic syndrome (HUS) is a multisystem disorder, which is triggered by bacterial infection with entero-hemorrhagic Escherichia coli (EHEC). HUS sporadically affects infants and young children and is characterized by the trias of acute renal failure, thrombocytopenia, and microangiopathic hemolytic anemia. Central nervous system complications may occur in up to 50 % and pediatric neuroimaging usually demonstrates bilateral, symmetric lesions of basal ganglia or extensive cortical and/or subcortical lesions which might resemble Posterior Reversible Encephalopathy Syndrome (PRES). The clinical outcome is generally good.

In adults, however, HUS occurs only rarely and is not associated with neurological complications. Having said that, the recent EHEC epidemic in Northern Germany in May/June 2011 affected as many as 3,800 patients. Those who developed HUS were mainly female adults, who developed neurological complications in about 50 %. Neuroimaging revealed mainly transient vasogenous edema of the pons as well as (persistent) supratentorial signal changes in the thalamus, mesolimbic structures and subcortically (Wengenroth et al. 2012; Fig. 17).

References

Aksel S (2001) Vasculitis of the nervous system. J Neurol 248:451–468

Berlit P (2004) Cerebral vasculitis. Nervenarzt 75:817–830

Birnbaum J, Hellmann DB (2009) Primary angiitis of the central nervous system. Arch Neurol 66:704–709

Bley TA, Wieben O, Uhl M, Thiel J, Schmidt D, Langer M (2005) High-resolution MRI in giant cell arteritis: imaging of the wall of the superficial temporal artery. Am J Roentgenol 184:283–287

di Comite G, Sabbadini MG (2005) Neurological involvement in rheumatological diseases. Neurol Sci 26(Suppl 1):S9–S14

Ducros A, Fiedler U, Porcher R, Boukobza M, Stapf C, Bousser MG (2010) Hemorrhagic manifestations of reversible cerebral vasoconstriction. Stroke 41(11):2505–2511

Ertl-Wagner B (2007) Pädiatrische Neuroradiologie. Springer, Berlin, pp 200–201

Ferro JM (1998) Vasculitis of the central nervous system. J Neurol 245:766–776

Giannini C, Salvarani C, Hunder G, Brown R (2012) Primary central nervous system vasculitis: pathology and mechanisms. Acta Neuropathol 123(6):759–772 (*this recent review by authors from the Mayo Clinic gives a very detailed overview about clinical and imaging signs of PCNSV*)

Jennette JC, Falk RJ, Andrassy K, Bacon PA, Churg J, Gross WL, Hagen EC, Hoffman GS, Hunder GG, Kallenberg CG et al (1994) Nomenclature of systemic vasculitides. Proposal of an international consensus conference. Arthritis Rheum, vol 37, pp 187–192

Kelley RE (2004) CNS vasculitis. Front Biosci 9:946–955

Kueker W (2007) Cerebral vasculitis: imaging signs revisited. Neuroradiology 49:471–479

Kueker W, Gaertner S, Nagele T, Dopfer C, Schoning M, Fiehler J, Rothwell PM, Herrlinger U (2008) Vessel wall contrast enhancement: a diagnostic sign of cerebral vasculitis. Cerebrovasc Dis 26:23–29

Moore PM, Richardson B (1998) Neurology of the vasculitides and connective tissue diseases. J Neurol Neurosurg Psychiatry 65:10–22

Pipitone N, Versari A, Salvarani C (2008) Role of imaging studies in the diagnosis and follow-up of large-vessel vasculitis: an update. Rheumatology (Oxford) 47:403–408

Salvarani C, Brown RD Jr, Calamia KT, Christianson TJ, Weigand SD, Miller DV, Giannini C, Meschia JF, Huston J 3rd, Hunder GG (2007) Primary central nervous system vasculitis: analysis of 101 patients. Ann Neurol 62(5):442–451

Salvarani C, Brown RD Jr, Hunder GG (2012) Adult primary central nervous system vasculitis: an update. Curr Opin Rheumatol 24:46–52 (*A nice review providing an extensive description of several subsets of PCNSV including neuroimaging and disease management*)

Sattar A, Manousakis G, Jensen MB (2010) Systematic review of reversible cerebral vasoconstriction syndrome. Expert Rev Cardiovasc Ther 8(10):1417–1421

Younger DS (2004b) Vasculitis of the nervous system. Curr Opin Neurol 17:317–336

Wengenroth M, Hoeltje J, Repenthin J, Meyer TN, Bonk F, Becker H, Faiss S, Stammel O, Urban PP, Bruening R (2013) Central nervous system involvement in adults with epidemic hemolytic uremic syndrome (HUS). AJNR

Zuccoli G, Pipitone N, Haldipur A et al (2011) Imaging findings in primary central nervous system vasculitis. Clin Exp Rheumatol 29(Suppl. 64):S104–S109

Pyogenic Cerebritis and Brain Abscess

Joachim Spreer

Contents

Abstract

Despite essential proceedings in diagnosis and therapy during the past decades, pyogenic cerebritis and brain abscesses remain severe, potentially life-threatening diseases of the CNS that should be diagnosed without delay. The spectrum of pathogens differs considerably depending on the route of infection, on the one hand, and the status of the immune system of the host, on the other. In addition to the clinical examination, imaging studies are the main diagnostic clues for an early diagnosis. The different histological stages of abscess formation from early cerebritis to a mature encapsulated abscess are reflected in nonenhanced and contrast-enhanced CT and MR imaging findings. Magnetic resonance imaging is the imaging procedure of choice, not only in the primary diagnosis, but also in planning surgical or stereotactic procedures, and in the follow-up of patients with pyogenic brain infections. In addition to the morphological information, DWI, PerfMRI, and MRS add valuable metabolic information that may help to differentiate pyogenic infections from other disease processes. The main differential diagnoses of cerebritis include arterial or venous infarction, and nonpyogenic inflammations. Abscesses have to be discriminated from autochthonous and metastatic brain tumors.

1 Epidemiology, Clinical Presentation, Therapy

1.1 Definition

In the literal sense the terms "cerebritis" (from Latin: cerebrum) and "encephalitis" (from Greek: encephalon) mean exactly the same, that is, an inflammation of the brain, irrespective of the etiology; however, in accordance with common clinical practice, in this chapter the term "cerebritis" is used in a more restricted sense to describe the early stage of a pyogenic infection of the brain.

J. Spreer (✉)
Department Neuroradiology, Cologne Medical Center,
Ostmerheimer Strasse 200, 51109 Köln, Germany
e-mail: spreerj@kliniken-koeln.de

S. Hähnel (ed.), *Inflammatory Diseases of the Brain*, Medical Radiology. Diagnostic Imaging,
DOI: 10.1007/174_2012_639, © Springer-Verlag Berlin Heidelberg 2012
Published Online: 21 June 2012

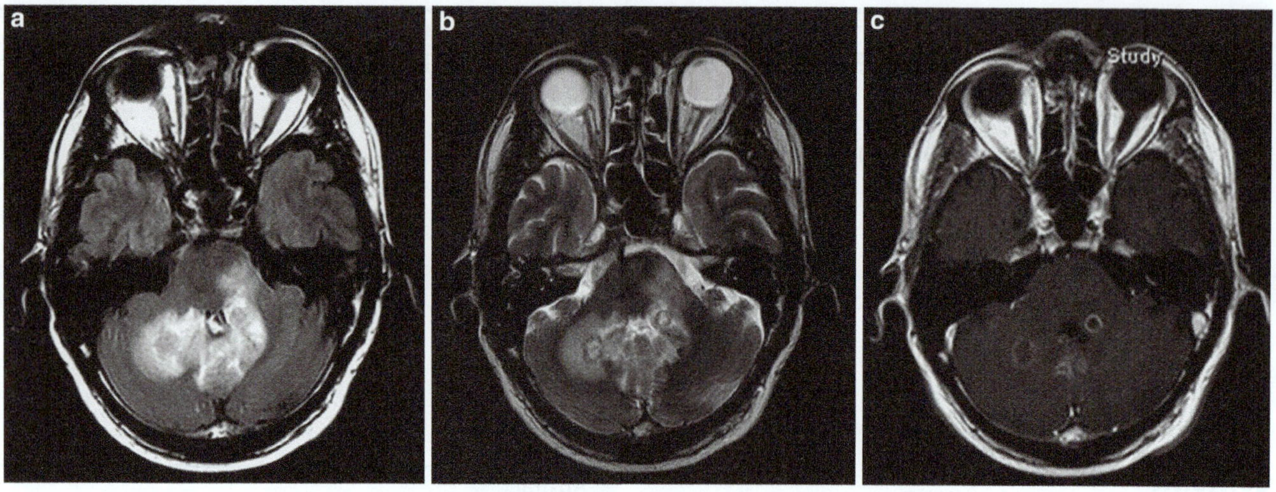

Fig. 1 Rhombencephalitis in brain infection with listeria monocytogenes. **a** Axial FLAIR image. **b** Axial T2-weighted image. **c** Axial T1-weighted image after contrast administration. Multiple infratentorial abscesses with ringlike enhancement (**c**) and perifocal edema (**a, b**). (Courtesy of W. Huber-Hartmann)

Table 1 Typical clinical findings in brain abscess

Headache	70–95
Nausea, vomiting	50–85
Impaired consciousness	50–70
Focal deficits	40–70
Fever	45–60
Seizures	20–30
Meningeal signs	15–25

Values are percentages

1.2 Epidemiology

Brain abscesses occur in all age groups; men are affected approximately twice as much as women. Abscesses are solitary lesions in 70 %, and multiple in 30 % (Berlit et al. 1996). Most commonly (30–60 %), they are caused *per continuitatem* from adjacent inflammatory foci, i.e., as a complication of infections of the paranasal sinuses and/or mastoid cells, dental infections, osteomyelitis, or purulent meningitis.

About 20–30 % of pyogenic brain infections are caused hematogenously. Predisposing factors are bronchiectasia, pneumonia, endocarditis, valvular heart defects, pulmonary AVM, and intravenous drug abuse. Large septic emboli may occlude major cerebral arteries and produce territorial infarcts. Small emboli typically result in multiple small abscesses that are characteristically located at the junction between gray and white matter.

Formation of cerebritis and abscesses induced by direct inoculation of bacteria in the course of a craniocerebral injury or following craniectomy/surgery (neurosurgery/others) is seen in about 10 % of cases. Posttraumatic abscesses may develop early and may also evolve years or even decades after an open craniocerebral injury.

In 10–20 % of cases, the cause of a brain abscess remains cryptogenic. During the past decades the pathogenetic spectrum of brain abscesses has changed. The number of cases secondary to otitis media and congenital heart disease has decreased, whereas the number of brain abscesses following brain surgery or trauma has increased (Carpenter et al. 2007).

Concerning localization, abscesses may occur in all parts of the brain; however, most often they are found in the frontal, parietal, and temporal lobes, and in the cerebellum. The occipital lobes, basal ganglia, thalami, and brain stem are affected less frequently. Some pathogens show a preference for certain brain areas, e.g., infections with listeria monocytogenes often are localized preferentially in infratentorial regions (rhombencephalitis) (Fig. 1).

1.3 Etiology and Pathogenesis

The spectrum of pathogens of bacterial infections of the brain depends on several extrinsic and intrinsic factors: local and/or regional distribution of pathogens, route of

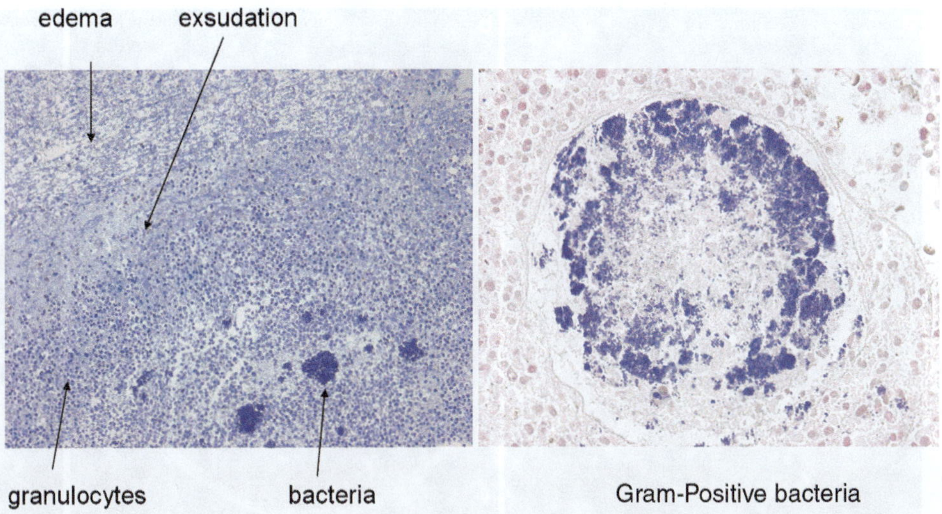

Fig. 2 Early cerebritis. Histological preparation. Infiltrates of inflammatory cells, exudation of protein-rich fluid, edema. (Courtesy of F. Feuerhake)

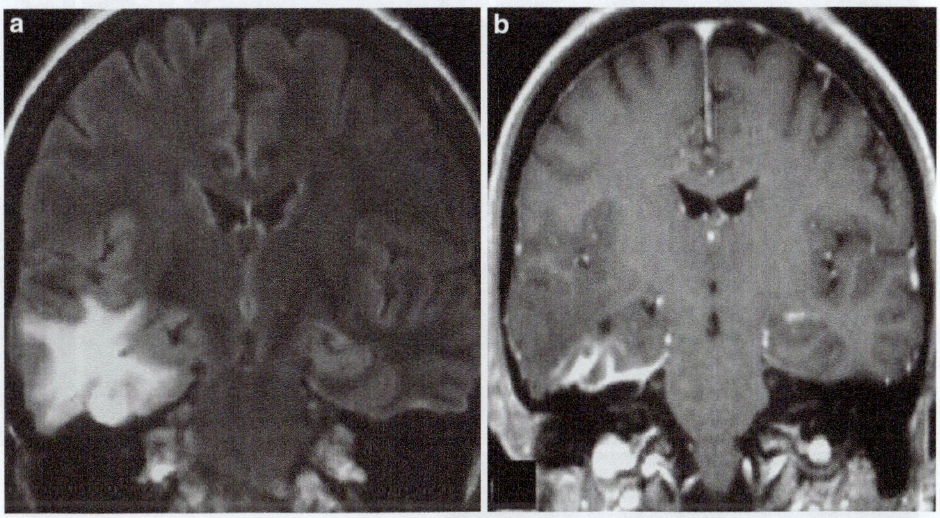

Fig. 3 Right temporal cerebritis by local spread of an infection of the adjacent mastoid cells. **a** Coronal FLAIR image. **b** Coronal T1-weighted image after contrast administration. Excessive edema with sulcal effacement (**a**). Only sparse enhancement of the infected brain, but thickening and enhancement of the adjacent meninges (**b**)

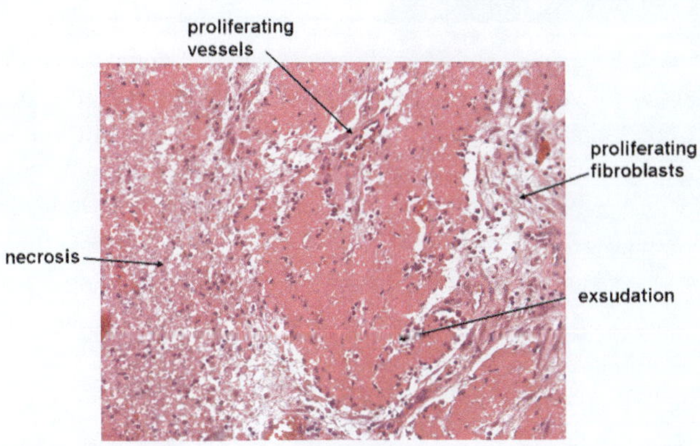

Fig. 4 Late cerebritis stage with early capsule formation. Histological preparation. Necrotic center; proliferating blood vessels, and fibroblasts in the periphery

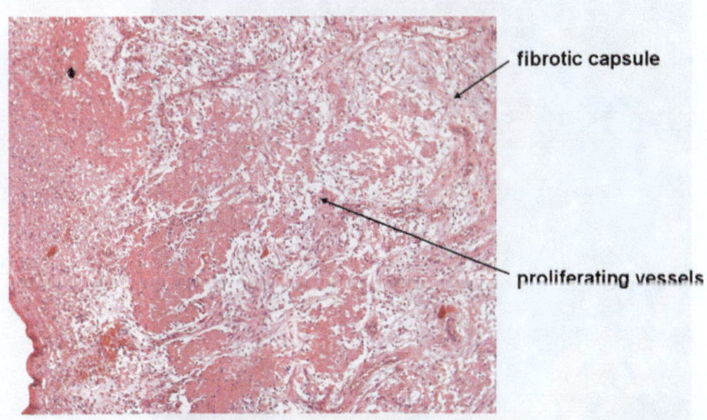

Fig. 5 Late capsule abscess stage. Histological preparation. Decreasing necrosis and edema, increasing thickness of the fibrotic capsule

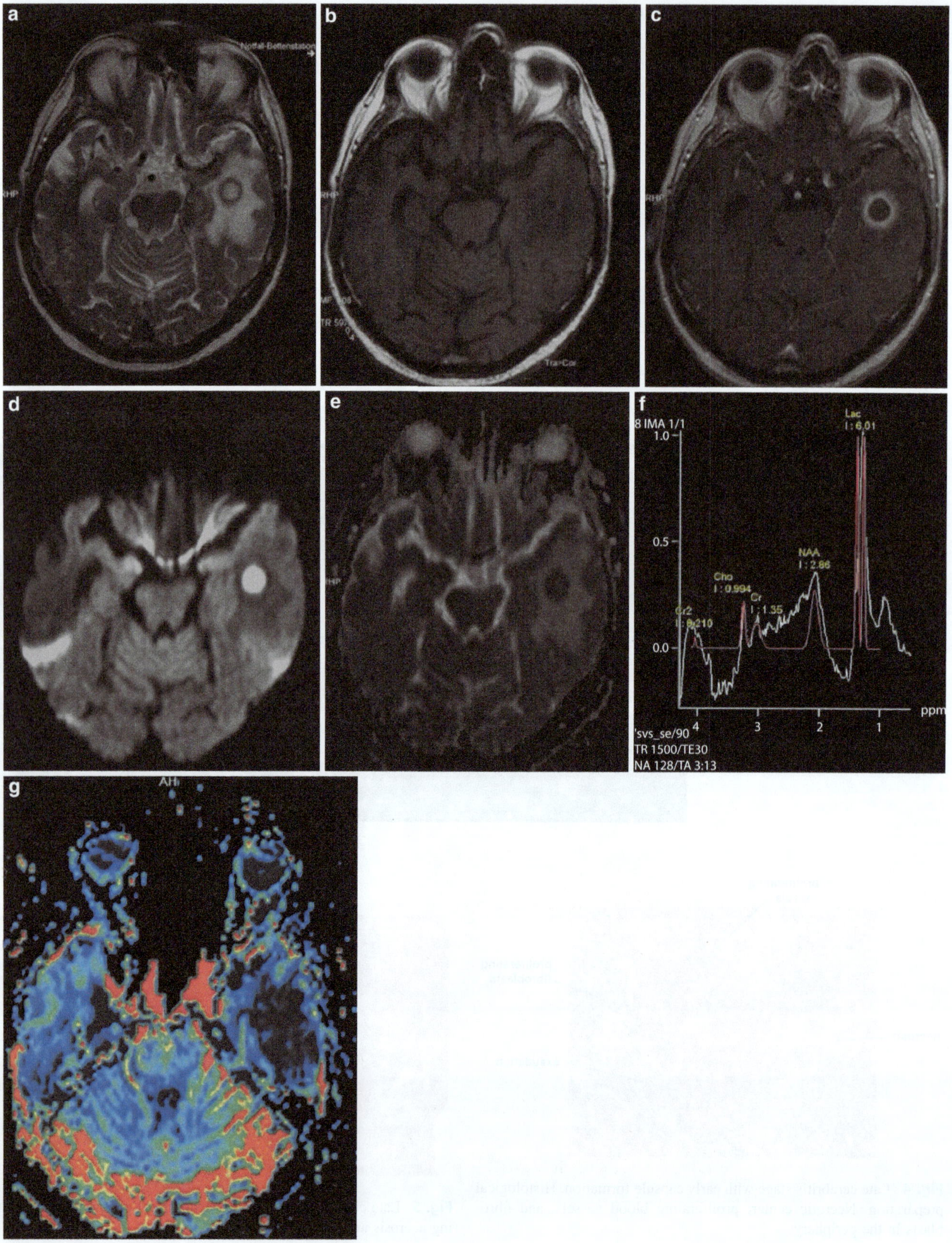
a
b
c
d
e
f
g
Notfall-Bettenstation
RHP
Tra-Cor
AH
8 IMA 1/1
Lac
I : 6.01
NAA
I : 2.86
Cho
I : 0.994
Cr
I : 1.35
Cr2
I : 0.210
1.0
0.5
0.0
ppm
4
3
2
1
svs_se/90
TR 1500/TE30
NA 128/TA 3:13

◂**Fig. 6** Mature abscess, late capsule stage. An 80-year-old man, immunosuppressed because of colitis ulcerosa. **a** Axial T2-weighted image. **b** Axial T1-weighted image before contrast administration. **c** Axial T1-weighted image after contrast administration. **d** Axial DWI. **e** Axial ADC map. **f** MR spectrogram. **g** rrCBV map (PerfMRI). The capsule presents as a regular ring structure with low signal on T2-weighted images (**a**), slightly hyperintense signal on nonenhanced T1-weighted images (**b**) and marked enhancement (**c**). Strongly restricted diffusion in the necrotic core of the abscess due to high viscosity of the pus (**d, e**). Elevated lactate (1.33 ppm) and lipids (0.9 ppm); Cho, Cr, and NAA are reduced with Cho/NAA not elevated (**f**). **g** rrCBV map (PerfMRI). The capsule presents as a regular ring structure with low signal on T2-weighted images (**a**), slightly hyperintense signal on nonenhanced T1-weighted images (**b**) and marked enhancement (**c**). Strongly restricted diffusion in the necrotic core of the abscess due to high viscosity of the pus (**d, e**). Elevated lactate (1.33 ppm) and lipids (0.9 ppm); Cho, Cr, and NAA are reduced with Cho/NAA not elevated (**f**). **g** In contrast to malignant tumors, rrCBV is not elevated

infection, and patient characteristics (age, medical conditions, status of the immune system).

Generally, the most common pathogens in bacterial brain abscesses in Western Europe and the U.S. are *Streptococci*, followed by *Staphylococcus*, *Pseudomonas*, *Enterobacteriaceae*, and *Bacteroides* species. Infections with several different pathogens are common.

In newborns the spectrum of pathogens includes *Citrobacter*, *Proteus*, *Pseudomonas*, and *Serratia* (see also "Neurolues").

In immunocompromised patients more uncommon pathogens, such as *Mycobacteriaceae*, *Klebsiella*, *Listeria*, and *Nocardia*, also have to be taken into consideration. In addition, non-bacterial pathogens, i.e., viruses (e.g., CMV, PML), fungi (aspergillosis, candida, etc.), and parasites (e.g., toxoplasmosis, cysticercosis) may be found, solely or in combination.

In brain abscesses following neurosurgical procedures and in posttraumatic abscesses, *Staphylococci* are the most common pathogens (Carpenter et al. 2007). In abscesses derived from otitic foci *Proteus*, *Enterobacteriaceae*, *Pseudomonas*, *Pneumococcus*, and *Haemophilus* predominate (Penido Nde et al. 2005).

In hematogenous abscesses, the spectrum of pathogens differs according to the site of the primary infection (heart, lung, intestine, etc.).

1.4 Clinical Presentation

The most common symptoms in patients with brain abscesses are listed in Table 1. Unspecific symptoms, such as headache and nausea, prevail. Only 40–55 % of the patients present with fever.

1.5 Laboratory Findings and Other Diagnostic Procedures

Blood examinations may reveal inflammatory signs, and C-reactive protein is increased in 80–90 % of cases; however, normal laboratory findings do not exclude a brain abscess.

The CSF may be normal (about 25 %) or show unspecific changes as increased protein and mild pleocytosis. In most cases it is not possible to isolate the pathogens from the CSF, because there is no communication of the abscess with the CSF spaces; thus, the value of CSF puncture in patients with brain abscess is limited. In cases with mass effect the risk of brain herniation has to be considered.

1.6 Therapy

Cerebritis is generally treated with antibiotics, accompanied by prompt medical and/or surgical therapy of the underlying focus, if possible. Once an abscess capsule has formed, in most cases combined surgical, i.e., stereotactic drainage or open surgical resection, and antibiotic therapy is mandatory. Antibiotics are chosen depending on the respective pathogen. Patients with multiple, small, and/or deeply situated abscesses may be treated with antibiotics without prior surgery. Additional corticosteroids may be required in cases with considerable edema and in patients with infratentorial abscesses, since the posterior fossa is prone to excessive edema formation. Prophylactic anticonvulsive therapy for about 2 years is generally recommended; however, some authors propose to restrict anticonvulsive medication to patients with manifest seizures induced by the inflammatory process.

1.7 Prognosis

Before the invention of computed tomography, the mortality of brain abscesses has been about 40 % (Rosenblum et al. 1978); however, despite the improvements in diagnosis and therapy in the past decades, the mortality of brain abscesses is still considerable, about 10 (Carpenter et al. 2007)–20 % (Blanco García et al. 1998). Not surprisingly, the prognosis is worse in patients with underlying brain tumors or severe medical problems (Carpenter et al. 2007).

2 Imaging in Correlation with Histopathological Findings

Compared with CT, MRI is much more sensitive in the early detection of small inflammatory foci. MRI allows to discriminate or exclude additional small lesions, and the involvement of important adjacent structures as venous sinuses or the meninges. Complications, such as spread of the inflammatory process into the ventricular system or the subarachnoid space, can be detected easier and earlier; thus, MRI is the imaging method of choice in the diagnosis of pyogenic cerebritis and brain abscesses. An additional CT examination may be helpful in depicting bony erosions, e.g., in infections arising from adjacent paranasal sinuses or mastoid cells.

The imaging features accompanying the formation of brain abscesses have been studied in detail in animal experiments (Obana et al. 1986; Enzmann et al. 1986; Britt et al. 1981; 1984, Flaris and Hickey 1992). According to those experiments, the development of brain abscesses may be divided into four stages: early cerebritis; late cerebritis; early capsule formation; and late capsule formation (Britt et al. 1981).

The early cerebritis stage (days 1–3) is characterized by perivascular infiltrates of inflammatory cells, exudation of protein-rich fluid, excessive edema, petechial hemorrhages, and necrosis (Fig. 2). On plain CT or MRI studies, the early cerebritis stage is characterized by an ill-defined area of low attenuation (CT) or high signal on T2-weighted images, respectively. On nonenhanced T1-weighted images, the early inflammatory changes are difficult to discriminate and may present with isointense or slightly hypointense signal. Mass effect in the form of narrowing of sulci and ventricular compression may be present. Following contrast injection there is no, or only sparse, inhomogeneous enhancement (Fig. 3).

In the late cerebritis stage (days 4–9) the necrotic center increases. Foam cells and fibroblasts appear in the periphery and new vessels are formed. The edema persists; astrocytes start to proliferate in the surroundings (early reactive astrocytosis; Fig. 4). On imaging studies, the blood–brain barrier (BBB) becomes disrupted in the tissue adjacent to the emerging necrotic center (abscess cavity), resulting in a ringlike enhancement. The thickness of the ring varies strongly depending on the delay between contrast administration and the time of image acquisition. On delayed scans the enhancement progresses from the periphery toward the center of the ring. As long as no larger necrosis has formed, this may result in a nodular appearance in scans obtained long after contrast infusion (>1 h). In the cerebritis stage, the intensity of the ring enhancement persists on delayed scans. With advancing necrosis the center of the inflammatory process liquefies. The CT density of the emerging necrosis may vary between strong hypodensity to nearly isodensity to normal brain parenchyma. On T1-weighted images, the signal of the liquid center is higher than that of CSF, depending on the content of proteins and other macromolecules. On T2-weighted images, the signal of the core may be similar to that of the surrounding edema or slightly lower.

During early capsule formation (day 10–13), the necrotic center decreases and the number of fibroblasts forming the capsule increases. The amount of reticulin produced by the fibroblasts is larger on the cortical side (directed to the brain surface) compared with the ventricular side of the abscess (Britt et al. 1984). Whereas the edema decreases, the reactive astrocytosis advances.

In the late capsule stage (day 14 and later), the volume of the necrotic center and the number of inflammatory cells decrease. The capsule becomes thicker and now consists of fibroblasts, reticulin, and collagen (Fig. 5).

The developing capsule may be visible already on plain CT or MRI as a ring structure. On CT the ring at the margin of the necrotic center is slightly hyperdense. On nonenhanced T1-weighted images the capsule may be slightly hyperintense, on T2-weighted images hypointense as compared with the necrotic core and the surrounding edema (Fig. 6).

There has been considerable discussion about the mechanisms underlying the MR signal characteristics of the rim. The formation of collagen could account for the low signal on T2-weighted images, but it cannot explain the hyperintensity on nonenhanced T1-weighted images. In addition, collagen formed in the capsule persists for months or even years, i.e., much longer than the rim is present on MRI. The signal characteristics of the ring, i.e., shortening of T1 and T2, could be explained by paramagnetic substances, for instance, blood degradation products. However, blood degradation products could not be found histologically, and the time course of the blood degradation process does not fit to the sequelae of the MRI signal changes; thus, it has been suspected that free radicals produced by macrophages in the periphery of the abscess during phagocytosis are responsible for the observed signal changes. Free radicals are strongly paramagnetic and therefore could account for the T1 and T2 shortening; however, since these substances are unstable and short-lived, continuous production during active phagocytosis has to be proven.

The localization of the hypointense rim on T2-weighted images corresponds to the ring enhancement following contrast administration; however, whereas the ring enhancement of brain abscesses may persist several months after successful treatment, the disappearance of the hypointense rim is better correlated with the clinical improvement and thus is better suited to monitor the effects of therapy.

Following contrast administration, the capsule of the mature abscess strongly enhances. During maturation of the abscess the enhancing ring becomes thicker, and the width may exceed 5 mm. Often the medial part (directed to the ventricle) of the ring is thinner than the lateral part (directed to the brain surface), in accordance with the histopathological findings (see above). This fact has been attributed to

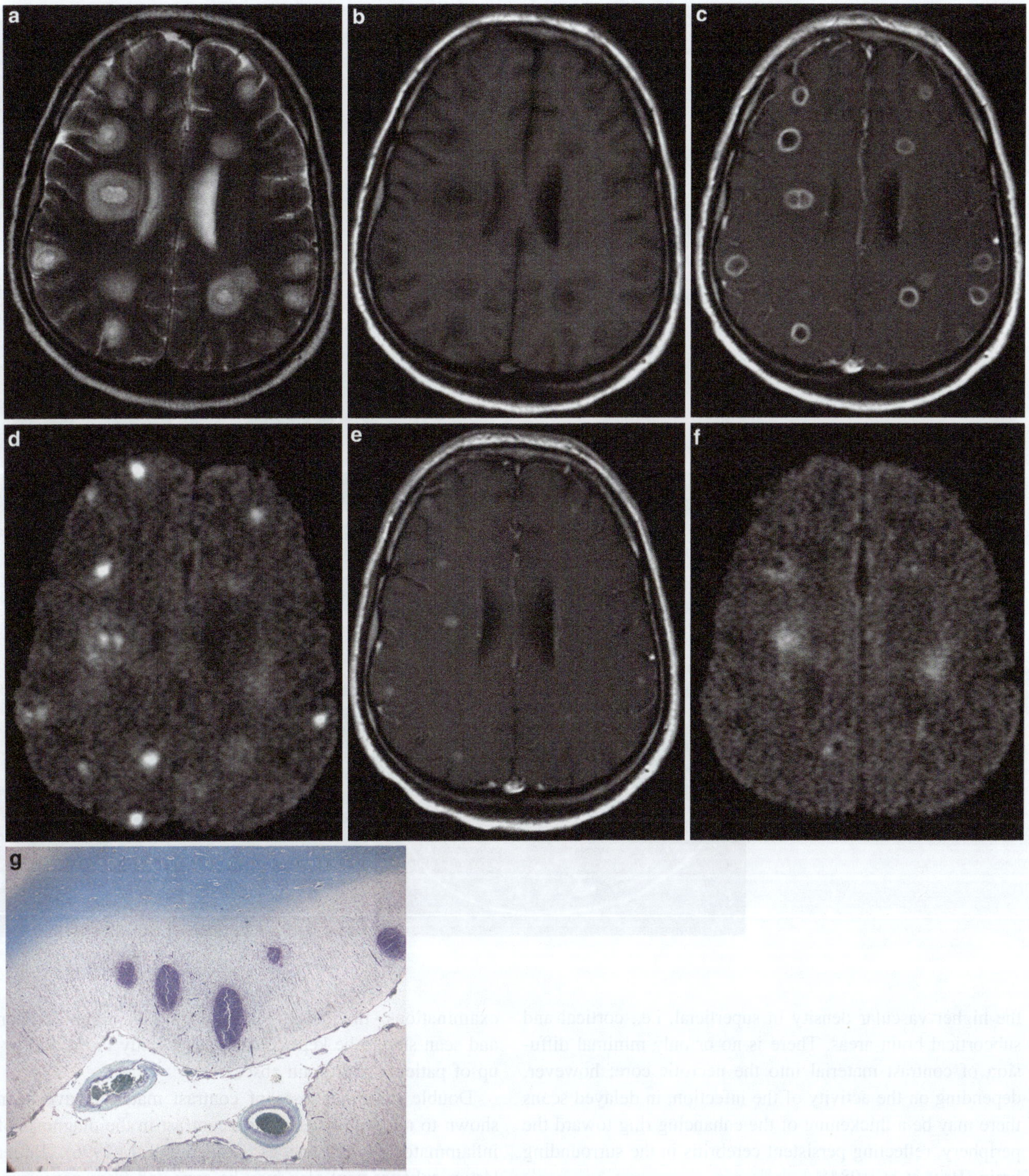

Fig. 7 Multiple hematogenous brain abscesses. A 43-year-old man; sepsis in the course of a complicated perianal abscess; headache, focal seizures, diplopic images. Initial examination. **a** Axial T2-weighted image. **b** Axial T1-weighted image before contrast administration. Initial examination. **c** Coronal T1-weighted image after contrast administration. **d** Axial DWI. Three-month follow-up after specific antibiotic therapy. **e** Axial T1-weighted image after contrast administration. **f** Axial diffusion-weighted MR image. **g** Histological preparation (different patient). Multiple ring-enhancing lesions (**c**) with perifocal edema (**a**) and hypointense rim on T2-weighted images (**a**). Note bright signal in DWI, suggestive of pus (**d**). Reduced, but still persistent, contrast enhancement and diffusion restriction despite complete clinical remission at 3-month follow-up (**e, f**). Histological preparation shows multiple intracortical microabscesses in the early stage. (Courtesy of B. Volk)

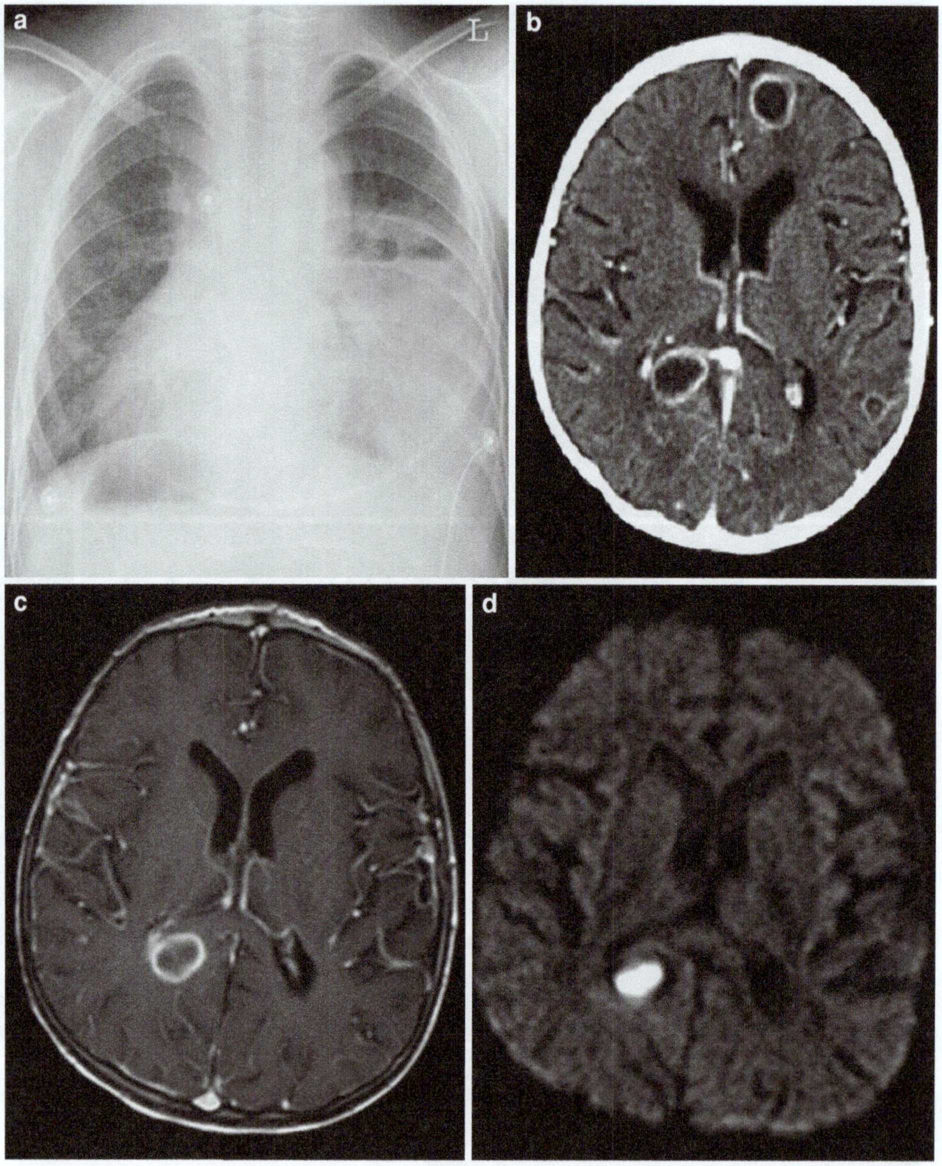

Fig. 8 A 6-year-old boy; complex heart malformation (Situs inversus, single inlet/double outlet ventricle with transposition); after surgical correction. **a** Chest X-ray. **b** Contrast-enhanced CT. **c** Axial T1-weighted image after contrast administration. **d** Axial DWI. Situs inversus (**a**). Multiple ring-enhancing lesions (**b, c**) with bright signal on DWI (**d**) indicative of pus with restricted diffusion

the higher vascular density in superficial, i.e., cortical and subcortical brain areas. There is no or only minimal diffusion of contrast material into the necrotic core; however, depending on the activity of the infection, in delayed scans there may be a thickening of the enhancing ring toward the periphery, reflecting persistent cerebritis in the surrounding brain (Britt et al. 1984).

The time delay between contrast infusion and scan strongly influences the intensity as well as the pattern of enhancement in bacterial brain infections. A longer delay may improve the contrast of the capsule of abscesses. In the early stages, i.e., before a large necrotic center has formed, with increasing delay the enhancement progresses from the periphery toward the center of the inflammatory lesion; however, to maintain comparability between different examinations, the delay between contrast administration and scan should be kept constant, especially in the follow-up of patients with brain abscesses.

Double or triple doses of contrast material have been shown to result in better lesion contrast in the diagnosis of inflammatory brain lesions (Runge et al. 1996). Better lesion enhancement also may be expected from new paramagnetic MR contrast media (Maravilla et al. 2006).

Brain enhancement following injection of common paramagnetic contrast media reflects an unspecific disruption of the BBB, irrespective of the cause and stage of the underlying process. Interesting new aspects concerning the imaging of brain infections may be expected from the clinical application of USPIO, which are phagocytosed by activated macrophages and thus presumably will enable a more specific diagnosis of

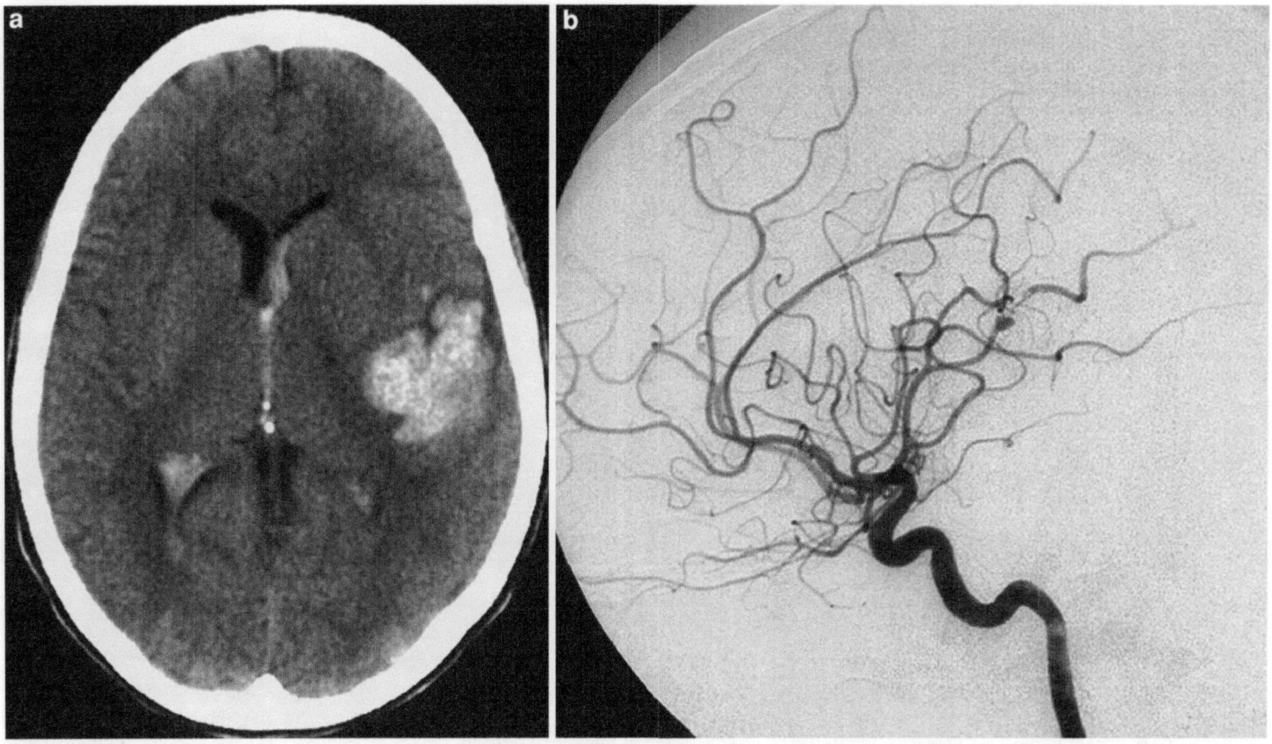

Fig. 9 Infectious aneurysm. A 27-year-old woman, acute headache and aphasia; endocarditis. **a** Axial computed tomogram without contrast enhancement. **b** Digital subtraction angiogram. Left sylvic/perisylvic SAH and intraparenchymal hemorrhage (**a**). Fusiform aneurysm of a parietal branch of the MCA (**b**)

inflammatory brain processes and a better differentiation between the different stages of abscess formation (Stoll and Bendszus 2009).

In the follow-up of patients with brain abscesses under therapy, it has to be considered that the imaging findings may show a substantial delay compared with the clinical development. Even with appropriate antibiotic therapy ring enhancement and edema may persist for weeks or even months, despite considerable clinical improvement (Fig. 7); thus, the imaging findings always have to be interpreted in the clinical context.

Eventual residual collagen in a completely healed abscess without surrounding edema cannot be depicted in CT, because it is isodense to brain parenchyma and does not enhance; however, in MRI the area of a former abscess may remain visible in form of subtle residual hyperintensities on T2-weighted images.

The time course and the degree of the morphological changes are influenced by the virulence of the pathogenic agent, e.g., experimental abscesses induced by *Staphylococcus* and *Bacteroides* species tend to be large; inflammatory changes outside the capsule, and complications, such as ependymitis, are found more frequently than in abscesses caused by less virulent pathogens (Enzmann et al. 1986).

On the other hand, the status of the immune system of the host is of crucial importance, not only concerning the type of pathogens, but also the clinical course and imaging features. Many ubiquitous pathogenic agents with low virulence may cause severe cerebritis and abscesses in the immunocompromised patient. On the other hand, inflammatory tissue responses, such as reactive astrocytosis and formation of the capsule, require a sufficient immunological capacity of the host. Reduced inflammatory responses following immunosuppression have been shown in experimental brain abscesses in dogs (Obana et al. 1986). The number of polymorphonuclear leukocytes and macrophages is reduced, the formation of collagen is decreased and delayed, and the bacteriae persist longer in the immunocompromised host. Accordingly, in patients with severe immunodeficiency, as in the terminal stages of AIDS, typical inflammatory changes may be missed even in advanced brain infections. The pathogens may multiply almost undisturbed without the typical histological and imaging findings of abscess formation. In such constellations, imaging studies may show paradoxical or pseudonormal findings.

Bacterial endocarditis, congenital heart disease, and intravenous drug abuse are common risk factors in the pathogenesis of septic emboli (Fig. 8). Large septic emboli

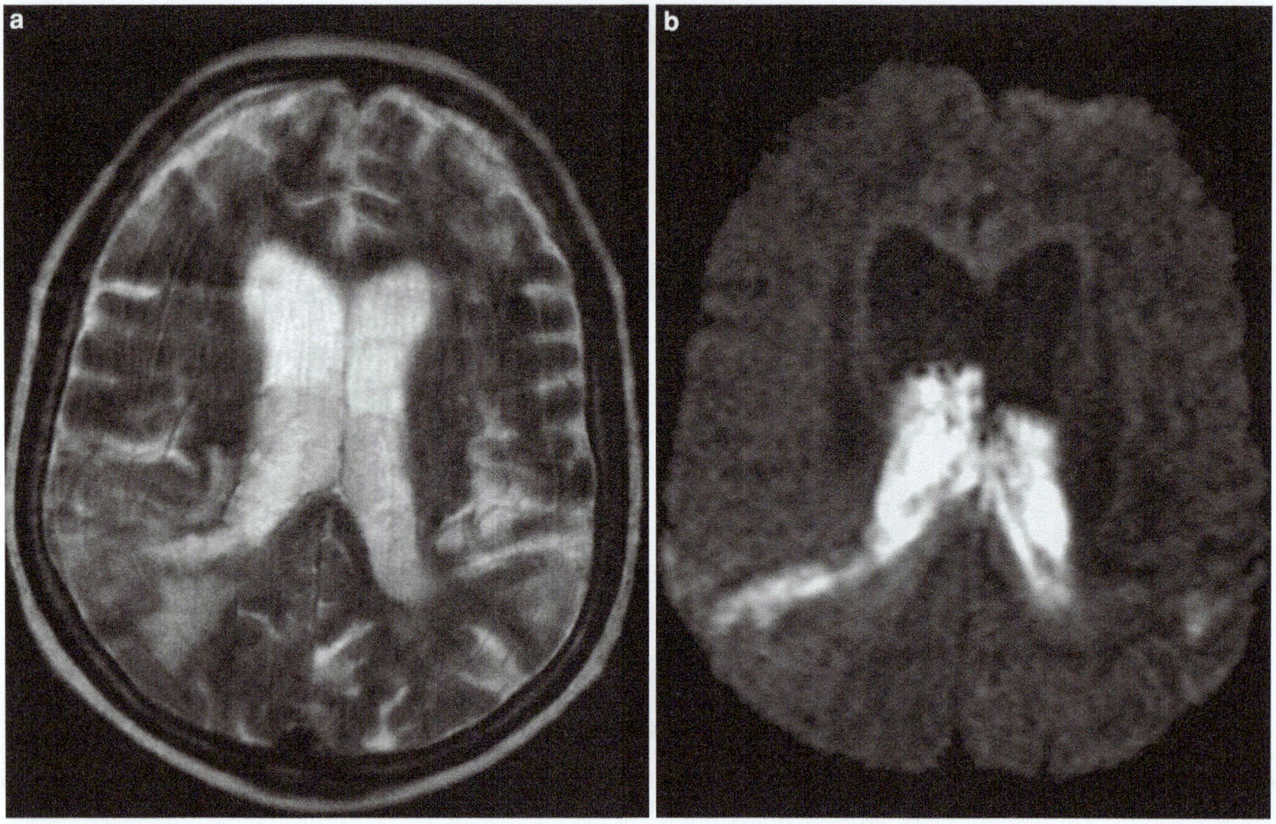

Fig. 10 Ventriculitis as a complication of meningoencephalitis. A 79-year-old man, severe meningoencephalitis (*streptococci*). **a** Axial T2-weighted image. **b** Axial DWI. Pathological substrate with intermediate to hypointense signal on T2-weighted images (**a**) and strongly hyperintense signal on DWI due to restricted diffusion (**b**) in the lateral ventricles, suspicious for pus. Periventricular hyperintensity (**a, b**), the correlate of vasogenic edema due to encephalitis

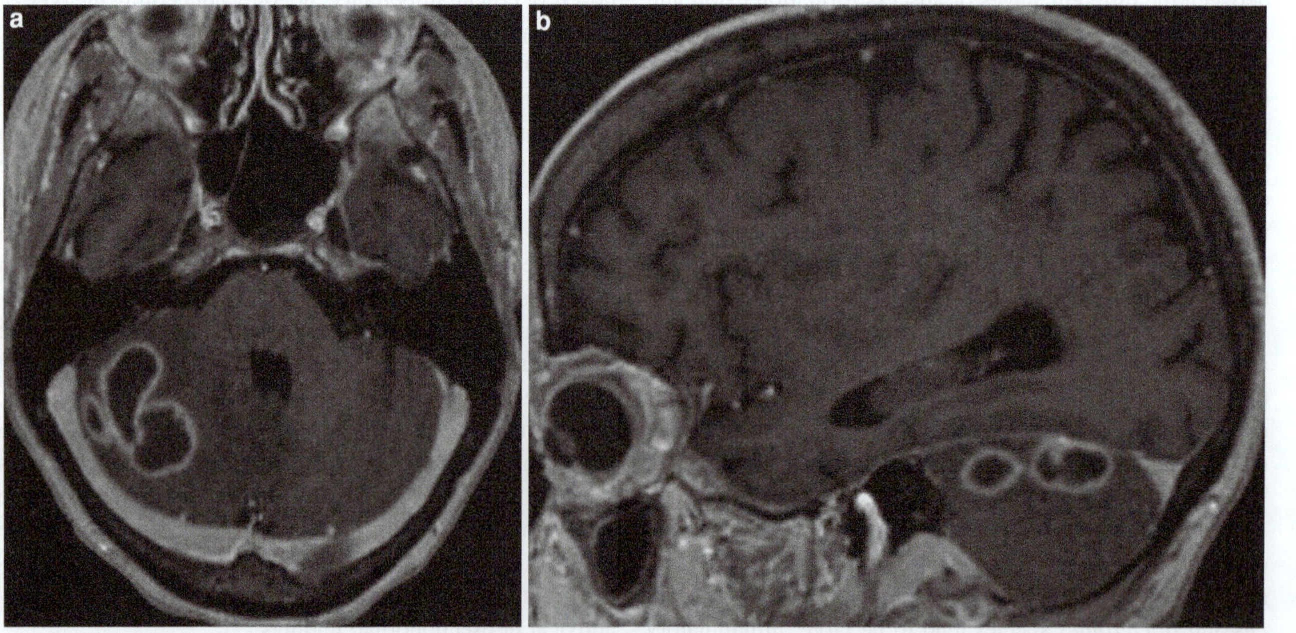

Fig. 11 Subacute arterial cerebellar infarct mimicking abscesses. Infarction was histologically verified by stereotactic biopsy. A 72-year-old woman with subacute ataxia. **a** Axial T1-weighted image after contrast administration. **b** Sagittal T1-weighted image after contrast administration. Ring-enhancing cerebellar lesions with perifocal edema

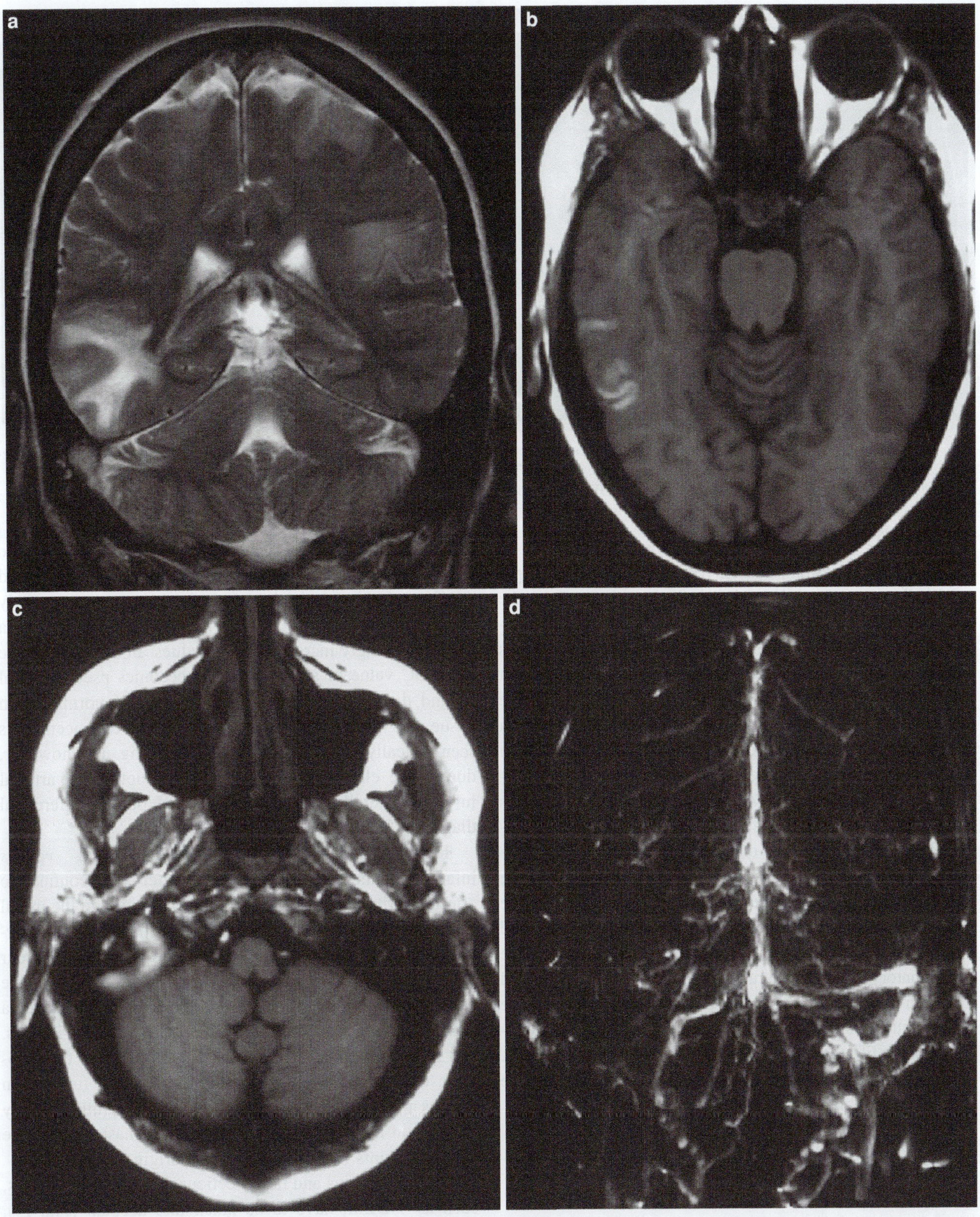

Fig. 12 Vasogenic edema due to sinus thrombosis as differential diagnosis of cerebritis. A 36-year-old woman, headache, seizures for 10 days. **a** T2-weighted image. (**b, c**) Axial T1-weighted images without contrast administration. **d** MIP of venous TOF MRA. Right temporooccipital edema (**a**) with subacute cortical hemorrhage (**b, c**). Subacute thrombosis with high signal on T1-weighted images of transverse and sigmoid sinuses (**b, c**). Absent venous flow in the transverse and sigmoid sinuses (**d**)

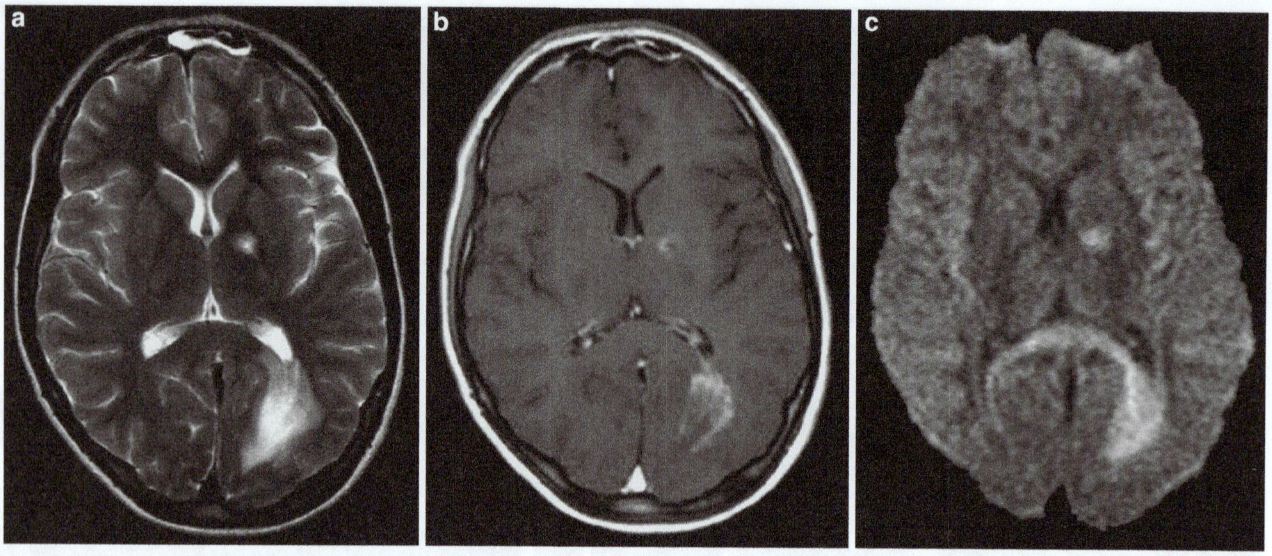

Fig. 13 ADEM mimicking cerebritis. A 19-year-old woman, headache, seizures for 10 days. **a** Axial T2-weighted image. **b** Axial T1-weighted image after contrast administration. **c** Axial DWI. Multifocal left hemispheric lesions with restricted diffusion and contrast enhancement. Similar changes can be seen in late stage of cerebritis

may occlude major cerebral arteries and may result in ischemic infarcts. Small emboli typically result in multiple small abscesses that characteristically are located at the junction between cerebral gray and white matter (corticomedullary junction). The localization of septic abscesses is similar to that of widespread cerebral metastases. Often, but not always, the abscesses are surrounded by extensive perifocal edema. A possible complication of septic emboli is the formation of infectious ("mycotic") aneurysms. In contrast to the much more common noninfectious aneurysms at the main branches of the circle of Willis, infectious aneurysms are located in small-sized arteries located distally to the main branches of the circle of Willis (Fig. 9).

Regarding complications, as pointed out previously, the medial wall of cerebral abscesses is generally thinner than the lateral circumference; thus, growing abscesses tend to expand in the corticofugal direction, i.e., toward the ventricles. If the inflammatory process penetrates the brain parenchyma toward the ventricles, ependymitis and ventriculitis result, and the inflammation may spread rapidly via the CSF spaces. Ventriculitis is a life-threatening condition with serious prognosis. If intravenous antibiotic therapy fails, antibiotics may be applied directly into the ventricular system (Fig. 10).

3 Differential Diagnosis

3.1 Cerebritis

The main differential diagnosis of cerebritis is venous or arterial infarction. Arterial infarcts can be attributed to an arterial territory, whereas cerebritis does not respect the limits of vascular areas. In arterial ischemic stroke diffusion is severely restricted due to cytotoxic edema with decreased ADC values already in the acute phase; however, the early phase of cerebritis is characterized by interstitial edema with accordingly increased ADC values. In the later course the ADC value of arterial infarcts becomes pseudonormal around day 10 and increases above that of normal brain tissue afterward. In infarcts, a dense cortical enhancement is seen typically from day 5 to the 8 week (Fig. 11); however, due to the clinical context and the abrupt onset, arterial infarcts generally will be easily ruled out as differential diagnosis for cerebritis.

The differentiation between cerebritis and *venous* infarction is more difficult, since the latter is not confined to arterial territories. The clinical characteristics and the initial course of both entities may be very similar (Fig. 12). Furthermore, venous infarction and cerebritis may occur combined in cases of infectious venous thrombosis. In the early phase of both entities, predominant interstitial edema will produce high signal on DWI and T2-weighted images, and the ADC values are increased. In contrast to the cytotoxic edema of arterial infarction, these early findings in venous infarction are potentially reversible. Inflammatory changes in adjacent paranasal sinuses or mastoid cells are important hints for an inflammatory origin.

Other infectious and noninfectious forms of encephalitis, such as ADEM, have to be taken into account (Fig. 13). Vasculitis is a challenging differential diagnosis, since clinical symptoms and the morphological appearance are extremely variable. Especially vasculitis in the course of collagen diseases, such as lupus erythematosis, may mimic the early stages of bacterial brain infection. Neither contrast

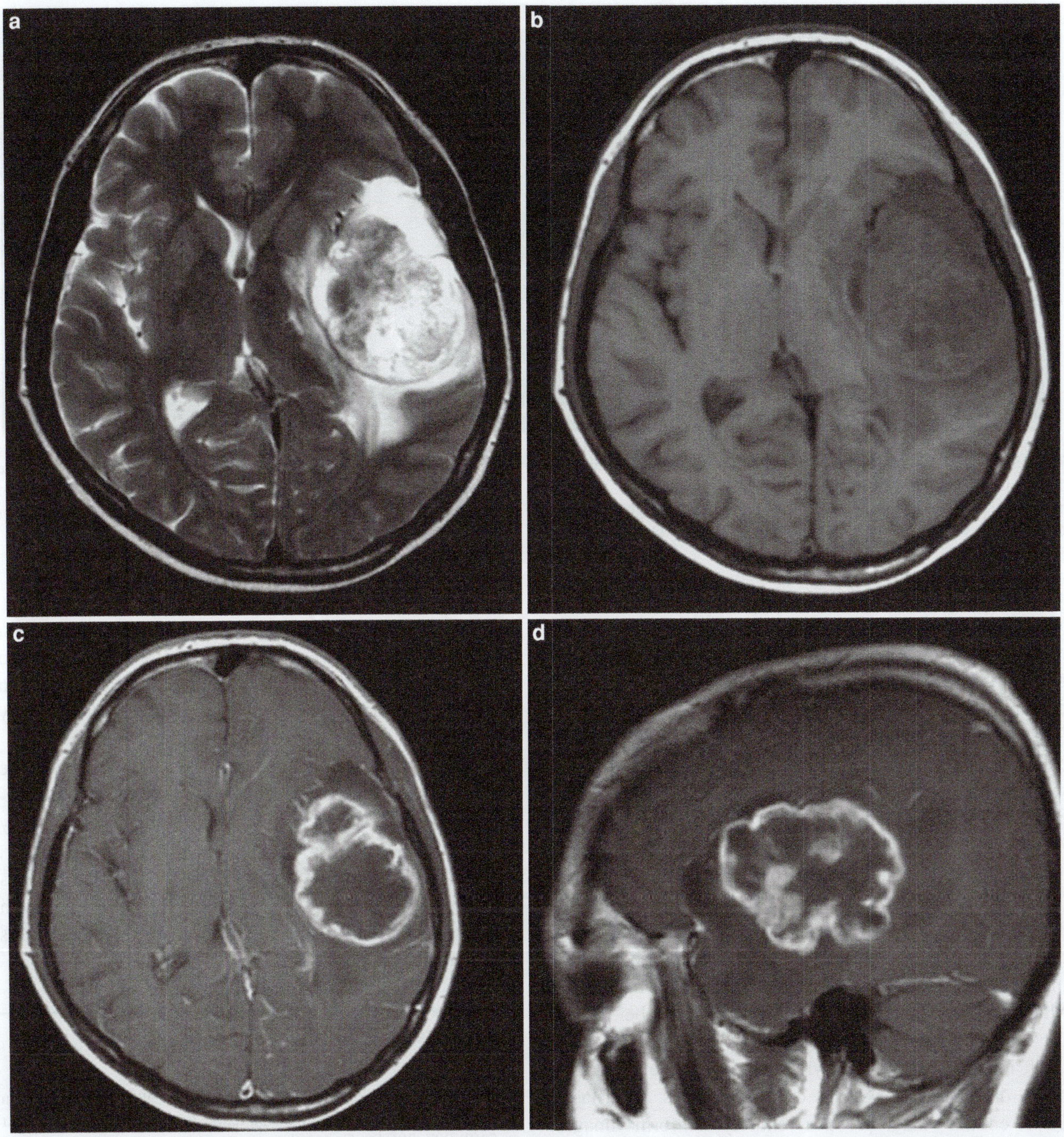

Fig. 14 Glioblastoma multiforme as differential diagnosis of solitary brain abscess in a 54-year-old man, rapid progressive headache, aphasia, hemiparesis. **a** Axial T2-weighted image. **b** Axial T1-weighted image before contrast administration. **c** Axial T1-weighted image after contrast administration. **d** Sagittal T1-weighted image after contrast administration. Left temporal mass lesion with perifocal edema, ring enhancement, and central necrosis. In contrast to brain abscess, the ADC (not shown) in the necrotic center of the mass was not reduced, and the wall thickness of the enhancing rim is more irregular than in brain abscess

administration nor advanced MR techniques allow for an unambiguous discrimination of these diseases. In many cases the differential diagnosis will be possible by additional laboratory tests such as blood or CSF analysis; if not, histological clarification is mandatory.

3.2 Abscess

All cerebral lesions with central necrosis and peripheral contrast enhancement may mimic brain abscesses. If the lesion is solitary, malignant glioma or solitary metastasis

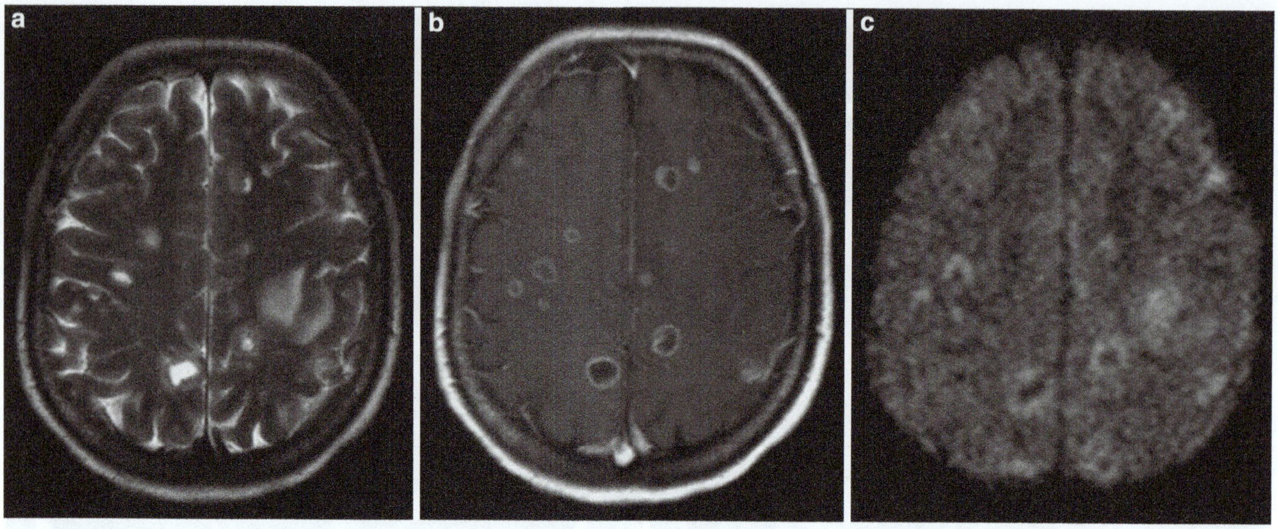

Fig. 15 Multiple metastases (bronchial carcinoma) as differential diagnosis of multiple brain abscesses in a 55-year-old woman; headache, no focal neurological deficits. **a** Axial T2-weighted image. **b** Axial T1-weighted image after contrast administration. **c** Axial DWI. Multiple ring-enhancing lesions in both hemispheres, moderate perifocal edema. Only slightly restricted diffusion, indicative of neoplastic rather than inflammatory process (**c**). See Fig. 7 for comparison

are the main differential diagnoses. In most cases, the rim enhancement of autochthonous brain tumors will be more irregular, with focal thickenings, and less well demarcated as the enhancement of an abscess capsule (Fig. 14). Metastases generally are equally well demarcated as abscesses. A regular, hypointense rim on T2-weighted images points to an inflammatory origin; however, not all abscesses exhibit this criterion. Reduced ADC within the liquid core of a ring-enhancing lesion is a strong hint for an inflammatory origin, but not absolutely specific. The suspicion is further supported by normal or only slightly increased PerfMRI parameters in the solid portions of the lesion, whereas strongly increased perfusion is a sign of a neoplastic origin. Magnetic resonance spectroscopy may also be helpful for differentiation (see also "Chap. 5").

If multiple space-occupying lesions are evident, the main differential diagnosis of abscesses is metastases. Both entities may produce entirely uniform images. Metastases as well as abscesses preferentially are located in the border zone between gray and white matter (corticomedullary junction). In both entities, perifocal edema will be found often, but also may be lacking completely. Diffusion-weighted imaging, diffusion tensor imaging (Toh et al. 2011), PerfMRI, and MRS may help to differentiate between inflammatory and neoplastic lesions (Fig. 15); however, in the single case the results of the imaging studies are not unequivocal. Often the clinical context will help to establish the final diagnosis; however, patients with malignancies or severely compromised immune system are prone both to multifocal tumors, lymphoma or metastases, and to abscesses; thus, due to the completely different therapeutic implications and prognosis, in most cases a histological clarification by stereotactic or open surgical biopsy is necessary.

Especially in immunocompromised patients multiple toxoplasma foci have to be considered as differential diagnosis of bacterial abscesses. Toxoplasma foci preferentially are deeply located, e.g., in the basal ganglia; however, atypical localizations are possible. The toxoplasmosis cysts typically reveal high ADC values as compared with abscesses according to the lower viscosity of the hydrous cyst content.

References

Berlit P, Fedel C, Tornow K, Schmiedek P (1996) Bacterial brain abscess: experiences with 67 patients. Fortschr Neurol Psychiatr 64(8):297–306 [in German]

Blanco García A, García Vázquez E, Benito N, Górgolas M de, Muñiz J, Gadea I, Ruiz Barnés P, Fernández Guerrero ML (1998) Brain abscess. Clinicomicrobiologic study and prognostic analysis of 59 cases. Rev Clin Esp 198(7):413–419 [in Spanish]

Britt RH, Enzmann DR, Yeager AS (1981) Neuropathological and computerized tomographic findings in experimental brain abscess. J Neurosurg 55(4):590–603

Britt RH, Enzmann DR, Placone RC Jr, Obana WG, Yeager AS (1984) Experimental anaerobic brain abscess. Computerized tomographic and neuropathological correlations. J Neurosurg 60(6):1148–1159

Carpenter J, Stapleton S, Holliman R (2007) Retrospective analysis of 49 cases of brain abscess and review of the literature. Eur J Clin Microbiol Infect Dis 26(1):1–11

Enzmann DR, Britt RR, Obana WG, Stuart J, Murphy-Irwin K (1986) Experimental *Staphylococcus aureus* brain abscess. Am J Neuroradiol 7(3):395–402

Flaris N, Hickey W (1992) Development and characterization of an experimental model of brain abscess in the rat. Am J Pathol 141:1299–1307

Maravilla KR, Maldjian JA, Schmalfuss IM, Kuhn MJ, Bowen BC, Wippold FJ 2nd, Runge VM, Knopp MV, Kremer S, Wolansky LJ, Anzalone N, Essig M, Gustafsson L (2006) Contrast enhancement of central nervous system lesions: multicenter intraindividual crossover comparative study of two MR contrast agents. Radiology 240(2):389–400

Obana WG, Britt RH, Placone RC, Stuart JS, Enzmann DR (1986) Experimental brain abscess development in the chronically immunosuppressed host. Computerized tomographic and neuropathological correlations. J Neurosurg 65(3):382–391

Penido Nde O, Borin A, Iha LC et al (2005) Intracranial complications of otits media: 15 years of experience in 33 patients. Otolaryngol Head Neck Surg 132:37–42

Rosenblum ML, Hoff JT, Norman D, Weinstein PR, Pitts L (1978) Decreased mortality from brain abscesses since the advent of computerized tomography. J Neurosurg 49:658–668

Runge VM et al (1996) The use of gadolinium-BOPTA on magnetic resonance imaging in brain infection. Invest Radiol 31:294

Stoll G, Bendszus M (2009) Imaging of inflammation in the peripheral and central nervous system by magnetic resonance imaging. Neuroscience 158:1151–1160

Toh CH, Wei KC, Ng Sh et al (2011) Differentiation of brain abscesses from necrotic glioblastomas and cystic metastatic brain tumors with diffusion tensor imaging. AJNR Am J Neuroradiol 32:1646–1651

Neurolues

Bodo Kress

Contents

Abstract

Since 1980 the incidence of syphilis has continuously increased. In the same way also an increase of neurolues is registered. *Treponema pallidum*, the causative agent of neurolues affects in stage III the central nervous system. Neurolues can take a serious course with a granulomatous or vasculitis form. Magnetic resonance imaging is able to detect both forms, but mostly usually allows no specific diagnosis.

1 Epidemiology, Clinical Presentation, Therapy

The causative agent of neurolues is the spirochaete *Treponema pallidum*. The course of the disease consists of three stages (Table 1). In the second stage the CNS may be involved with the symptoms of a "meningeal catarrh". The typical symptoms of the CNS manifestation of neurolues (progressive paralysis, meningovascular neurolues, tabes dorsalis) are assigned to the tertiary or late stage. Although the incidence of syphilis decreased with the discovery of penicillin around 1940, the incidence increased with the beginning of the HIV epidemic at the beginning of the 1980s strongly into the late 1990s. In Central Europe there has been a dramatic increase in neurolues at the beginning of the twenty-first century. In Germany alone, the incidence increased in the years 2001–2004 from 2.4/100,000 to 4.1/100,000, an increase of almost 100 %. It is more prevalent in urban areas, both in men and, generally, in people of African descent. Neurolues is transmitted by unprotected sexual intercourse. The diagnosis is usually made by means of medical history and the serological *T. pallidum* hemaglutination (TPHA) test and the absorption fluorescent treponemal antibody (FTAabs) test. The mean accuracy of these tests is below 95 %, and a negative test does not secure the exclusion of the disease. In addition, the specificity of the FTAabs test is low. From the chancre

B. Kress (✉)
Department Neuroradiology,
Central Institute of Radiology and Neuroradiology,
Steinbacher Hohl 2-26, 60488 Frankfurt, Germany
e-mail: kress.bodo@khnw.de

S. Hähnel (ed.), *Inflammatory Diseases of the Brain*, Medical Radiology. Diagnostic Imaging,
DOI: 10.1007/174_2012_623, © Springer-Verlag Berlin Heidelberg 2012
Published Online: 14 June 2012

Table 1 Stages of neurolues

Stage 1	Infection is restricted to the primary infection site. About 3 weeks after exposure a solitary painless chancre is seen
Stage 2	Without antibiotic treatment T. pallidum is spreading through blood over a few weeks. Numerous clinical manifestations are the result: fever; lymphadenopathy; condylomata lata
Stage 3 (late stage)	Years after, the infection can involve any organ system. Main concern is the cardiovascular complication and the involvement of the CNS

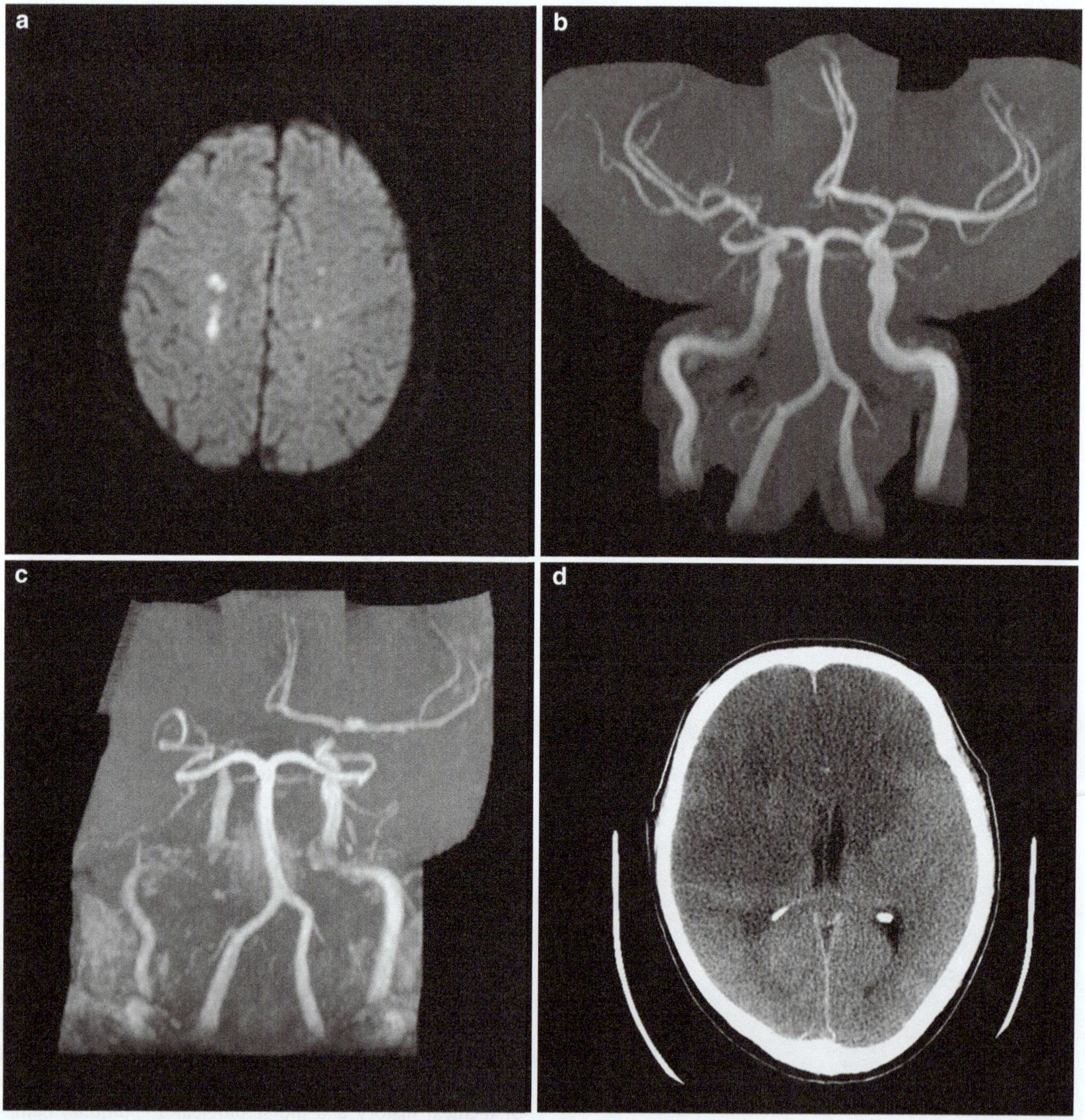

Fig. 1 Luetic vasculitis. **a**, **b** Early stage of the disease: Axial DWI (**a**); MIP of a arterial TOF MRA (**b**). **c**, **d** Later stage of the disease: MIP of a arterial TOF MRA (**c**). Axial computed tomogram (**d**). Luetic vasculitis affects mainly the larger arteries of the circle of Willis and causes stenosis of the distal segments of both ICAs (**b**) followed by hemodynamic infarction in both hemispheres with restricted diffusion in the early stage (**a**). Despite aggressive treatment with steroids and immunosuppressive cytostatics, the patient suffered rapidly progressive clinical course and further vessel narrowing and the consequence of vessel occlusion of the right MCA (**c**) followed by territorial infarction and death (**d**)

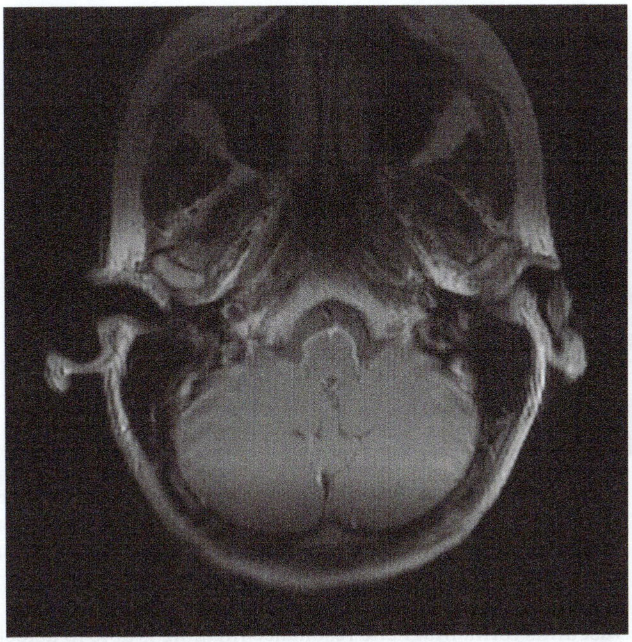

Fig. 2 Neurolues. Axial T1-weighted image after contrast administration. Thickened and contrast-enhancing leptomeninges around the medulla oblongata

T. pallidum can be detected using dark-field microscopy. Meningovascular neurolues may be associated with brain infarctions, vasculitic aneurysms, and SAH. Typical microscopic findings of luetic meningitis are lymphoplasmatic infiltrates thickening the meninges. In the vasculitic form the infection affects the connective tissue of blood vessels, and especially small- and medium-sized arteries. The diagnosis cannot be made by the description of the vascular lesions alone. In particular, the pioneering serum and CSF findings make the classification of the vascular lesions possible. Penicillin G is still the first choice of treatment; second-line treatments are tetracyclines, Ceftriaxone (combination), or azithromycin.

2 Imaging

Parenchymal infection manifests as cerebral gummae 2 mm to several centimeters in size with strong contrast enhancement. Preferred locations of gummae are the brain stem, the cerebellum, and the skull base. Gummae have the typical appearance of granulomatous diseases with centrally hypo- to isointense signal on T2-weighted images. Vasculitic vessel stenoses or occlusions in the territories of middle-sized or larger arteries (Heubner arteriitis) or, less commonly, smaller arteries (Nissl Alzheimer arteriitis) with the consequence of brain infarction (Fig. 1) may be detected by the use of DSA or MRA (Fig. 1). A diffuse, basal leptomeningitis may be found involving the cranial nerves and the craniocervical junction (Fig. 2). In some cases, the spinal cord is involved with monstrous thickening of the meninges and secondary (edema) and sometimes primary (vasculitis) involvement of the myelon (Fig. 3). Sometimes separated arachnoidal spaces occur which causes CSF circulation problems.

3 Differential Diagnosis

The granulomatous history form of neurolues must be differentiated especially from tuberculosis. The CSF findings for cells and proteins are unspecific; only the antibody detection confirms the diagnosis. Magnetic resonance imaging alone does not allow the differentiation between neurolues and tuberculosis (TB). Other important differential diagnoses are Lyme disease and neurosarcoidosis. Most of the granulomas at the time of diagnosis, in Lyme disease and also in sarcoidosis, are smaller than those in neurolues. In addition, Lyme disease may induce white matter lesions. Also, the differential diagnosis from other causes of vasculitis and from arteriosclerotic vascular disease might be difficult. The vasculitis form has to be differentiated from other forms of vasculitis, especially from Moyamoya disease (younger patients) and Takayasu arteritis (larger vessels, such as aorta). The other possible arteriosclerotic vascular diseases do not have such a rapidly progressive and malignant course as neurolues vasculitis.

4 Summary

Since 1980 the incidence of syphilis has continuously increased. In the same way also an increase of neurolues is registered. *Treponema pallidum*, the causative agent of

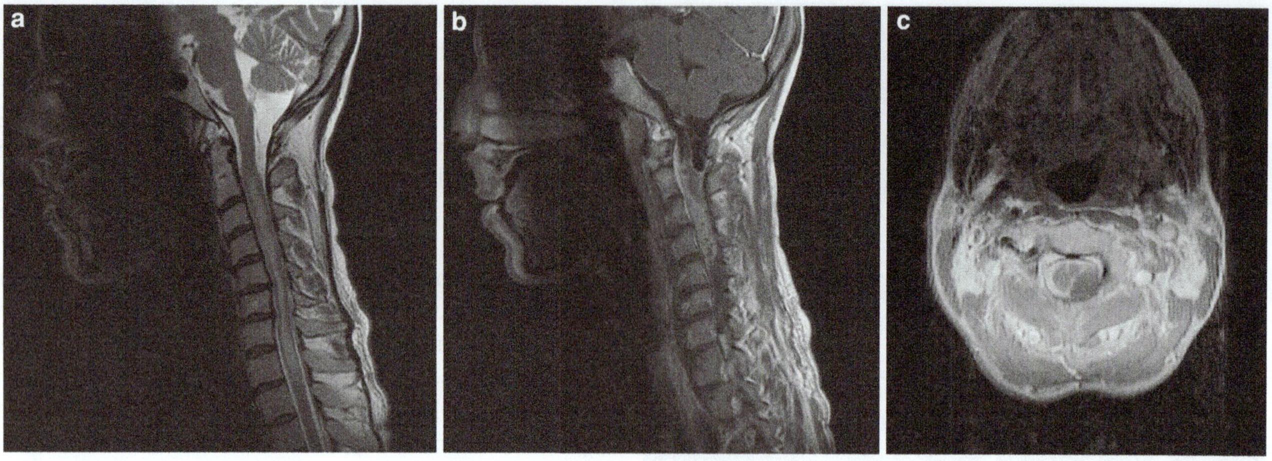

Fig. 3 Neurolues. The leading symptom of this patient was tetraparesis. **a** Sagittal T2-weighted image. **b** Sagittal T1-weighted image after contrast administration. **c** Axial T1-weighted image after contrast administration. The contrast-enhancing granulomatous tissue (**b**) causes edema of the cord due to mass effect (**a**). By septation additional rooms were created (**c**), which impedes the CSF circulation

neurolues affects in stage III the central nervous system. Neurolues can take a serious course with a granulomatous or vasculitis form. Magnetic resonance imaging is able to detect both forms, but mostly usually allows no specific diagnosis.

Neurotuberculosis

Stephan G. Wetzel and Thilo Kollmann

Contents

S. G. Wetzel (✉)
Department of Diagnostic and Interventional Neuroradiology, University Hospital Basel, Petersgraben 4, 4031 Basel, Switzerland
e-mail: stephan.wetzel@hirslanden.ch

T. Kollmann
Department of Psychiatry, University Hospital Basel, Wilhelm Klein-strasse 27, 4012 Basel, Switzerland

Abstract

Tuberculosis is still one of the leading causes of death worldwide: one-third of the world population is believed to be infected with *Mycobacterium tuberculosis*. Neurotuberculosis, which affects mainly young patients, is considered the most dangerous complication as it often leads to severe neurological sequelae or death. The clinical presentation of neurotuberculosis can be quite variable and laboratory investigations, e.g. CSF studies, have a limited sensitivity. On the other hand, tuberculostatic therapy is effective and treatment should not be delayed. Imaging, therefore, plays an important role for the workup of this disease. In most cases, a haematogenous spread of the bacteria leads to a meningeal or parenchymal affection, whereby both compartments are commonly affected. Meningeal tuberculosis is characterised by a thick basal exudate most pronounced in the basal cisterns that is best appreciated on contrast-enhanced T1-weighted images. Complications due to this infectious process include cranial nerve affection, hydrocephalus, and ischaemic infarctions. Tuberculous granulomas (tuberculomas) are the most common parenchymal manifestation of neurotuberculosis. They represent circumscriptive, inflammatory lesions affected by mycobacteria that are surrounded by a granulomatous reaction. These mass lesions are usually located at the corticomedullary junction and are hypodense on CT and hypointense on T1-weighted images on native scans. After contrast administration they show, depending on the stage of maturation, a homogenous (non-caseating tuberculoma) or rim enhancement. On T2-weighted images a caseating tuberculoma with solid centre shows characteristically a low signal in the centre. Non-caseating tuberculoma or caseating tuberculoma with a liquid centre is hyperintense. A tuberculous abscess might be indistinguishable from a caseating tuberculoma with liquid centre. Typically, however, an abscess is larger and patients are more severely sick. The

S. Hähnel (ed.), *Inflammatory Diseases of the Brain*, Medical Radiology. Diagnostic Imaging,
DOI: 10.1007/174_2012_691, © Springer-Verlag Berlin Heidelberg 2012
Published Online: 18 September 2012

differential diagnoses of tuberculous meningitis include other infectious diseases, sarcoidosis and meningeal carcinomatosis. Tuberculomas and tubercular abscesses primarily have to be differentiated from primary and secondary brain tumours and other granulomatous/infectious processes.

1 Epidemiology, Clinical Presentation, Therapy

Approximately one-third of the world population is infected with *Mycobacterium tuberculosis*, the most common pathogenic agent of tuberculosis (TB) in men. The bacteria are spread from one person to another by airborne infection while coughing or even speaking. In an immunocompetent person primary infection with *Mycobacterium tuberculosis* usually does not cause an immediately active TB; however, mycobacteria are able to survive within hilar lymph nodes of the lung, a state known as latent TB. In case the immune defence weakens, e.g. following HIV infection, malnutrition or old age, the dormant tubercle bacilli within macrophages can cause reactivation of TB. Approximately 5–10 % of the infected individuals develop active TB during their lifetime, leading annually to approximately 3 million deaths worldwide. TB is still one of the leading causes of death.

Infection of the central nervous system by *Mycobacterium tuberculosis* is the most dangerous form of systemic TB, due to its high rates of fatal outcomes and possible risk of serious neurological sequelae. Of all patients with systemic TB, 2–5 % suffers the complication of neurotuberculosis. This number increases to 10 % in patients with HIV co-infection. Neurotuberculosis can occur in all age groups. In underdeveloped countries mainly children are affected, whereas in developed countries adults are predominantly affected.

With an unfavourable prognosis of neurotuberculosis, on one hand, and potent causal and symptomatic treatment options, on the other hand, the early diagnosis of this disease is essential. As clinical symptoms are often unspecific, the observation of signs of extra-neural TB, which is reported in a significant percentage of patients, can be a first hint.

Neurotuberculosis causes first and foremost an inflammation of the meninges. Parenchymal tuberculosis is more common in HIV-infected persons and can occur with or without tuberculous meningitis. The meningeal infection will most often present as a basal exudative leptomeningitis. Intraparenchymal neurotuberculosis presents preferentially with localised granulomas (tuberculomas), and more rarely as an abscess; however, in many patients both compartments are more or less affected, as the tuberculous leptomeningitis often leads to parenchymal lesions, and vice versa.

Table 1 Clinical stages of tuberculous meningitis (Adapted from criteria developed by the British Medical Research Council)

Stage	Characteristics
I	Non-specific symptoms (fever, headache, irritability, anorexia, nausea)
	No alterations in consciousness
II	Altered consciousness (coma or delirium)
	Meningism, cranial nerve dysfunction, minor focal neurological signs
III	Stupor or coma
	Severe neurological disorders

Tuberculous meningitis potentially leads to severe neurological sequelae or death. A complete recovery rate after 1 year of treatment is seen in around 20 % of patients. About half of patients with tuberculous meningitis suffer life-long neurological deficits. A long duration of illness and higher age are factors that are related to a worse outcome. Initially, symptoms often develop over a long period of time, starting with headache, apathy and nausea, which aggravate over weeks or even months (Table 1, stage I). During the meningeal stage, the clinical presentation of the disease is mostly fulminant. Nearly, all patients present with high fever and the majority with a disturbance of consciousness (Table 1, stage II); the latter indicates an infectious involvement of brain parenchyma, which stresses the fact that meningeal and parenchymal affliction influence each other. Seizures are common, especially in children. Dysfunctions of cranial nerves are characteristic for tuberculous meningitis, and are due to the preferentially basal inflammation site. They are found in approximately one-third to half of all patients with tuberculous meningitis. Cranial nerves II, III, IV, VI and VII are affected most frequently, with the nerve dysfunction thought to be related to vascular compromise. The most common visual affection of tuberculous meningitis, papilledema, leads to impairment of vision. In adults, secondary optic atrophy may occur following chronic papilledema. In paediatric cases, papilledema may progress to primary optic atrophy and blindness resulting from involvement of the optic nerves and the chiasm by basal exudates. Basal inflammatory changes may also lead to pituitary dysfunction, which is often encountered. Approximately half of the patients with tuberculous meningitis show a mild-to-moderate hyponatraemia. Various mechanisms, including an inappropriate antidiuretic hormone secretion, are discussed. Sudden onset of focal neurological deficits, such as hemiparesis, tetraparesis or aphasia, has been reported and is most often due to vasculitic changes resulting in ischaemia; however, these symptoms can sometimes be postictal (Todd's paresis) or less likely following hydrocephalus.

Laboratory studies play the major role for the workup of patients suspected to suffer from neurotuberculosis; however, all tests have certain limitations in sensitivity and specificity that should be known. The purified protein derivative test (Mantoux test), a skin test, does not rule out TB, and is often negative in patients with neurotuberculosis. It must also be kept in mind that this test will be positive in patients with a history of BCG vaccination. Interferon-γ release assays, which measure a component of cell-mediated immune reactivity to *M. tuberculosis*, are more specific, easy to handle, give no positive results due to BCG vaccination and are increasingly used; however, the exact role of this test yet remains to be determined. Cerebrospinal fluid (CSF) studies are the key to the diagnosis. In tuberculous meningitis, unspecific meningitic CSF alterations, such as higher CSF pressure, elevated protein levels, reduced glucose concentration, pleocytosis (initially polymorphs then lymphocytes) are commonly observed. In co-morbid HIV patients, normal cell count or even no cells at all have been reported. Distinctive protein levels for the tuberculous meningitis condition range between 1 and 8 g/l, with a higher level frequently being related to a poor outcome. Specific CSF investigations include detection of acid-fast bacilli using Ziehl-Neelsen stain and fluorochrome tissue stain. Even if the Ziehl-Neelsen stain with a sensitivity of only up to 40 % does not show the causative agent in every case of tuberculous meningitis, immediate evidence of acid-fast bacilli occasionally may settle the diagnosis instantly. Fluorochrome tissue stains require special microscopes and are usually not instantly available. The highest specificity (close to 100 %) in detection of mycobacteria in CSF samples is provided by polymerase chain reaction (PCR). This technique detects mycobacteria DNA in roughly 50–80 % of CSF samples from patients with tuberculous meningitis and has a latency of about 2 days. The growth of *M. tuberculosis* in culture proves the pathogen in 50–80 % of cases but takes several weeks.

Parenchymal TB is usually seen in conjunction with tuberculous meningitis but may as well occur as an isolated entity. HIV patients in particular may present with isolated tuberculous granuloma (tuberculoma) within the brain parenchyma following a pulmonary tuberculous primary. The clinical appearance of isolated intracerebral tuberculomas is less fulminant than that of tuberculous meningitis. Seizures are often a first symptom. Focal neurological signs depend on the location of tuberculomas and include aphasia, pyramidal and cerebellar syndromes, for instance. Visual disturbances, such as photophobia and intracranial hypertension with papilledema and headache, are also described to be widespread. The CSF diagnostics may show an unspecific elevated protein concentration indicating a disturbance of the blood–brain barrier. Previously mentioned CSF studies will only exceptionally be able to verify mycobacteria or their DNA in samples; therefore, diagnosis in these cases has to be based on factors besides clinical appearance and anamnestic information on neuroimaging findings and response to antituberculous therapy. Unlike tuberculomas, tuberculous abscesses present with an accelerating clinical appearance such as acute high fever, headache and severe focal neurology; however, abscesses often develop from a possibly asymptomatic tuberculoma over time.

The therapeutic armamentarium for a successful treatment of neurotuberculosis includes tuberculostatic chemotherapy, neurosurgery and symptomatic measures. The exact duration of chemotherapy is still a matter of debate. In tuberculous meningitis, at least 6–9 months of antituberculous medication are required, with some authors recommending as much as 24 months of therapy. Proven, classical antimicrobial agents in treatment of neurotuberculosis are isoniazid, rifampicin, pyrazinamide, and streptomycin, which enter CSF readily in the presence of meningeal inflammation. Second-line agents include ethionamide, cycloserine and para-amino salicylic acid. Usually, a combination of three first-line substances plus a fourth agent, selected by the local physician, is used. According to recent studies, corticosteroids should be routinely used in HIV-negative patients with tuberculous meningitis to reduce death and disabling neurological deficits. An anticonvulsive strategy is an important part of an effective symptomatic therapy.

Neurosurgical interventions mostly consist of placement of a ventricular drain. Ventricular shunting has to be discussed early, as studies have shown that an early shunting significantly improves the outcome of patients, in particular in patients with few neurological deficits.

Surgical treatment may further appear to be necessary when tuberculomas have a mass effect on vital structures. Usually, however, tuberculomas are not an indication for neurosurgery.

2 Imaging

For the primary workup, patients still often undergo a CT examination as the initial imaging modality. Clearly, an MRI examination is superior to CT in detection and assessment of neurotuberculosis. Apart from imaging of the brain, imaging of the spine should be considered as a concomitant affection of the spinal compartments and is seen in about 10 % of the

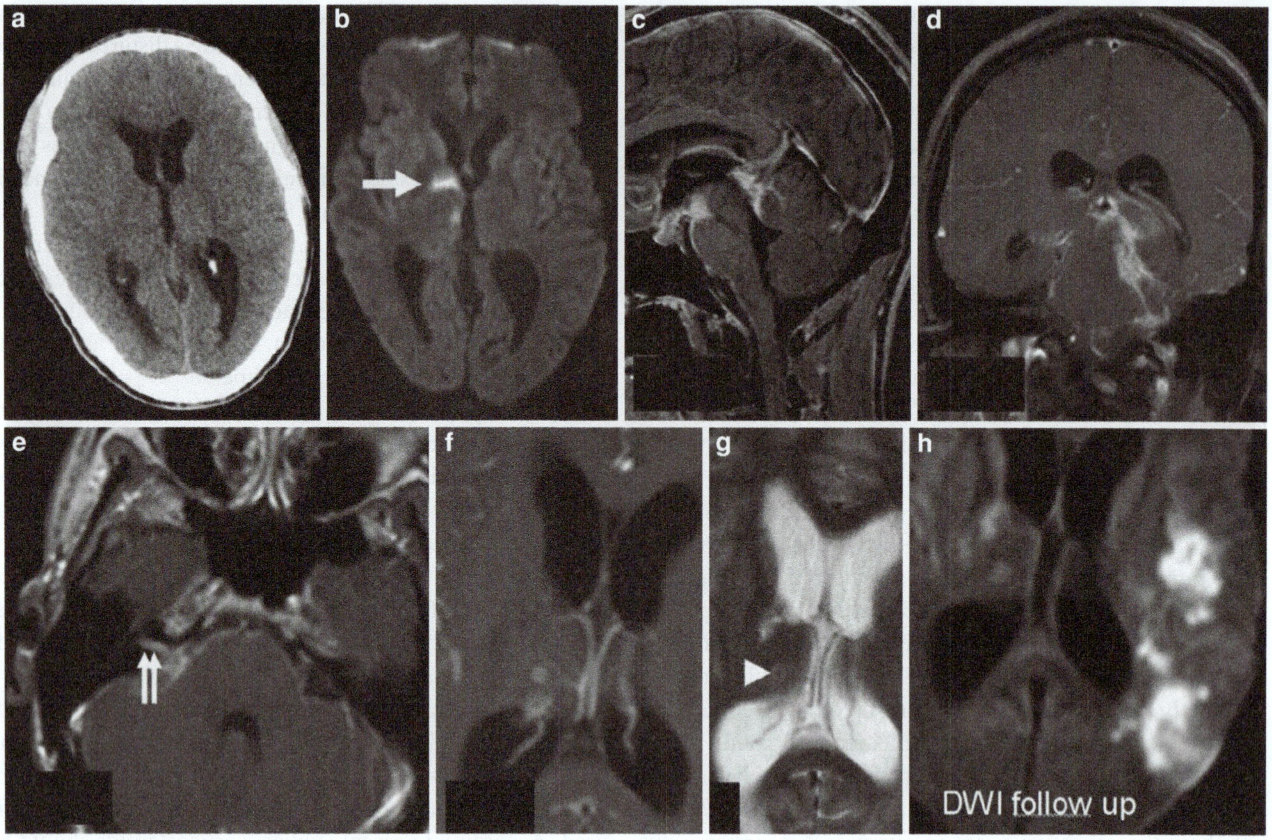

Fig. 1 A 24-year-old man who suffered from fever, headache and weight loss for several weeks and came to admission after a seizure. **a** Non-enhanced CT. **b** Axial DWI. **c** Sagittal T1-weighted image after contrast administration. **d** Coronal T1-weighted image after contrast administration. **e**, **f** Axial T1-weighted image after contrast administration. **g** Axial T2-weighted image. **h** Axial DWI (follow-up). (**a**) Enlarged ventricles. On DWI (**b**) focal hyperintensities are seen at the level of the right thalamus and the basal ganglia (*arrow*) with reduced ADC values, reflecting acute infarcts. Key to the diagnosis is the severe basal meningeal enhancement as seen on the sagittal and coronal reconstruction of 3D T1-weighted images (**c**, **d**). Marked contrast enhancement of the right seventh and eighth cranial nerves is seen (*arrows*; **e**). Note a small ring-enhancing lesion (**f**) with hypointense centre on the T2-weighted image (**g**; *arrowhead*), reflecting a tuberculoma with solid centre. This lesion as well as a larger infarct in the territory of the middle cerebral artery, as shown on the DWI image, became apparent during the course of the disease

Table 2 Imaging hallmarks in tuberculous meningitis

Basal meningeal enhancement	Hydrocephalus	Infarctions
Around brain stem and Sylvian fissure	Communicating > obstructive; consider early shunting	Basal ganglia and thalami predominantly affected

patients. The cognition of characteristically pathological changes in neurotuberculosis enables an improved interpretation of the neuroradiological examination.

2.1 Meningeal Tuberculosis

Tuberculous meningitis is a granulomatous, exudative inflammation that predominantly affects the leptomeninges. Although there is controversy among authors as to whether or not tuberculous meningitis is obligatory secondary to primary extracranial active TB, there is agreement over the fact that tuberculous meningitis is triggered by the outward extension of tiny *M. tuberculosis*-containing foci into the subarachnoid or ventricular space. These microscopic noduli, which are not visible on CT or MR, are commonly referred to as "Rich foci". They are located in subpial or subependymal regions and are mostly derived from haematogenous spread. Once mycobacteria have accessed the subarachnoid space in sufficient numbers, the mainly exudative and fibrinous inflammation develops fast and may even spread towards the spinal meninges. On unenhanced CT this inflammatory process, which leads to a thickening of the basal meninges and consequently obliteration of the basal cisterns, might be visible as hyperdense substrate. The

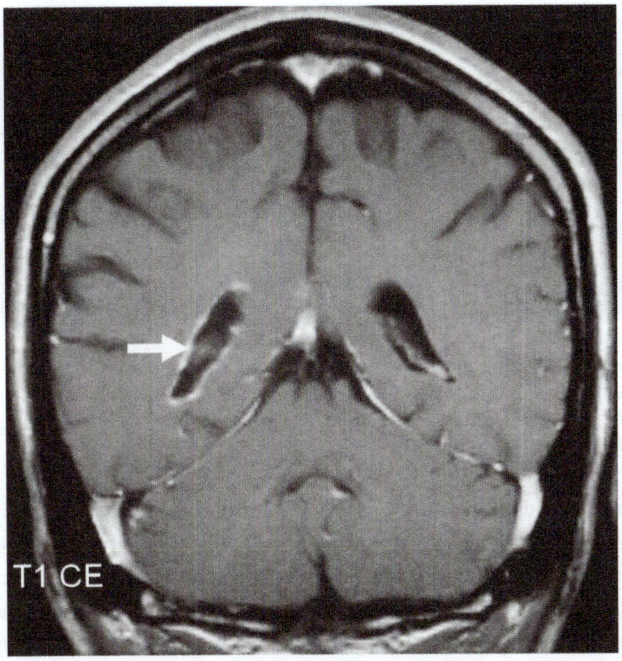

Fig. 2 Tuberculous ependymitis (ventriculitis) in a 53-year-old patient with tuberculous meningitis. Coronal T1-weighted image after contrast administration. Ependymal enhancement (*arrow*). (Courtesy of J. Spreer)

most consistent clue and decisive feature diagnosing tuberculous meningitis is, however, predominantly the basal enhancement of the meninges on contrast-enhanced CT and MRI (Fig. 1). As generally stated, contrast-enhanced MRI displays the abnormal meningeal enhancement with a higher sensitivity as compared to contrast-enhanced CT. The enhancement is visualised not only at the level of the subarachnoid basal cisterns, as often the meninges of the sylvian fissures (Table 2) enhance and the cerebellar sulci might be affected as well. The enhancement is caused by increased permeability of the basal vessels due to inflammation. Some authors have recognised a reduced or even absent meningeal enhancement on contrast-enhanced CT or MRI images in patients with AIDS-related tuberculous meningitis. Ependymitis and inflammatory affection of the choroid plexus might be caused by extension of the infection to the ventricles via the CSF pathways. A transdural invasion from or into calvarian tissue in tuberculous meningitis is very uncommon; in the majority of the cases the dural barrier remains intact. However, tuberculous empyemas following a tuberculous osteitis or tuberculous meningitis have been described. In this context, it has to be mentioned that neurotuberculosis can manifest as well as a focal dural-based en-plaque mass (Fig. 2).

According to most studies on tuberculous meningitis, hydrocephalus is the most frequently observed complication (Fig. 1a). Untreated hydrocephalus is the major reason for a fatal outcome of tuberculous meningitis and there is clear evidence that early ventricular shunting reduces the mortality. Although hydrocephalus is not at all specific, it has therefore to be regarded as an important diagnostic item, in particular when encountered in combination with the previously mentioned clinical symptoms. Hydrocephalus usually presents as the communicating type due to impaired CSF resorption by inflammatory exudates in the basal subarachnoidal cisterns in early phases of the disease, or secondary to obstruction of CSF absorption pathways by fibrous tissues in the latter course of the disease; however, in some cases an obstructive hydrocephalus may be encountered. Possible mechanisms include entrapment of a ventricle due to ependymitis (Fig. 3), narrowing of the aqueduct due to compression by inflammatory fibrous exudates or CSF pathway obstructions by large tuberculomas. Once, having correctly established the diagnosis of tuberculous meningitis, the detection of a probable disturbance of CSF circulation is one of the radiologist's major tasks in follow-up studies; therefore, attention has to be paid in particular to the width of the inferior temporal horns of the lateral ventricles whenever analysing tomograms of patients with tuberculous meningitis. Moreover, a hyperintense periventricular signal on T2-weighted images or a hypodensity in the brain tissue adjacent to the ventricles on CT might indicate a transependymal migration of CSF following increased intraventricular pressure. Ultrasonography can be used to display and monitor the ventricular dilatation in babies. Although rarely used in developed areas, plain radiography may help the less equipped radiologist to show suture diastasis owing to a rise in intracranial pressure in small children.

Cerebral infarctions (Fig. 1b) are a second possible complication of tuberculous meningitis, occuring in approximately one-third to half of the patients, and are mainly responsible for neurological sequelae. The basal meningeal exudates that are typical for meningitis primarily affect the vessel wall of the basal perforating arteries, especially the lenticulostriate arteries, which lead to infarcts of the basal ganglia and the internal capsule. Histologically, the exudate affects first the adventitia but, eventually, a panarteritis occurs with secondary thrombosis and vessel occlusion. Entrapment and vasculitic occlusion of larger arteries, such as the MCA, may occasionally occur and can result in larger, territorial infarction. Even an occlusion of the internal carotid artery, due to the inflammatory processes, has been described.

The cytotoxic oedema of early ischaemic infarction is detected with high sensitivity and specificity on DWI as a focal hyperintensity on trace images (Fig. 1b), with a reduced ADC. Healing of tuberculous meningitis may be recognised by the lack of meningo-vascular enhancement; however, despite adequate treatment, some patients might

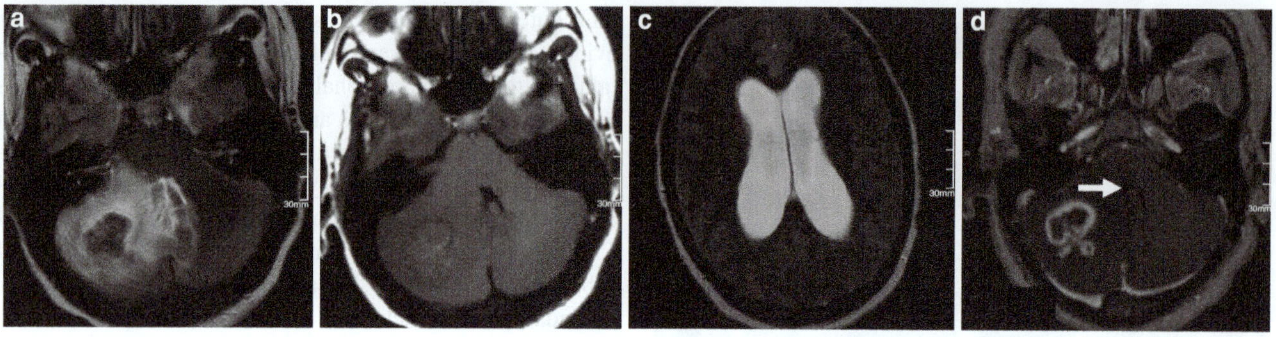

Fig. 3 Cerebellar tuberculous abscess in a 21-year-old woman. Clinically, a papilledema and paresis of the trigeminal and facial nerve was the leading focal symptomatology. **a**, **c** Axial T2-weighted images. **b** Axial T1-weighted image before contrast administration. **d** Axial T1-weighted image after contrast administration. Ring-enhancing lesion in the left cerebellum with a considerable oedema (**a**) and mass effect on the fourth ventricle (*arrow*; **d**). **c** Beginning hydrocephalus. (Courtesy of J. Spreer)

show an initial increase in enhancement, and an enhancement might persist in some cases of tuberculous meningitis.

2.2 Parenchymal Tuberculosis

2.2.1 Tuberculoma

A tuberculoma is a circumscriptive, inflammatory lesion of parenchyma affected by mycobacteria. This focus is surrounded by a wall of epithelioid cells, lymphocyte-like cells and giant cells of the Langerhans type (granulomatous reaction), that may transform into a collagenous capsule. The centre of these lesions most often shows a caseation, or even liquefies which refers to necrotic tissue with only few TB bacilli remaining. A parenchymal oedema surrounds the capsule. The majority of tuberculomas result from haematogenous spread of mycobacteria: conglomerates of microgranuloma in an area of cerebritis join to form a mature noncaseating tuberculoma. However, tuberculomas might as well result from contiguous spread of the infectious process from the CSF via cortical veins or perivascular Virchow-Robin spaces.

In most cases, subsequent central caseous necrosis develops which is at first solid but may liquefy over time. Tuberculomas can affect the central nervous parenchyma in a disseminated fashion affecting both the brain and spine, or might be visualised as solitary lesions. In children, tuberculomas are often found in an infratentorial location. In adults the tuberculoma is most often found in the frontal or parietal lobes, predominantly situated at the corticomedullary junction.

On non-enhanced CT non-caseating tuberculoma are isodense or sometimes slightly hypodense and have a round to oval shape. On MR, these lesions appear hypointense on T1-weighted images and hyperintense on T2-weighted images.

A homogeneous contrast enhancement of the lesion is the hallmark for non-caseating granuloma for both imaging modalities. On the contrary, the caseating granuloma will display a strong ring-like enhancement in the periphery. The ring enhancement of the capsule is thereby usually unbroken and of uniform thickness. The centre of the lesion can be either solid or liquid (Fig. 1). If the centre of the caseating granuloma is solid, it is iso- or hypointense to normal brain tissue on T1-weighted and T2-weighted images, and might enhance heterogeneously. Finally, with the advent of liquefaction, the centre of the caseating granuloma will appear hypodense on unenhanced CT, with MRI displaying a hypointensity on T1-weighted and hyperintensity on T2-weighted images. Occasionally, new tuberculomas may be observed despite appropriate therapy. This might be due to liberation of tuberculoprotein that results in an inflammatory reaction of the focus. However, roughly 4–6 weeks after beginning of tuberculostatic therapy, a clinical and radiological improvement should be monitored when therapy is effective. In case of failure, either drug resistance or misdiagnosis has to be considered. Most lesions leave no radiologically visible traces, but regional atrophy and calcifications might occur following successful medical treatment.

The so-called target sign, defined as a lesion with peripheral enhancement followed by a zone of isodense tissue that contains an enhancing or calcified nidus in its centre, was once considered to be pathognomonic for a tuberculoma; however, this sign has also been observed, for example, in pyogenic abscess and metastatic adenocarcinoma.

In miliary TB numerous round, very small enhancing lesions that are scattered throughout the brain are encountered. Only few patients with this form of CNS TB have a severe clinic, and usually a primary pulmonary focus of TB is present. In infants and young children with pulmonary TB extensive damage to the white matter may occur in the setting of tuberculous encephalopathy. An "allergic" hypersensitivity mechanism is believed to be causative for this disorder that leads to drowsiness and coma and which has a poor prognosis.

2.2.2 Tuberculous Abscess

Tuberculous abscesses occur in approximately 10 % of all patients with neurotuberculosis. This complication may either develop secondarily from a parenchymal tuberculoma or result from a tuberculous spread from the meninges in patients with tuberculous meningitis. Unlike tuberculomas, tuberculous abscesses contain masses of vivid mycobacteria, with the wall lacking the giant cell granulomatous reaction of TB granulomas. The clinical presentation is often more severe than with tuberculomas; however, the imaging findings do not differ markedly from caseating tuberculomas, with a ring-enhancing wall surrounding a hyperintense centre on T2-weighted images. In such cases, indicators might be a tendency for a larger size (over 3 cm in diameter), a thinner wall and the fact that they are often solitary (Fig. 2).

3 Differential Diagnosis

Radiological findings in neurotuberculosis are not specific. TB, with its variable imaging appearance, is known to mimic other pathological entities; therefore, one has to be aware of a wide differential diagnosis.

3.1 Meningeal Tuberculosis

The differential diagnosis of the MR appearance of meningeal tuberculosis includes other infectious diseases, non-infectious inflammatory disease affecting the leptomeninges, such as neurosarcoidosis or manifestations of rheu matoid arthritis and meningeal carcinomatosis. Non-tuberculous bacterial meningitis can be caused by a wide variety of pathogenic agents. *Haemophilus influenzae* in particular poses a challenge, as it may cause both basal enhancement of the meninges as well as infarctions. Neonates, who are hardly affected by tuberculous meningitis, will often suffer meningitis caused by group-B *Streptococcus, Escherichia coli* and *Listeria monocytogenes*. Particularly, in immunocompromised patients, fungal meningitis must also be considered. Coccidioidomycosis has to be considered in AIDS patients from Central- or South America. The disease is likely to show an even stronger basal enhancement than seen in tuberculous meningitis; however, focal granulomas and infarctions are rare in coccidioidomycosis. *Cryptococcus neoformans* may give rise to both basal enhancement as well as arteriitis, leading to infarctions of the basal ganglia. A clear distinction from tuberculous meningitis may thus not be possible; however, CSF studies usually allow an isolation of the pathogenic agent. Aspergillosis and mucormycotic infections usually have their origin in the nasal cavity or paranasal sinuses. They can spread towards brain parenchyma along vessel walls and might cause infarctions which, however, are typically found in a cortical or subcortical location. Viral meningitis often improves quickly and, overall, the illness is usually much less severe than in tuberculous meningitis; however, for example, the herpes zoster virus meningitis, which may have an aggressive course if encephalitis is present, has to be differentiated. The parenchymal affection, mainly of the temporal brain structures, is the key for the imaging diagnosis. Spirochaetal diseases, namely Lues and Lyme, may present with both basal meningitis and granuloma. Contrary to neurotuberculosis, syphilitic granulomas appear in a more peripheral distribution and are often even attached to the meninges. Granulomas in Lyme disease will lack ring enhancement on contrast-enhanced images and can thus be distinguished. The clinical awareness of erythema migrans and a detailed history will help in finding the right diagnosis. Neurosarcoidosis occurs in approximately 5 % of cases of pulmonary sarcoidosis. It has usually a more prolonged and less severe clinical course as compared with tuberculous meningitis; however, neurosarcoidosis produces a similar basal enhancement of the meninges as seen in tuberculous meningitis. In leptomeningeal carcinomatosis a basal meningeal enhancement is usually patchy and irregular, in contrast to the more homogeneous appearance in tuberculous meningitis.

3.2 Parenchymal Tuberculosis

The characteristic shortening on T2-weighted images seen in caseating tuberculomas with a solid centre is very rarely found in other space-occupying lesions and may be helpful to establish the correct diagnosis; however, non-caseating and caseating tuberculomas with a liquid centre can especially pose diagnostic problems. The differential diagnosis includes primary and secondary neoplasms of the brain and inflammatory or granulomatous processes of a different origin.

If a ring-enhancing lesion is present, the main differential diagnoses are necrotic tumours or pyogenic or fungal cerebral abscess. The distinction between any kind of abscess and a tumour is frequently impossible on conventional contrast-enhanced CT or MR images. An incomplete wall that shows a variable and irregular thickness is indicative of a tumour, in particular if a surrounding oedema has an emphatic mass effect; however, this allows no highly reliable distinction. Advanced MR imaging techniques, such as DWI, PerfMRI, MTR and MRS, improve the diagnostic accuracy of conventional CT and MR imaging. It is beyond the scope of this chapter to discuss all aspects of these techniques and to discuss the possible findings for all ring-enhancing mass lesions, but a few key findings are given. On DWI, a restricted diffusion in the centre (necrotic cavity) of the lesion is highly indicative of an abscess, whereas apart from rare exceptions, this is not the case in the necrotic cavity of tumours; however, a low ADC value does not enable one to differentiate between a tubercular and a fungal or pyogenic abscess. On PerfMRI, solid portions of ring-enhancing tumours usually show a markedly elevated rrCBV in contrast to the abscess wall. Yet, very little data on findings from PerfMRI studies, specifically in tuberculous abscesses or tuberculomas, are currently available. Determination of MTR, although not widely used, has to be considered another promising MR technique. In general, abscesses have markedly increased MTR compared with neoplastic ring-enhancing lesions in the centre of the lesion. The high viscosity of the protein-rich cystic fluid in abscesses is probably responsible for that difference.

Particularly in AIDS patients, toxoplasmosis and lymphoma have to be differentiated. The distribution in the corticomedullary junction and the basal ganglia is similar in both tuberculoma and toxoplasmosis, and in both diseases mostly multiple lesions are present. On conventional images a point of discrimination may be a thicker and more irregularly shaped wall of toxoplasmotic lesions. In lymphoma, often a reduced ADC is observed.

Both metastases and tuberculomas often appear as numerous lesions with different sizes, are localised near the corticomedullary junction, and reveal homogenous contrast enhancement. Both entities pose an important differential diagnosis particularly in elderly patients; however, tuberculoma rarely show signs of haemorrhage. For the distinction, advanced imaging techniques are helpful: Tuberculomas usually reveal reduced ADC with hyperintense signal on DWI, whereas the majority of solid metastases are isointense or hypointense on DWI. In practice, however, the history of primary malignancy will primarily help to determine the diagnosis. For sarcoid parenchymal granulomas, only small surrounding oedema has been described with a usual solid enhancement. Destructive lesions of the calvarium might occur in neurosarcoidosis that is unusual in neurotuberculosis due to the intact dural barrier. Moreover, several infectious diseases have to be kept in mind when encountering tuberculoma-suspected lesions. For example, cysticercosis and tuberculosis have similar geographic distributions and might share the same clinical type of onset. In particular, at the stage of circumferential inflammatory reaction of neurocysticercosis, a differentiation from tuberculomas is difficult. Cysticerci may be more numerous than tuberculomas, yet both a tuberculoma and a cysticercal cyst can be present as singular lesions. Although there is no basal meningeal enhancement in neurocysticercosis, a marked cyst formation can occur in the basal CSF cisterns and the sylvian region.

Solitary tuberculomas or abscesses may be mistaken for tumefactive MS when contrast enhancement is present and the MS plaques are surrounded by vasogenic oedema. Usually the clinical presentation will enable discrimination, as patients with MS are likely to show a history of previous neurological deficits.

Finally, it has to be acknowledged that the consideration of the clinical history, laboratory findings and follow-up investigations remains indispensable for an optimised treatment, as the imaging signs and patterns of tuberculomas are nonspecific.

References

Al-Okaili RN, Krejza J, Woo JH et al (2007) Intraaxial brain masses: MR imaging-based diagnostic strategy: initial experience. Radiology 243(2):539–550

Bernaerts A, Vanhoenacker FM, Parizel PM et al (2003) Tuberculosis of the central nervous system: overview of neuroradiological findings. Eur Radiol 13(8):1876–1890

Dastur DK, Manghani DK, Udani PM (1995) Pathology and pathogenetic mechanisms in neurotuberculosis. Radiol Clin North Am 33(4):733–752

Luthra G, Parihar A, Nath K et al (2007) Comparative evaluation of fungal, tubercular, and pyogenic brain abscesses with conventional and diffusion MR imaging and proton MR spectroscopy. Am J Neuroradiol 28(7):1332–1338

Gupta RK, Kumar S (2011) Central nervous system tuberculosis. Neuroimaging Clin N Am 21(4):795–814

Medical Research Council (1948) Streptomycin treatment of tuberculous meningitis. Lancet 1:582–596

Prasad K, Singh MB (2008) Corticosteroids for managing tuberculous meningitis. Cochrane Database Syst Rev 23(1):CD002244

Yaramis A, Gurkan F, Elevli M et al (1998) Central nervous system tuberculosis in children: a review of 214 cases. Pediatrics 102(5):E49

Other Bacterial Infections

Michael Lettau

Contents

M. Lettau (✉)
Division of Neuroradiology, Department of Neurosurgery,
University of Freiburg Medical Center, Breisacher Strasse 64,
79106 Freiburg, Germany
e-mail: michael_lettau@gmx.de

Abstract

This chapter focuses on a number of rare bacterial infections that affect the central nervous system. The most common manifestations as well as the characteristic features of these infectious processes, as displayed on imaging studies, are stressed.

1 Summary

This chapter focuses on a number of rare bacterial infections that affect the central nervous system. The most common manifestations as well as the characteristic features of these infectious processes, as displayed on imaging studies, are stressed.

2 Introduction

Infections of the CNS pose an ever-growing worldwide public health problem. Widespread immigration means that infectious diseases once relatively confined to certain geographic areas are now everywhere. Prompt detection and accurate diagnosis of CNS infection is critical because most of these disorders are readily treatable. In brain abscesses, a broad spectrum of bacteria are involved. The incidence of brain abscesses has decreased since the 1970s because of better care of the predisposing factors, but bacterial epidemiology has been dramatically modified. Brain abscess puncture often reveals several microbial strains and recent reports stress the increasing frequency of anaerobes (Le Moal et al. 2003). This chapter focuses on a number of bacterial infections (Table 1) that affect the CNS. The characteristic features of these infectious processes on imaging studies are stressed.

S. Hähnel (ed.), *Inflammatory Diseases of the Brain*, Medical Radiology. Diagnostic Imaging,
DOI: 10.1007/174_2012_624, © Springer-Verlag Berlin Heidelberg 2012
Published Online: 27 May 2012

Table 1 Other bacterial infections that affect the CNS

Bacterium	Most common CNS manifestations	Other most common manifestations
Mycoplasma pneumoniae	Encephalitis	Respiratory diseases
Listeria monocytogenes	Meningitis	Bacteremia
Borrelia burgdorferi	Meningitis, meningoencephalitis, cranial neuritis, meningoradiculitis	Erythema migrans, arthritis, cardiac myositis
Leptospira species	Meningitis, meningoencephalitis	Fever, thrombocytopenia, coagulopathy
Brucella species	Meningitis, meningoencephalitis, myelitis, polyradiculoneuritis, cranial nerve palsies	Multisystemic disease with non-specific manifestations
Legionella pneumophila	Encephalopathy	Severe pneumonia
Tropheryma whipplei	Supranuclear ophthalmoplegia, confusion and dementia, psychiatric signs, myoclonic signs	Abdominal pain, malabsorption with diarrhea and weight loss, migratory arthralgias
Nocardia species	Cerebral abscess(es)	Respiratory diseases
Salmonella typhii	Encephalopathy, meningitis (mainly affecting children)	Enteric disease
Neisseria meningitidis	Meningitis	Bacteremia, fulminant meningococcal sepsis
Francisella tularensis	Meningitis	Ulceroglandular, oculoglandular, oropharyngeal, pneumonic, or typhoidal syndromes
Actinomyces species	Cerebral abscess(es)	Cervicofacial, thoracic, or abdominal infections
Fusobacterium species	Meningitis	Gingivitis, peridontal disease, bacteremia

3 *Mycoplasma Pneumoniae*

Mycoplasma pneumoniae is endemic in most areas of the world. The highest incidence is seen in school-aged children and adolescents. Respiratory diseases ranging from mild upper respiratory tract illness to severe pneumonia are most common. Infections of the middle ear, muscles, kidneys, and heart can occur.

The CNS complications are the most frequent extrapulmonary complications, which occur in about 1 per 1,000 patients with *M. pneumoniae* respiratory infections but occur in as many as 7 % of patients who are hospitalized for such infections. Central nervous system complications were seen between 3 days and 4 weeks after the onset of respiratory symptoms. Encephalitis is most frequent, but meningoencephalitis, meningitis, neuropathies with cranial nerve palsies, myelitis, and polyradiculitis are reported as well. Strokes are a rare complication and are reported in children and adults, mainly affecting the middle cerebral artery. Posterior cerebral artery occlusion and internal carotid artery occlusion have been reported in children. Vasculitis as etiology is discussed. Another rare complication is basal ganglia syndromes. Bilateral striatal necrosis has been reported in several patients aged from 5 to 17 years (van Buiren and Uhl 2003). Bilateral thalamic necrosis has been seen in children. Severe hemorrhagic leukoencephalitis (Hurst) has been reported in adults. Acute disseminated encephalomyelitis (ADEM) and Guillain–Barré syndrome have been reported in children and adults as rare complications.

4 Listeriosis

Listeria monocytogenes is a ubiquitous bacterium. About 5–10 % of all people in the United States carry the organism in their stool. Ingestion of *L. monocytogenes*-contaminated food is considered to be the source of nearly all listerial human infections. The annual incidence is about five cases per million population in the United States, excluding HIV infected patients and pregnant women, whereas among persons over 70 years of age that incidence rises to 21 cases per million per year. Males are more commonly infected than women with male-to-female ratio of 1.4 to 1. A bacteremia can occur in immunocompetent patients (Gerner-Smidt et al. 2005).

In the United States, between 55 and 75 % of all age groups with listeriosis present with meningitis, 25 % reveal bacteremia, 7.5 % endocarditis, and 6.5 % nonmeningitic cerebritis, meningoencephalitis, and rhombencephalitis. Brain abscess is

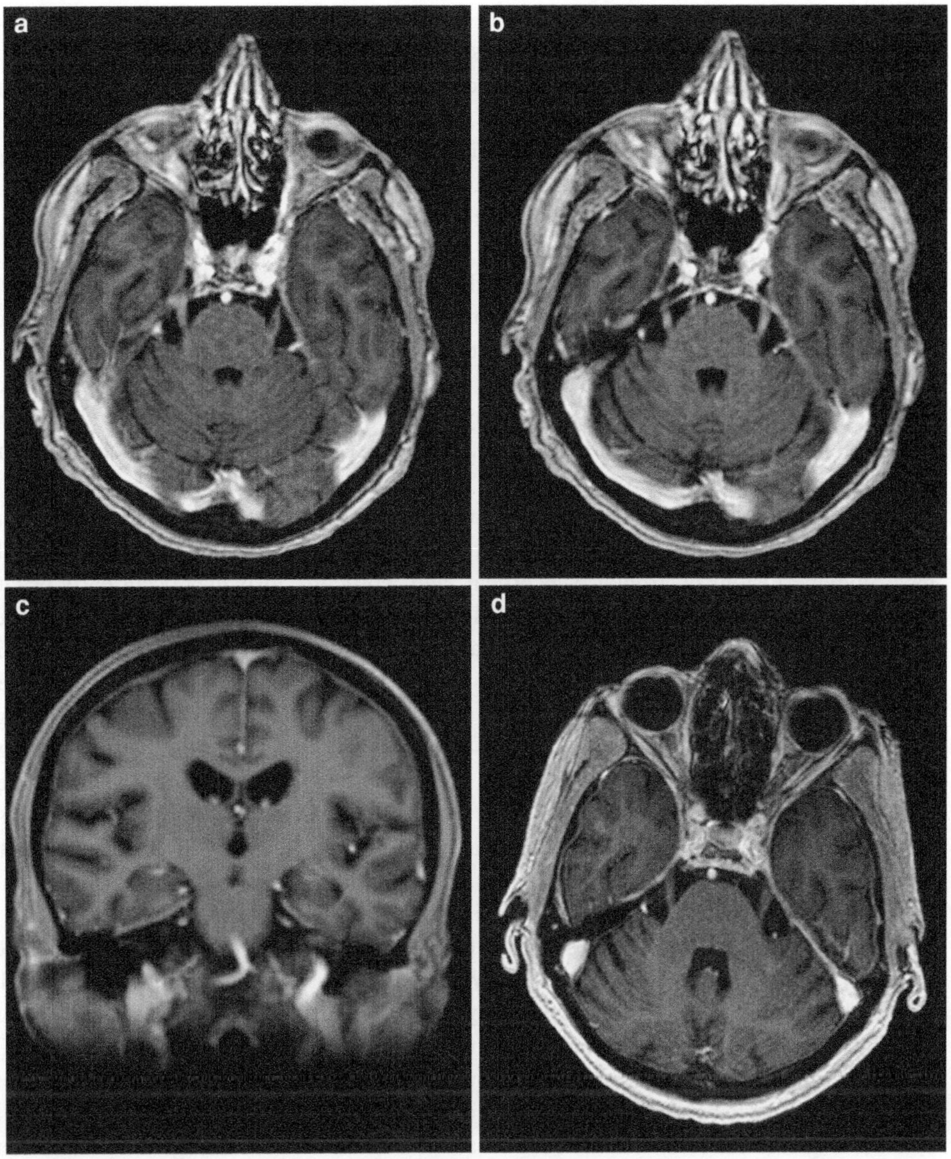

Fig. 1 Neuroborreliosis. Routine follow-up MRI scans of a 67-year-old immunocompromised woman. **a, b, d** Axial T1-weighted images after contrast administration. **c** Coronal T1-weighted image after contrast administration. Enhancement of both trigeminal nerves due to *Borrelia burgdorferi* infection (**a–c**). An MRI scan obtained 1 month later (**d**) after the patient had received effective antibiotic therapy demonstrates a reduction of contrast enhancement.

seen in 1 % of infections and is most often found in patients with organ transplants and hematological malignancies. Cerebellar and spinal cord abscesses are rare manifestations. Endophthalmitis, osteomyelitis, peritonitis, pleuritis, pneumonia, endometritis, and arterial infections constitute the remaining presentations. (*L. monocytogenes* infections in newborns and prematures are discussed elsewhere).

5 Borreliosis

Lyme disease, or borreliosis, is a zoonosis with an incubation period of 3–32 days, transmitted by *Borrelia burgdorferi*, a member of the family of spirochetes. Lyme disease involves skin, heart, joints, and, in 15 % of affected individuals, the CNS. Early manifestations of the disease include severe headache, neck pain, fever, chills, musculoskeletal pains, malaise, and fatigue.

Sometimes, the CNS is already involved at the onset of the clinical manifestations of borreliosis; however, most often the CNS is involved only months after onset, and the disorder appears as aseptic meningitis or fluctuating meningoencephalitis, and neuropathy of cranial nerves (Fig. 1) (Mygland et al. 2010). The seventh cranial nerve is most often involved. Involvement of peripheral nerves (radiculitis) is also possible. Cases with seizures, choreiform movements, cerebellar ataxia, dementia, and myelitic syndrome are rarely described. As another rare complication, cerebral vasculitis can be induced by *B. burgdorferi*, possibly leading to aneurysms, subarachnoid hemorrhage, intraparenchymal brain hemorrhage, or ischemic stroke. Vessel irregularities occur mainly in the vertebrobasilar territory and have mainly been observed in the third stage (chronic meningoencephalitis) of borreliosis. Some reports on large cerebral vessel disease in borreliosis have been published. Multifocal encephalitis has been reported. Focal encephalitis may be induced by direct invasion of the brain by spirochetes or occur secondary to vasculitis. Common imaging findings are multiple hyperintense lesions in the periventricular area on T2-weighted MR images, most probably corresponding to foci of demyelination. Lyme encephalopathy is a neuropsychiatric disorder beginning months to years after the onset of infection. Objective evidence of memory impairment is usually present on formal neuropsychological testing. Other symptoms may include mild depression, irritability, fatigue, and excessive daytime sleepiness. In these patients, brain MRI is usually normal, although in some patients, white matter lesions are seen. In SPECT studies, Lyme encephalopathy patients have hypoperfusion of frontal subcortical and cortical structures. Rare ophthalmic manifestations of borreliosis include external ocular and intraocular inflammations, retinal vasculitis, and optic neuropathy.

6 Leptospirosis

Leptospirosis is a worldwide zoonosis that occurs most commonly in tropical and subtropical areas. The lack of a pathognomonic syndrome hinders diagnosis. The clinical spectrum can range from an asymptomatic, subclinical infection to a fatal hepatorenal syndrome (Weil's disease). Fever, thrombocytopenia, and coagulopathy are frequent. Hepatorenal syndrome as well as pulmonary renal syndrome are seen in leptospirosis. Diffuse bilateral pulmonary hemorrhage was found to be a main cause of death in leptospirosis.

Neurological manifestations are seen in about 10–15 % of cases. It is not common for leptospirosis to present as a primary neurological disease. All of the neurological complications mostly develop in the late period of leptospirosis. Severe leptospirosis is frequently associated with neurological symptoms, such as headache, vomiting, focal neurological deficits, diminished level of vigilance, and seizures. Mathew et al. (2006) reported about 31 patients with neuroleptospirosis. Twenty-five patients (81 %) had altered sensorium, with four (12.9 %) being deeply comatose. Eleven (35.5 %) had acute symptomatic seizures at the time of presentation. A septic meningitis is the most common form of neurological complication. In one study, meningitis was diagnosed in 29 % and meningoencepalitis in 5 % of cases. Encephalitis, cerebellitis, myelitis, flaccid paraplegias including Guillain–Barré syndrome-like presentation, mononeuritis, neuralgia, facial palsy, and polymyositis are other reported complications of leptospirosis. Cerebral vasculitis and patients with multiple occlusive vascular disorders have been reported. Infarcts appeared in areas supplied by the middle cerebral artery. Intracerebral hemorrhage has been reported only sporadically.

7 Brucellosis

Brucellosis is an important systemic zoonotic infection with a worldwide distribution which is endemic in many parts of the world. It has variable and nonspecific clinical signs and symptoms, mimics many other diseases, can involve any organ or system of the body, and may have an acute, subacute, or chronic clinical course. The spectrum of systemic involvement includes hematological, gastrointestinal, cardiorespiratory, and musculoskeletal systems.

Central and peripheral nervous systems are involved in 3–13 % of patients. Neurological manifestations in Brucellosis may occur early or late in the disease. Late manifestations, which are more frequent, may last months or years after having occurred in the septicemic period, which many times is subclinical. Clinical presentations are diverse and may imitate many other neurological diseases. Acute, subacute, or chronic meningitis, meningoencephalitis, myelitis, polyradiculoneuritis, and cranial nerve palsies are the most frequent features of neurobrucellosis (Al-Sous et al. 2004, Karaoglan et al 2008). Brucella exhibits a great affinity for the meninges and most patients with neurobrucellosis present meningeal involvement at same stage. It is well-known that brucellosis can cause vasculitis. This disease shows no predilection of size or location of vascular structure and arterial and/or venous structures may be affected. Although, very rare, aortitis has been reported. Cerebrovascular involvement as vasculitis or mycotic aneurysm is a rare complications. Cerebral venous thrombosis, cerebral abscess, pituitary gland abscess, granulomatous encephalitis mimicking cerebral tumor, involvement of the white matter, and recurrent transverse myelitis have also been described. In case reports, brucella endocarditis and extensive aortic vegetations have provided a clear origin for septic emboli.

8 Legionellosis

Infection with *Legionella pneumophila* ranks among the three most common causes of severe pneumonia in the community setting and is isolated in 1–40 % of hospital-acquired pneumonia cases. Patients with an impaired immune system have a high risk of acquiring Legionnaires' disease, or legionellosis. There are no clinical features unique to legionellosis.

In patients with legionellosis, 40–50 % develop neurological signs and symptoms. The most common finding is encephalopathy, manifesting as confusion, disorientation, delirium, stupor, and coma. Brain abscess, myelitis, cerebellar or brain-stem

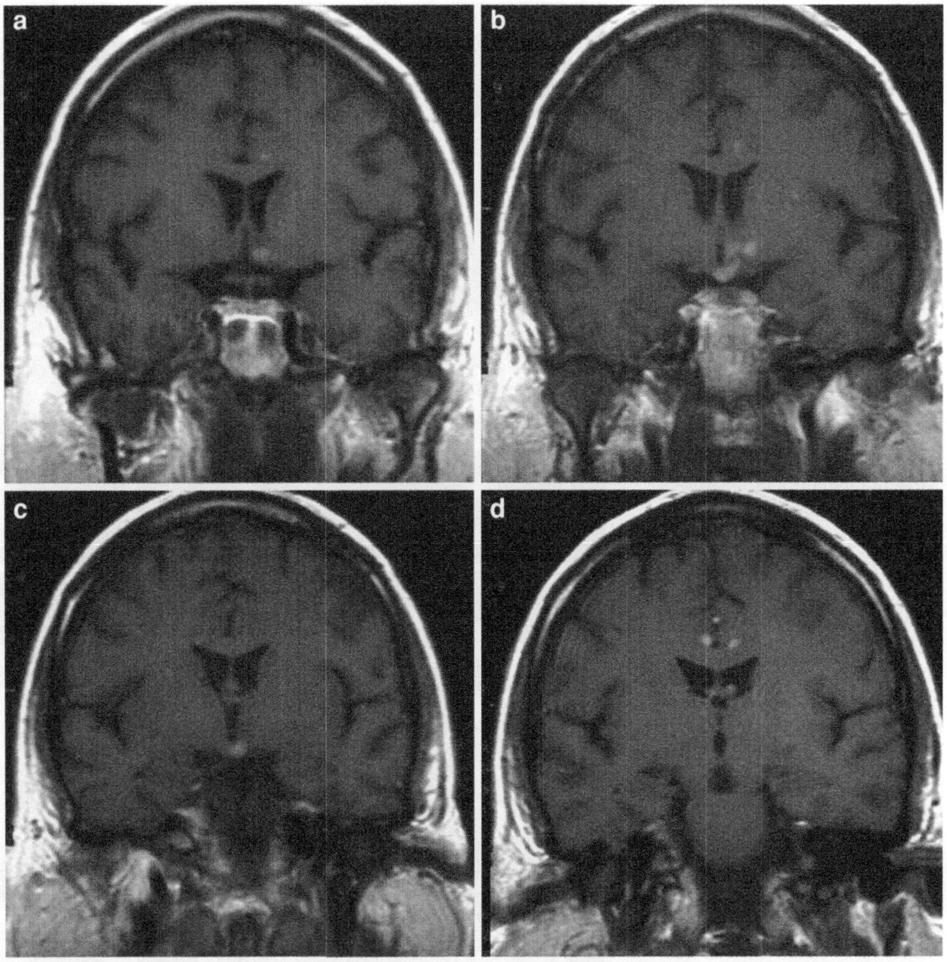

Fig. 2 Whipple's disease. **a–d** Coronal T1-weighted images after contrast administration. Multiple enhancing lesions in the hypothalamus, and the parasagittal frontal cortex (cingulate gyrus) above the corpus callosum

dysfunction, cranial nerve involvement, peripheral neuropathy, and ADEM have also occasionally been reported; however, evidence of vasculitis has not yet been detected. Neuroimages and neuropathological studies are typically normal. In a neuropathological evaluation of 40 confirmed cases of legionellosis (16 with neurological symptoms), Pendlebury et al. (1983) could not demonstrate lesions attributable to disseminated legionellosis in any patient. The pathogenesis of neurological dysfunction in legionellosis remains unclear.

9 Whipple's Disease

Whipple's disease is a multisystemic granulomatous infectious disease caused by *Tropheryma whipplei* which is ubiquitously present in the environment. The most common symptoms of Whipple's disease are abdominal pain, malabsorption with diarrhea and weight loss, and migratory arthralgias. Extraintestinal manifestations may also involve the ocular, pulmonary, cardiovascular, and hematological systems, and are often accompanied by general symptoms such as fever and lymphadenopathy.

Symptomatic CNS involvement occurs in 6–43 % of patients with Whipple's disease. The CNS involvement is observed mainly during relapse of the disease and has been reported particularly in patients who previously received antibiotic treatments that could not cross the blood–brain barrier. In as many as 5 % of cases, cerebral Whipple's disease may also occur without evidence of gastrointestinal infection. In many cerebral Whipple's disease cases, diagnosis is made after death. Gerard et al. (2002) reported neurological signs of cerebral Whipple's disease in 122 cases from the literature. All reviewed observations showed diffuse neurological signs. On average, four to five signs were observed. The following predominant clinical features, in decreasing order of frequency, were reported: supranuclear ophthalmoplegia; confusion, and dementia; psychiatric signs; myoclonic signs; seizures; hypothalamic involvement; cerebellar, and myorhythmic forms; cranial nerve involvement; peripheral neuropathies; and spinal cord involvement. Cerebral Whipple's disease should be included in the differential diagnosis of patients presenting with progressive dementia and cognitive decline. Hypothalamic manifestations, such as severe insomnia, hypersomnia,

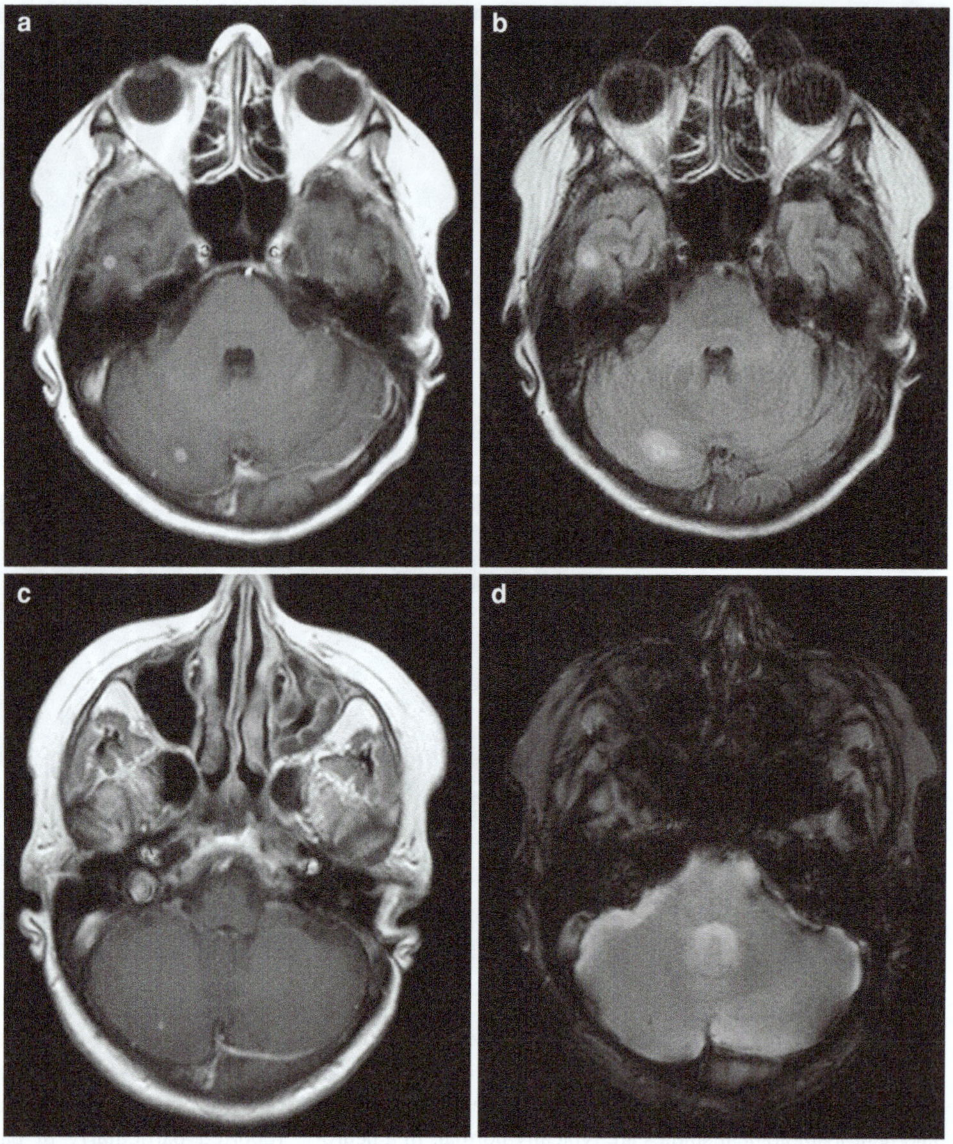

Fig. 3 Brain abscesses due to *Nocardia* infection. A 60-year-old woman with amyloidosis who was immunocompromised after heart transplantation. **a**, **c** Axial T1-weighted images after contrast administration. **b** Axial FLAIR image. **d** Axial T2*-weighted image. FLAIR image (**b**) reveals a hyperintense rim at the periphery of two small lesions with surrounding hyperintense edema in the right temporal lobe and the right cerebellar hemisphere. T1-weighted image after contrast administration demonstrates peripheral ring enhancement in both lesions (**a**). After the patient had received effective antibiotic therapy, the lesion in the right cerebellar hemisphere had decreased in size 1 month later (**c**) as compared with the initial examination (**a**). T2*-weighted image (**d**) after antibiotic therapy reveals a small hypointensity in the lesion in the right cerebellar hemisphere, suggestive of calcification or blood products

hyperphagia, and changes in libido, have been reported. Cerebral Whipple's disease resembling a stroke syndrome is rare. Preferential sites of the well-known neuropathological lesions, which consist of granulomatous polioencephalitis or panencephalitis, are the basal parts of the telencephalon, the hypothalamic nuclei, thalamus, the periaqueductal gray, and the tegmentum pontis. Radiologically, cerebral Whipple's disease has no characteristic appearance. On T2-weighted images, hyperintense lesions have been detected in several locations affecting, in decreasing order of frequency, the frontal cerebral cortex, the basal ganglia, the periventricular white matter, the hypothalamus, the temporal cortex, and the parietal cortex. Contrast-enhanced T1-weighted images (Fig. 2) may demonstrate ring or strongly enhanced high-signal, large-mass lesions. Vasculitis has been described in retinal Whipple's disease but has not been reported elsewhere in the CNS.

10 Nocardiosis

Nocardia species are ubiquitous in the environment. Nocardiosis is considered an opportunistic infection, primarily associated with defects in cell-mediated immunity. *Nocardia* infections are being reported with increasing frequency. Nocardiosis is primarily an infection of the respiratory tract. Subsequent hematogenous dissemination may lead to infection of almost any organ.

Nocardia species have a well-recognized predilection for invasion of the CNS, even when the primary site of infection is no longer evident. *Nocardia* accounts for 2 % of all brain abscesses and are 2.5 times more common in men. An analysis of 1,050 nocardial infections (Beaman and Beaman 1994) found that 23 % of infections involved the CNS, and 44 % of patients with systemic nocardiosis had CNS infections. In addition, 38 % of the infections described involved the CNS without evidence of infection elsewhere in the body. Of these CNS infections, 42 % occurred in previously healthy individuals with no identifiable predisposing factor. Infections of the brain by *Nocardia* species are often insidious in onset and difficult to diagnose. The lesions in the brain may be recognized as either granulomata or, more frequently, abscesses in any location within the brain (Fig. 3). Multiple lesions are not uncommon, being reported in 38 % of cases of cerebral nocardiosis. Less common manifestations, such as diffuse cerebral inflammation, meningitis, and spinal cord lesions, have also been reported. There have been numerous reports of CNS nocardiosis mimicking conditions, such as primary or secondary neoplasms, vasculitis, and stroke.

11 Typhoid Fever

Typhoid fever is caused by *Salmonella typhii* associated with enteric disease, with worldwide distribution. Neurological complications are not common, but any clinicopathological syndrome may appear. During epidemics approximately 5–35 % of all patients have symptoms related to CNS involvement. Neurological sequelae are rare. Encephalopathy, coma, meningitis, brain abscess, transient Parkinsonism, motor neuron disorder, seizure, cerebellitis, peripheral neuropathy, and Guillain–Barré syndrome have been reported to accompany typhoid fever. The pathogenesis of *Salmonella* encephalopathy is not totally understood. *Salmonella meningitis* mainly affects infants and children and rarely causes purulent meningitis. Mortality is highest in patients showing pronounced disruption of consciousness, with a rate of about 20–30 %.

12 Meningococcal Disease

Neisseria meningitidis is a strictly human bacterium. The human nasopharynx is the only known natural reservoir and transmission occurs directly. A history of recent upper respiratory tract infection is common. In individuals lacking humoral immunity to meningococci, proliferation of the organisms in the circulation leads to septicemia. Fulminant meningococcal sepsis, the most devastating form of sepsis with a mortality rate varying from 20 to 30 %, is characterized by circulatory collapse, multiple organ failure, and extensive coagulopathy.

A bacteremic phase is an essential preliminary stage for meningococci to gain access to the subarachnoid compartment and initiate meningitis. *N. meningitidis* is the most common pathogen associated with acute bacterial meningitis in young adult populations. Serogroup B is most common with mortality rate of 9 %. Alternatively, meningococcal meningitis can also develop in the absence of peripheral signs of sepsis. When treated, this form of meningitis has a relatively low rate of mortality and neurological sequelae. Complications, such as cranial nerve palsies, severe cerebral edema, hydrocephalus, or venous sinus thrombosis, may be associated with meningococcal meningitis. There are very few clinical reports of cerebral infarction, spinal cord injuries, transverse myelitis, infarction of the spinal cord, and arachnoiditis associated with meningococcal meningitis. Meningococcal meningitis at an extremely young age is associated with a greater risk of developing neurological complications.

13 Tularemia

Tularemia is a zoonotic disease caused by *Francisella tularensis*. This disease is commonly seen in five clinical syndromes: ulceroglandular; oculoglandular; oropharyngeal; pneumonic; and typhoidal.

Tularemic meningitis is a rare complication with only about 15 cases reported in the literature to date. In one case report tularemia meningitis was presented that was complicated by the formation of multiple cerebral microabscesses.

14 Actinomycosis

Actinomycosis, derived endogenously and not spread person to person, is a chronic suppurative infection seen mainly in the cervicofacial, thoracic, or abdominal regions which is characterized by abscess formation, tissue fibrosis, and draining sinuses. Disseminated infection has been reported. Actinomycotic infections usually occur both in immunocompetent persons and in persons with impaired host defenses.

Actinomycosis of the CNS is uncommon, affecting between 1 and 35 % of cases with actinomycotic infection. Although rare, brain abscesses are the commonest type of CNS actinomycotic lesions. They are generally singular, encapsulated, with a marked predilection for the temporal, frontal, or parietal regions, but multiple sites have been reported in 5.7 % of cases. Smego (1987) reviewed the literature on central nervous system (CNS) actinomycosis, and described the features of 70 cases. The most common CNS manifestation was cerebral abscess (67 %), followed by meningitis or meningoencephalitis (13 %), actinomycoma (7 %), subdural empyema (6 %), and epidural abscess (6 %). In the spinal canal, most of the reported cases presented with epidural abscesses that extended from the paravertebral infectious lesions. Spinal intrathecal actinomycosis is extremely rare. A diffuse form of brain actinomycosis has been reported. Extremely rare is the primary cerebral location of the disease.

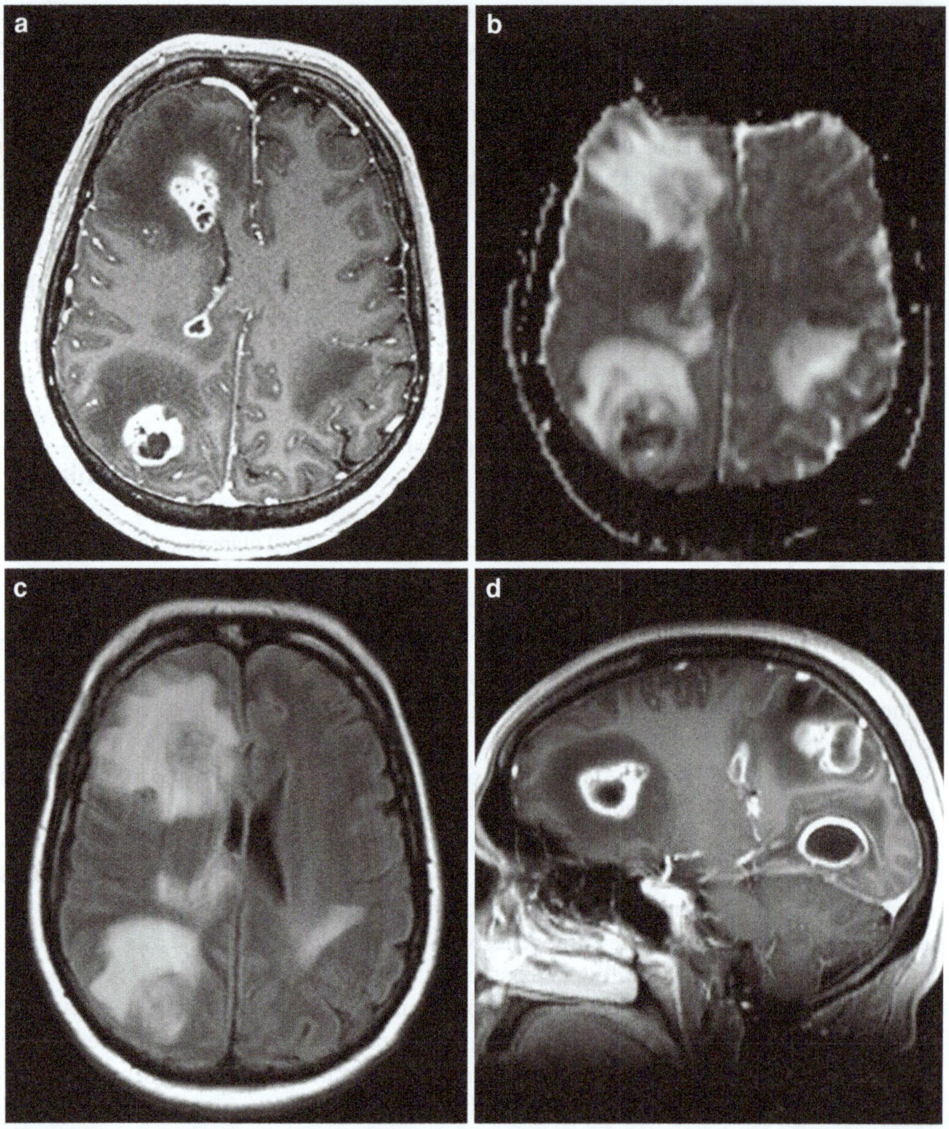

Fig. 4 Multiple brain abscesses caused by *Fusobacterium nucleatum* in a 51-year-old immunocompromised woman with seizures. **a** Axial T1-weighted MR image after contrast administration. **b** Axial ADC map. **c** Axial FLAIR image. **d** Sagittal T1-weighted image after contrast administration. T1-weighted MR images after contrast administration (**a, d**) demonstrate strong peripheral ring enhancement in multiple lesions. FLAIR image (**c**) reveals surrounding hyperintense edema predominantly in the right hemisphere. The ADC map (**b**) demonstrates restricted diffusion centrally in the lesion in the right parietal lobe, suspicious for pus

15 Fusobacterial Infection

Of the 15 *Fusobacterium* species recognized, *Fusobacterium nucleatum* and *Fusobacterium necrophorum* are the most frequently isolated species from clinical specimens. These species are most commonly found in the mouth but rarely give rise to severe disease. *Fusobacterium* species can form aggregates with other bacteria in peridontal diseases. Devitalized tissue may provide a suitable environment for the growth of these organisms. *Fusobacterium nucleatum* has been reported to be associated with gingivitis, peridontal disease, abscesses, and venous thrombosis in various anatomical locations associated with septicemia.

Le Moal et al. (2003) reported 46 patients with brain abscess (Fig. 4) and found *Fusobacterium nucleatum* as the predominant isolate in 14 patients. The production of proteolytic enzymes by *Fusobacterium* organisms may allow for invasion of regional veins. Unusual cases of fusobacterial infections caused by *Fusobacterium nucleatum* as well as *Fusobacterium necrophorum* with septicemia and meningitis complicated by cavernous sinus thrombosis, carotid artery stenosis, and ischemic stroke have been reported. Septic thrombophlebitis of the orbit and cavernous sinus was seen in a patient with severe peridontal disease caused by *Fusobacterium nucleatum*.

References

Al-Sous MW, Bohlega S, Al-Kawi MZ, Alwatban J, McLean DR (2004) *Neurobrucellosis*: clinical and neuroimaging correlation. AJNR Am J Neuroradiol 25:395–401

Beaman BL, Beaman L (1994) *Nocardia* species: host—parasite relationships. Clin Microbiol Rev 7:213–264

Gerard A, Sarrot-Reynauld F, Liozon E, Cathebras P, Besson G, Robin C, Vighetto A, Mosnier J-F, Durieu I, Durand DV, Rousset H (2002) Neurologic presentation of Whipple disease. Report of 12 cases and review of the literature. Medicine 81:443–457

Gerner-Smidt P, Ethelberg S, Schiellerup P, Christensen JJ, Engberg J, Fussing V, Jensen A, Jensen C, Petersen AM, Bruun BG (2005) Invasive *listeriosis* in Denmark 1994–2003: a review of 299 cases with special emphasis on risk factors for mortality. Clin Microbiol Infect 11:618–624

Karaoglan I, Namiduru M, Akcali A, Cansel N (2008) Different manifestations of nervous system involvement by *neurobrucellosis*. Neurosciences (Riyadh) 13:283–287

Le Moal G, Landron C, Grollier G, Bataille B, Roblot F, Nassans P, Becq-Giraudon B (2003) Characteristics of brain abscesses with isolation of anaerobic bacteria. Scand J Infect Dis 35:318–321

Mathew T, Satishchandra P, Mahadevan A, Nagarathna S, Yasha TC, Chandramukhi A, Subbakrishna DK, Shankar SK (2006) Neuroleptospirosis-revisited: experience from a tertiary care neurological centre from South India. Indian J Med Res 124:155–162

Mygland A, Ljøstad U, Fingerle V, Rupprecht T, Schmutzhard E, Steiner I (2010) EFNS guidelines on the diagnosis and management of European lyme *neuroborreliosis*. Eur J Neurol 17(8–16):e1–e4

Pendlebury WW, Perl DP, Winn WC Jr, McQuillen JB (1983) Neuropathologic evaluation of 40 confirmed cases of *Legionella* pneumonia. Neurology 33:1340–1344

Smego RA Jr (1987) Actinomycosis of the central nervous system. Rev Infect Dis 9:855–865

Van Buiren M, Uhl M (2003) Images in clinical medicine. Bilateral striatal necrosis associated with *Mycoplasma pneumoniae* infection. N Engl J Med 348:720

Viral Encephalitis

Stefan Hähnel

Contents

S. Hähnel (✉)
Division of Neuroradiology, University of Heidelberg Medical Center, Im Neuenheimer Feld 400, 69120 Heidelberg, Germany
e-mail: Stefan.Haehnel@med.uni-heidelberg.de

Abstract

With the exception of herpes simplex virus encephalitis type 1 involving preferentially limbic structures of the brain the imaging features of viral encephalitis are mostly unspecific. Typical features of viral encephalitis are vasogenic brain oedema and swelling, variable contrast enhancement of the involved structures and possibly haemorrhage. The major task of the neuroradiologist is to differentiate viral encephalitis from other noninflammatory entities such as neoplastic diseases or ischaemia.

1 Introduction

Over 100 viruses are known as possible causal agents of human encephalitis or meningoencephalitis. The occurrence depends on the immunization of the population, the geographical region, the contact with diseased people, animals, and so forth, with large differences seen between Europe, Asia and the U.S. For instance, St. Louis virus encephalitis, which is caused by a mosquito arbovirus, occurs in the midwestern and eastern states of the U.S., but not in the U.K., whereas Japanese encephalitis is an epidemiological problem in Asia, and is the most important cause of epidemic viral encephalitis worldwide with 15,000 deaths annually.

Tables 1 and 2 give an overview of the most important viruses and their MR imaging patterns. The most important causative agents of virus encephalitis are the viruses of the herpes group (herpes simplex viruses, humane herpes viruses' types 6 and 7, cytomegalovirus, Ebstein-Barr virus, Varicella zoster virus). Mumps encephalitis and poliomyelitis play only a subordinate role in developed countries. In a recent PCR-based Finnish study of over 3,000 patients it

S. Hähnel (ed.), *Inflammatory Diseases of the Brain*, Medical Radiology. Diagnostic Imaging,
DOI: 10.1007/174_2012_631, © Springer-Verlag Berlin Heidelberg 2012
Published Online: 19 June 2012

Table 1 Imaging patterns of viral encephalitis-DNA viruses

Disease	Kind of virus	Transmission	Imaging pattern
Herpes encephalitis or herpes meningo-encephalitis	HSV type 1	Droplet or lubrication infection, or infection from saliva, urine or excrement	Involvement of the inferior or mesial parts of the temporal lobes, of the insular cortex, of the thalamus, of the cingulate gyrus or of the frontobasal cortex (limbic pattern)
		Primary infection: gingivostomatitis; neuronal transmission, activation of a latent infection of the Gasserian ganglion (ganglion trigeminale)	Often haemorrhagic transformation and contrast enhancement
Herpes encephalitis of the newborn child	HSV type 2	Droplet or lubrication infection, or infection from saliva, urine or excrement	Early phase: diffuse brain oedema and haemorrhagic transformation; later: calcification
		Primary infection: herpes genitalis	Brain volume loss
		Uterine or perinatal infection of the newborn child	
Human herpes virus type 6 encephalitis	Human herpes virus type 6	Transmission by direct body contact	Cortical accentuated hyperintensity on T2-weighted images
		Primary infection: exanthema subitum	
		Transmission route into the CNS obscure	
CMV encephalitis in immunocompromised adults	CMV	Haematogenous transmission, e.g. by blood products, organ transplantations, droplet or lubrication infection	Hyperintensity on T2-weighted images in the subependymal (periventricular) white matter with slight space-occupying effect
			Brain volume loss
Congenital CMV encephalitis	CMV	Transplacental transmission	Parenchymal calcifications with preference for the periventricular region
			Brain volume loss
EBV encephalitis	EBV	Haematogenous transmission	Hyperintensity on T2-weighted images in the basal ganglia, rarely EBV cerebellitis
		Primary infection: infectious mononucleosis	
VZV encephalitis	VZV	Droplet or lubrication infection	Vasculitic and demyelinating lesions of brain parenchyma; (haemorrhagic) brain infarctions
		Primary infection: chickenpox	
		In the case of reactivation: herpes zoster (shingles), encephalitis	
		Haematogenous transmission of the virus into the CNS	
PML	JC virus (papova virus)	HIV infection	Irregular, round or ovoid confluent hyperintensity on T2-weighted images in the subcortical white matter with involvement of the deep cortical layers
			Preference for the parietal and occipital lobes
			Involvement of the subcortical U fibers
HIV encephalitis	Vaccine of the pox virus	HIV infection	Uni- or bilateral, asymmetric, irregular multifocal hyperintensity on T2-weighted images
			Brain volume loss

CMV cytomegalovirus, *EBV* Epstein-Barr virus, *VZV* Varicella zoster virus, *PML* progressive multifocal leukoencephalopathy

Table 2 Imaging patterns of viral encephalitis-RNA viruses

Disease	Kind of virus	Transmission	Imaging pattern
Meningitis, encephalitis	Rubella (German measles)	Droplet or lubrication infection	Microcephaly, parenchymal calcifications, preferred in the basal ganglia
		Primary infection: rubella	
		Haematogenous transmission of the virus into the CNS	
Tick born meningoencephalitis (spring – summer meningoencephalitis)	Tick-borne virus (arbovirus)	Tick bite Haematogenous transmission of the virus into the CNS	MRI mostly normal, rarely hyperintensity on T2-weighted MR images in the thalamus, cerebellum and caudate nucleus
Japanese B encephalitis	Arboviruses	Mosquitoes	Hyperintensity on T2-weighted MR images in the nuclei of the brain stem and of the thalamus, and of the basal ganglia
		Haematogenous transmission of the virus into the CNS	
Rabies encephalitis	Rhabdoviruses	Bites from dogs or wild living animals	Initial stage: preference for the grey matter
			Later stages: diffuse hyperintensity on T2-weighted MR images in the basal ganglia, the pulvinar thalami, in the periventricular white matter, in the hippocampus and in the brain stem
		Haematogenous transmission	End stage: diffuse brain oedema, haemorrhagic transformation
Acute measle encephalitis	Measle virus	Droplet or lubrication infection	Hyperintensity on T2-weighted MR images in the subcortical white matter, in the brain stem and in the cerebellum
		Primary infection: measles	
		Haematogenous transmission	
Subacute sclerosing panencephalitis (SSPE)	Measle virus	Droplet or lubrication infection	Findings initially normal, then diffuse swelling of the brain, hyperintensity on T2-weighted images in the periventricular white matter, in the brain stem, in the cerebellum, involvement of the putamen and the caudate nucleus
		Primary infection: measles	
		Haematogenous transmission	End stage: brain volume loss
Congenital HIV infection	HIV	Sexual intercourse, blood transfusion	Progressive loss of brain volume over months
			Mostly symmetrical and irregular-confluent focal lesions of the white matter, cortex and U-fibers mostly spared
Lymphozytic choriomeningitis or chorioencephalitis	Arenaviruses	Rodents	
Meningitis, encephalitis, myelitis	Mumpsvirus (paramyxoviruses)	Haematogenous transmission from primary infection (mumps)	
Meningitis, myelitis	Polio virus (enteroviruses)	Fecal – oral route	
Influenza encephalitis	Influenza viruses		

was found out that Varicella zoster virus, the causative agent of chickenpox and herpes zoster was the most frequently detected virus at 29 % of the patients, with HSV and enteroviruses accounting for 11 % of all cases.

As a matter of principle, the neurotropic viruses may reach the CNS by a haematogenous or neural route. Certain viruses have a special affinity for specific cells of the CNS due to their cell-surface properties. Meningeal cells, oligodendrocyte, astrocytes and nerve cells are all involved by different virus types. Herpes viruses multiply mainly in neuronal and glial cells of the limbic system. The JC virus, the causative agent of progressive multifocal leukoencephalopathy, involves mainly oligodendrocytes. Coxsackie-, echo- and mumps viruses often involve meningeal and ependymal cells, but rarely nerve cells.

Brain damage in virus encephalitis, on the one hand, results from the intracellular virus proliferation, and on the other hand, from inflammatory immunological response of the host. This immunological response may be directed humorally against the virus or cellularly against the infected cell. Certain encephalitic viral infections resemble each other with regard to their pathological features: Macroscopically, in the early stage the brain parenchyma is normal. Later the transparency of the meninges is reduced and vascular congestion as well as local or diffuse swelling is evident. Microscopically, an infiltration by inflammatory cells is typical for all encephalitic viral infections of the CNS.

With the exception of the HSV encephalitis showing an almost pathognomonic involvement of typical structures and a relatively specific MR imaging pattern, the radiological findings in viral encephalitis are unspecific. Common findings are focal or diffuse brain oedema in the acute phase and focal atrophy in the chronic stage; therefore, neuroradiological imaging techniques, such as MRI, CT, and DSA, may contribute important information for distinction between brain inflammation and others (e.g. neoplastic diseases or ischaemia), but contribute only little to the determination of the type of virus; however, there are some encephalitic viral infections with neuroradiological specifics which may help to isolate the differential diagnosis.

2 Herpes Simplex Virus Encephalitis

2.1 Epidemiology, Clinical Presentation, Therapy

Despite human infection with HSV, virus type 1 only rarely leads to inflammation of the CNS. The HSV type 1 encephalitis accounts for 95 % of all cases with herpes encephalitis, and the HSV type 1 virus is one of the most common causes of meningoencephalitis in immunocompetent adult persons. The incidence is 1/250,000–1,000,000 persons per year. Half of the patients are younger than 50 years. After primary infection, the virus spreads transneuronally to the bulbus olfactorius or along a branch of the trigeminal nerve into the gasserian ganglion. In the gasserian ganglion the virus persists in 70 % of the patients latently. Molecular analyses of paired oral/labial and brain sites have indicated that HSV type 1 encephalitis can be the result of a primary infection, a reactivation of latent HSV or of a re-infection; however, in about one-third of the patients HSV type 1 encephalitis occurs already during primary infection. The reactivation of the latent HSV infection being promoted by immunosuppression leads to further spreading of the virus across dural branches of cranial nerves into the anterior or middle cranial fossa. Reactivation of the virus is sometimes accompanied by labial herpes. The primary infection with HSV type 1 arises as a mostly asymptomatic infection of the oropharyngeal mucosa with gingivostomatitis or pharyngitis lasting for 2–3 weeks. Sometimes the involvement of the mucosa is manifested by fever or dysphagia. The prodromal stage of the herpes encephalitis lasts 1–4 days and is characterised by influenza-like complaints. The majority of the patients with HSV type 1 encephalitis suffers from fever and hemicranial holocephalic headache. Additional symptoms are confusion and personality change. Dysphagia, epilepsy and hemiparesis are typical focal neurological deficits. In immunocompromised patients the clinical course is rarely acute but instead is remitting-relapsing. In these patients synchronous labial herpes occurs only rarely.

The majority of cases with HSV encephalitis in newborn children are caused by the HSV type 2, whereas only 6–15 % of the cases with herpes encephalitis in adults are caused by HSV type 2. In adults HSV type 2 is mostly causative for benign lymphocytic meningitis. The incidence of HSV type 2 encephalitis is 1/200–1/5,000 births. The neonatal infection arises through intranatal contact of the newborn with the genital secretion of the mother, in the case that the mother suffers from genital herpes.

The risk of a fetal infection in cases of a primary genital infection of the mother is 30–50 % higher as compared with mothers suffering from relapsing genital infects (3 %). Intrauterine infection occurs only rarely.

The pathological correlation of HSV encephalitis is a fulminating haemorrhagic necrotizing meningoencephalitis with preference for limbic structures. Macroscopically, in HSV type 1 encephalitis bilateral, temporobasally and frontobasally located necrotic zones are evident; in HSV type 2 encephalitis more diffuse changes are found. Microscopically, perivascular infiltrations, gliosis, destroyed nerve cells and viral inclusion bodies are detected. In immunocompromised persons an inflammatory reaction may be absent at the beginning despite CNS involvement. In patients suffering from AIDS in the advanced stage the typical haemorrhagic encephalomyelitis is missing; instead, massive virus inclusions are detected in the infected cells. Therefore, in immunocompromised persons the neuronal damage results more or less only from direct toxic effects of the virus. Brain biopsy is nowadays unnecessary for diagnosis.

The CSF findings in HSV encephalitis include a lymphocytic pleocytosis of 50–500/3 cells mm^{-3}. The CSF proteins are increased to 0.5–2.5 g/l in more than 80 % of the cases. A fourfold increased HSV-specific antibody titer in the CSF relative to the initial titer is proof of the disease. The most reliable and rapid method for the confirmation of the diagnosis is the direct proof of virus DNA using PCR. Besides the clinical, radiological and CSF findings, also typical EEG findings may be observed.

Therapy in HSV encephalitis includes common medical treatment and specific therapy using acyclovir; thereby the

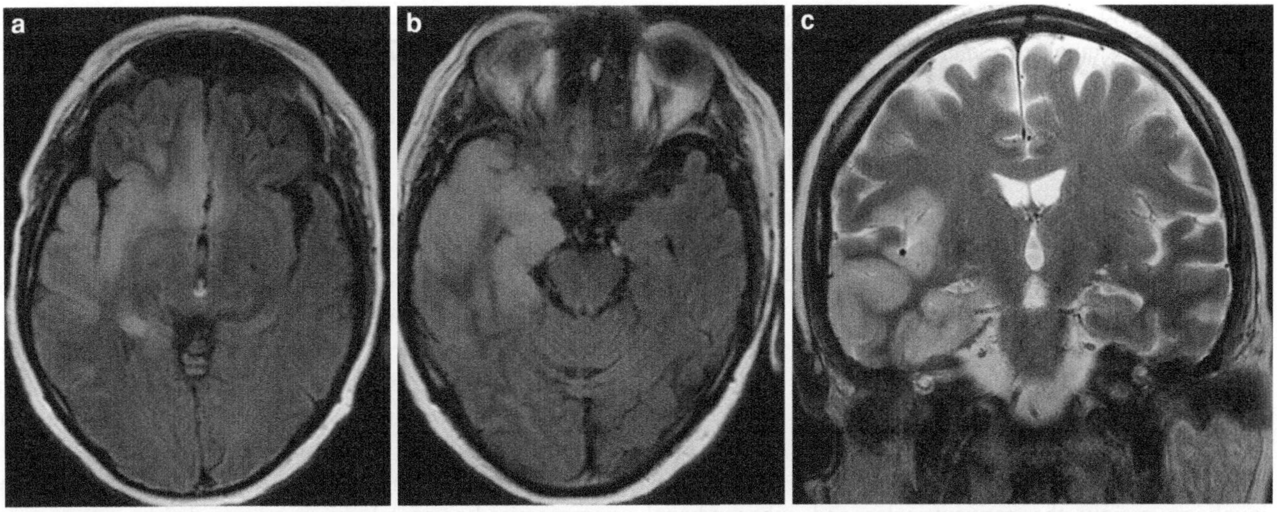

Fig. 1 Herpes simplex virus encephalitis type 1, in a 56-year-old woman with seizures. **a, b** Axial FLAIR images. **c** Coronal T2-weighted image. Slightly space-occupying oedema in the right superior, medial and inferior temporal lobe extending into the insula and the right cingulate gyrus, but also the left cingulate gyrus is involved

lethality of HSV encephalitis can be reduced from 70 % in untreated adults to 20 % in treated adults, and in children from 80 to 50 %.

2.2 Imaging

In contrast to other forms, the MRI pattern in HSV type 1 encephalitis is very specific: as the correlate of focal brain oedema hyperintensity on PD-weighted, T2-weighted and FLAIR images in the medial and inferior temporal lobe extending into the insula and the cingulate gyrus are evident (Fig. 1). Typically, the putamen is spared. Sometimes, the frontal, occipital and parietal lobes, as well as the thalamus, hypothalamus and brain stem, may also be involved. These signs are detectable reliably 48 h after onset of the clinical symptoms. The value of advanced MR imaging techniques, such as DWI, has not yet been proven sufficiently. According to our own experiences, in particular patients the initial cell damage may temporarily manifest as cytotoxic brain oedema with reduction of the ADC. Contrast enhancement is absent in the early stage of the disease, but later, on meningeal contrast enhancement and parenchymal contrast enhancement at the corticomedullary junction, it is visible. Not before 3 or 4 days after clinical onset are parenchymal petechial haemorrhages at the corticomedullary junction with initially high signal on T1-weighted images (methaemoglobin) detectable. Besides axial standard sequences, the optimal study protocol for the examination of herpes encephalitis includes coronal T2-weighted or FLAIR images and T1-weighted images before and after contrast application.

In the follow-up of days and weeks involvement of the contralateral hemisphere with the same predilection is evident. After the course of the acute inflammatory stage, a cystic-gliotic residual defect zone remains leading to focal or diffuse brain atrophy. Sometimes dystrophic calcifications may be visible, best on T2*-weighted images or by CT. The HSV type 2 encephalitis manifests as unspecific brain swelling, brain oedema and leptomeningeal enhancement. The diagnosis is difficult because the cerebral white matter is not completely myelinated in newborns and therefore is hyperintense on T2-weighted images also in healthy children. Like in HSV type 1 encephalitis, haemorrhage may occur also in HSV type 2 encephalitis.

3 Cytomegalovirus Encephalitis

3.1 Epidemiology, Clinical Presentation, Therapy

In immunocompromised adults, for instance, in patients with AIDS the CMV, encephalitis arises from reactivation of the CMV; however, recently, with the action of highly active antiretroviral therapies in this patient group CMV encephalitis has become rarer again. CMV encephalitis is the most common congenital infection of the CNS, being more common than toxoplasmosis, rubella (German measles) and HSV type 2 encephalitis. In the U.S. 1 % of newborns are involved; 50–80 % of all women with childbearing potential are seropositive for CMV. Of all pregnant women, 5 % excrete the virus by urine. In these cases the foetus is infected by a transplacental route.

In more than 60 % of the infected newborns more than one organ system is involved, including CNS. Later the children become apparent with deafness, epilepsy, mental retardation, chorioretinitis, microcephaly, optic neuritis and malformation of the eye. Therapeutic attempts by the administration of ganciclovir are reported. In newborns the CMV has an exceptional affinity for the subependymal germinal matrix. Extended periventricular tissue necrosis is evident. Histologically, eosinophil inclusion bodies can be found.

3.2 Imaging

For adults, hyperintensity on T2–weighted MR images involving mainly the periventricular and subependymal supratentorial white matter is evident. The lesions are often blurred and slightly space occupying. On native MR images CMV lesions may have the same appearance as lesions from HIV encephalitis; however, whereas CMV encephalitis is mostly characterised by contrast enhancement, HIV lesions commonly do not enhance. In newborns and children microcephaly, brain atrophy with dilated CSF spaces, migration disorders and delayed myelination are typical findings. For the detection of periventricular calcifications CT is superior to MRI. A complicating ventriculitis is characterised by ependymal contrast enhancement and hydrocephalus.

4 Epstein-Barr-Virus Encephalitis

4.1 Epidemiology, Clinical Presentation, Therapy

The primary infection of Epstein-Barr-Virus encephalitis is infectious mononucleosis. Both during primary infection and during virus reactivation encephalitis or Guillain-Barré syndrome may arise. The EBV infection is associated with Burkitt lymphoma and nasopharyngeal carcinoma. According to serological examinations, 90 % of the healthy population has experienced EBV infection before the fortieth year of age. Patients become clinically apparent with meningism, failure of cranial nerves (e.g. Bell's palsy) and epilepsy. Standard therapy consists of acyclovir or ganciclovir.

4.2 Imaging

Hyperintensity in the basal ganglia on T2-weighted images are typical.

5 Varicella-Zoster-Virus Encephalitis

5.1 Epidemiology, Clinical Presentation, Therapy

The incidence of Varicella zoster virus (VZV) is 1–2/10,000 persons per year. The primary infection is chickenpox. The reactivation of the virus leads to herpes zoster (shingles) or to infectious encephalitis (*Varicella*). Other manifestations in the CNS are a para- or postinfectious encephalomyelitis or cerebellitis subsequent to a chickenpox infection in 4/4,000 children, Guillain-Barré syndrome or Reye syndrome. The majority of the patients with *Varicella-zoster*-virus encephalitis have experienced shingles. Immunocompromised persons have an increased risk.

The patients typically have headache, ailment and confusion for days to months (average 9 days) after exacerbation of the shingles; however, encephalitis may also occur without shingles in the history. Specific standard therapy is performed using acyclovir. Modern drugs, such as valaciclovir or famiciclovir, are effective in herpes zoster (shingles) but have not been proven for the treatment of *Varicella-zoster*-virus encephalitis. Lethality of the encephalomyelitis subsequent to chickenpox is about 30 %, that of cerebellitis only 0–5 %. In adults the prognosis is good. Pathologically, different oligodendrocytes, ependymal cells and endothelial cells are preferentially infected. Histologically, inflammatory changes, haemorrhagic necroses and vasculitic lesions can be found. Subsequently, secondary ischaemic brain infarctions may develop. In the postinfectious form, besides directly viral-induced tissue damage, also secondary immunomediated mechanisms are potential causes for inflammatory reaction. Intrauterine infection may lead to a severe necrotizing encephalomyelitis.

5.2 Imaging

In immunocompromised persons three involvement patterns are characteristic: (1) haemorrhagic or non-haemorrhagic infarcts in the territories of large- or middle-size arteries; (2) ischaemic or demyelinating lesions in the deep white matter as a result of the involvement of small-size arteries and (3) ventriculitis or periventriculitis. Multiple, spherical lesions of the white matter are found with high signal on T2-weighted images, preferentially located in the periventricular region, the cerebellum and the cervical cord. Partly haemorrhagic transformed cortical and subcortical infarcts can be found in the territory of small- and large-size vessels as a result of vasculitis. Ventriculitis or periventriculitis

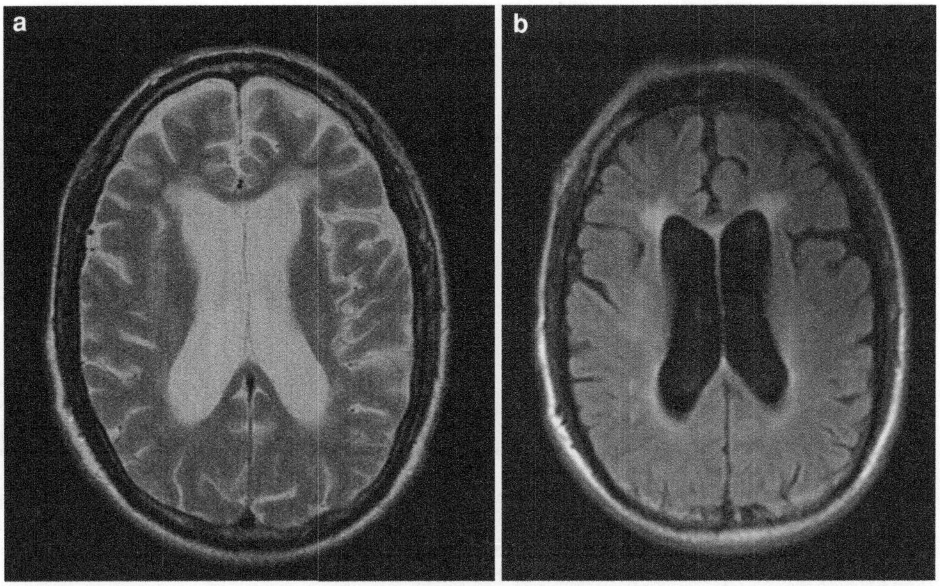

Fig. 2 HIV encephalopathy (progressive diffuse leukoencephalopathy) in a 36-year-old man. **a** Axial T2-weighted image. **b** Axial FLAIR image. Brain atrophy and confluent hyperintensity in the supratentorial periventricular white matter. In contrast to progressive multifocal leukoencephalopathy (PML), the hyperintense lesions spare the subcortical U-fibres

may mimic CMV encephalitis when high signal on T2-weighted images and homogeneous contrast enhancement is evident. Magnetic resonance angiography may reveal irregularities of the cerebral arteries.

6 Human-Immunodeficiency-Virus Encephalitis and Encephalopathy

6.1 Epidemiology, Clinical Presentation, Therapy

The terms HIV encephalitis and HIV encephalopathy are used synonymously in the medical literature. Of the patients with AIDS, 60 % develop HIV encephalitis or HIV encephalopathy through direct infection by the HIV. In 3–10 % of all AIDS patients, HIV-encephalitis or HIV encephalopathy is the first manifestation of the disease. Besides HIV encephalitis, immunocompromised persons may suffer from a variety of other, opportunistic infections. Clinically, the disease is characterised by slowly progressive demential reduction, tiredness, impulselessness and memory deficit. Disturbance of the motor coordination, such as tremor and gait disturbance may develop.

Children with HIV encephalitis show retardation, behavioural disturbances and motor deficits. A specific therapy currently does not exist. By the use of antiretroviral drugs the course of the disease can be influenced positively, at best. The infection of the CNS leads to an inflammatory parenchymal reaction with the formation of multinuclear giant cells and glial nodules. In time demyelination, axonal loss and brain atrophy develop. The cortex may be histopathologically involved, even in cases without radiologically proven cortical lesions. Damage to the limbic system and striatum are probably the result of the toxic effects of Quinoline acid, released by activated macrophages and microglial cells after infection by HIV.

6.2 Imaging

As with other viral infections of the CNS, the imaging findings are unspecific: in the *first stage*, mostly at the time point of the initial HIV infection, multiple, approximately 10-mm-large hyperintense lesions are visible in the white matter on T2-weighted images. These changes can be detected in 20 % of the cases. The lesion pattern is almost symmetrical: lesions are irregular in shape and confluent. The cortex and the U-fibres (subcortical fibres) are spared. This phenomenon can be used as a diagnostic criterion for the differentiation between PML and HIV; in PML the U-fibres are typically involved. Additionally, magnetisation transfer measurements may be helpful: whereas in lesions of HIV encephalitis a reduction of the magnetization transfer ratio of only 20 % relative to normal values is observed, the magnetization transfer ratio in PML is the correlate of more intense demyelination and is reduced by 45 % relative to normal values. The *second stage* of HIV encephalitis is characterised by progressive subacute encephalitis with brain atrophy (Fig. 2). A central atrophy (ventricular enlargement) preponderates relative to cortical atrophy (sulcal enlargement). The course of the brain atrophy is slowly progressive over months. In the course of the disease calcifications of the basal ganglia, the frontal lobes and the cerebellum may occur. In children HIV encephalitis may be associated with vasculitis and the

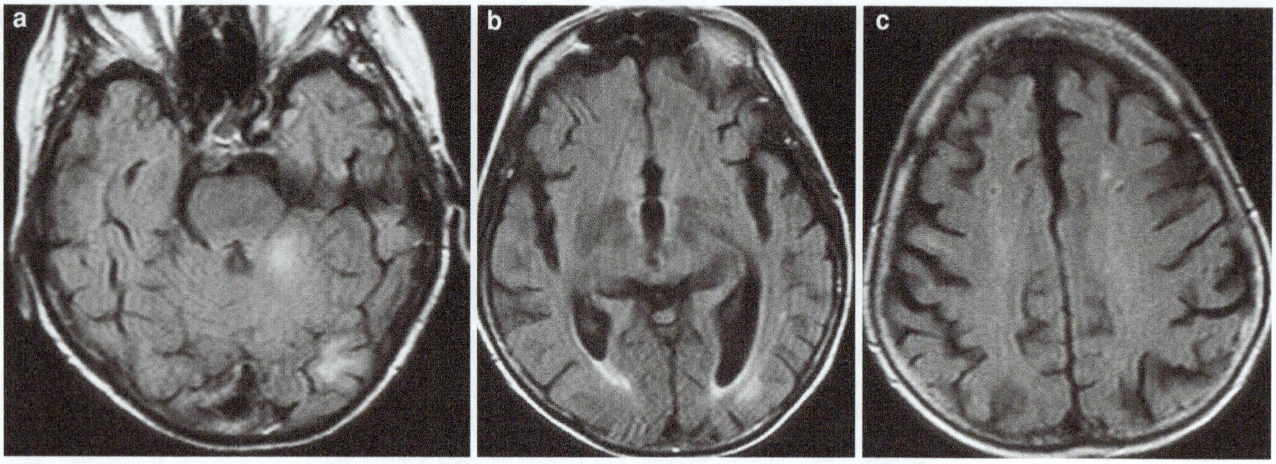

Fig. 3 PML in a 37-year-old immunocompromised woman with AIDS. Initial imaging at the time of admission. **a – c** Axial FLAIR images. Hyperintensity in the left cerebellar hemisphere (**a**) and in the left occipital lobe (**a**). Only discrete hyperintensity in the right central region (**c**). The right temporal lobe appears normal (**b**). In contrast to HIV encephalopathy, the hyperintense lesions in PML typically involve the subcortical U-fibres

development of cerebral aneurysms. A variant of the HIV encephalitis is progressive diffuse leukoencephalopathy (PDL). This variant is characterised by signal changes predominately in the deep frontal cerebral white matter always sparing the U-fibres (Fig. 2).

7 Progressive Multifocal Leukencephalopathy

7.1 Epidemiology, Clinical Presentation, Therapy

In progressive multifocal leukoencephalopathy (PML) the causative agent is the JC virus, a DNA-containing papilloma virus, which was named for the initials of the patient (J.C.), in whom the disease was first described. The incidence of PML is 4–7 % in all patients with AIDS with increasing frequency during the last years. The PML is the most frequent opportunistic viral infection of the CNS. In addition, PML occurs preferentially in persons with severe cellular immunodeficiency such as leukemia, Hodgkin's disease and disorders of the autoimmune system. Depending on the involved structure, the clinical picture includes headache, cognitive deficits and defects of the visual field or ataxia. Sometimes hemipareses may develop. Mostly the disease leads to death within 3–24 months after diagnosis. By the administration of cidofovir the neurological condition may be improved. Particular cases with spontaneous cessation of the disease have been described; therefore, with AIDS as the base disease an optimal antiviral therapy with respect to HIV has to be implemented. Oligodendrocytes are infected via the JC virus. Demyelination is the histological correlate of damage and destruction of oligodendrocytes.

Recently, a variety of diseases have been reported which are related to JC-Virus apart from classical PML. (1) PML may occur under the treatment with highly effective immunosuppressive therapy with monoclonal antibodies. (2) A PML-immune reconstitution inflammatory syndrome (PML-IRIS) is the result of an intensive immune response against antigens of opportunistic infectious agents. In association with the treatment of HIV-positive patients with highly active antiretroviral therapy an IRIS may develop during rapid increase of the CD4 cells and a rapid decrease of the viral load. (3) The monoclonal antibodies natalizumab, efalizumab and rituximab—used for the treatment of multiple sclerosis, Crohn's disease, psoriasis, haematological malignancies and rheumatic diseases—have been associated with PML. An abrupt finishing of the therapy with such a highly effective immunsuppression may result in IRIS.

7.2 Imaging

Most often, the posterior centrum semiovale is involved. Typically, the disease begins in the posterior subcortical lobar white matter. In contrast to HIV encephalopathy, the U-fibres (fibrae arcuatae) are almost always affected being an important differential diagnostic criterion. The cortex, however, is spared. In progressed cases confluent and enlarging white matter lesions with high signal on T2-weighted images are evident. Also the thalamus, basal ganglia, corpus callosum and infratentorial structures may be affected. Involvement of the brain stem and the cerebellum may also often occur.

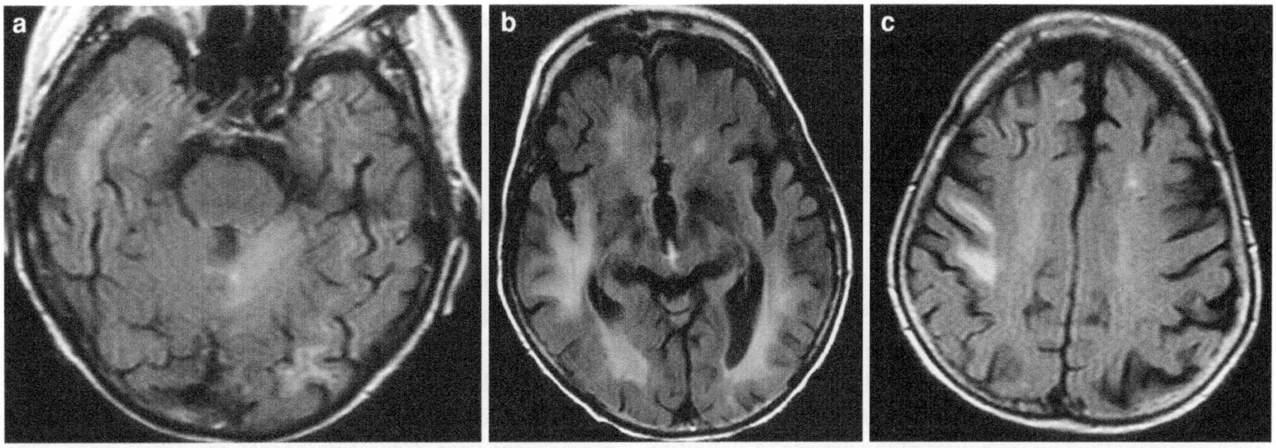

Fig. 4 PML. Same patient as in Fig. 3. Follow-up imaging 4 weeks after the initial examination. Axial FLAIR images. The hyperintensity in the cerebellar hemisphere (**a**), in the left occipital lobe (**a, b**) and in the right central region (**c**) have markedly increased. Now, extensive hyperintensity also in the right temporal lobe is present (**a, b**)

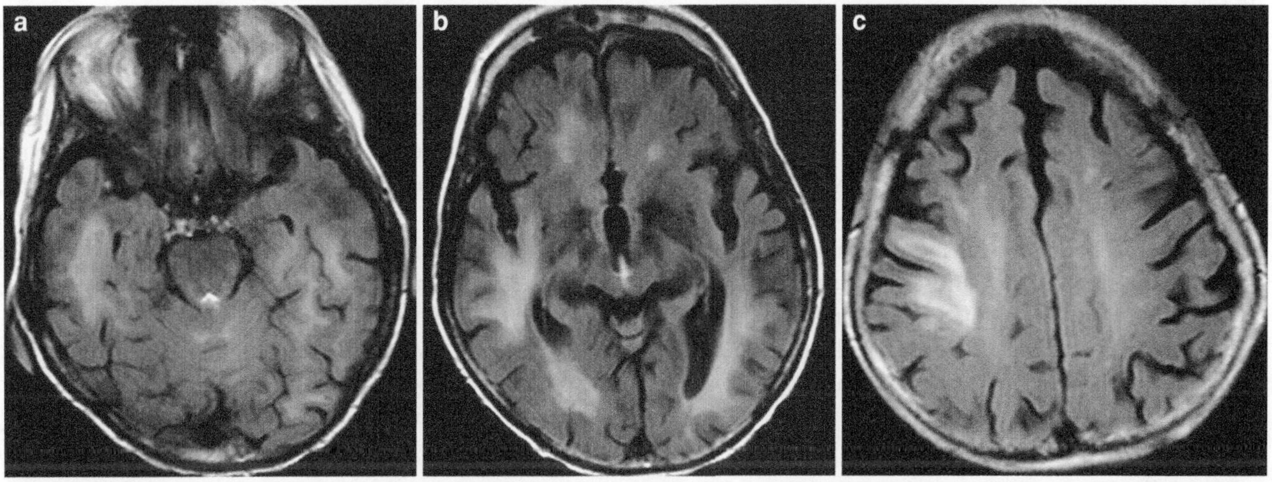

Fig. 5 PML. Same patient as in Fig. 3. Follow-up imaging 7 weeks after the initial examination. **a–c** Axial FLAIR images. The lesions have further markedly increased

Contrast enhancement is not typical. The lesions may be space occupying (Figs. 3, 4, and 5).

In contrast to classical PML contrast enhancement is reported in PML occuring under the treatment with highly effective immunosuppressive therapy with monoclonal antibodies, in PML-IRIS, and in PML due to the monoclonal antibodies such as natalizumab, efalizumab and rituximab.

8 Measle Encephalitis

8.1 Epidemiology, Clinical Presentation, Therapy

Measle infection may result in three forms of encephalitis:

1. Before the introduction of the measle vaccination, an acute postinfectious auto immunological measle encephalitis develops in 10/100,000 children below the age of 16 years. It begins shortly after the measle exanthema or as acute progressive encephalitis months later. The possibility to become diseased from an encephalitis after immunization accounts for 8/100,000 vaccinations.

2. A subacute measle encephalitis, which typically manifests 1–10 months after measle infection in immunocompromised persons.

3. Subacute sclerosing panencephalitis (SSPE) occurs at the earliest 6 years after measle infection and affects mostly children and adolescents who had been diseased with measles before the second year of life. The typical age of manifestation is before the thirtieth year of life, the average being the

age of 7 years. The causative agent is a mutational variant of the measle virus. The incidence is 1/1,000,000 persons of the non-immunized people per year. The acute post infectious encephalitis is characterised by recurrence of fever, reduced consciousness, epilepsy and focal neurological deficits a few days or weeks after experienced measle infection during convalescence. The resistance of epilepsy to therapy is typical for the subacute measle encephalitis. Fever is not a symptom of this type of encephalitis. The SSPE is accompanied by myoclonia, epilepsy and psychic conspicuousness. According to recent reports, a combination therapy consisting of high-dose intrathecally administered alpha-interferon and intravenously administered ribavirin given in the early stage has a positive effect on the course of the disease. A definitive therapy of SSPE has not been established. Histopathologically, for SSPE nerve cell damage, astrogliosis, demyelination and infiltration by inflammatory cells are typical findings. Intranuclear cell inclusions are found in neurons, oligodendrocytes and astrocytes. Using the electron microscope, nucleocapsids are detected.

8.2 Imaging

The acute encephalitis is characterised by hyperintensity on T2-weighted images in the subcortical white matter, brain stem and cerebellum. In SSPE, the initial imaging findings are commonly normal. Later, diffuse brain swelling and focal hyperintensity on T2-weighted images in the central white matter, cortex, basal ganglia and cerebellum are found. The end stage of SSPE is characterised by brain atrophy.

9 Congenital Rubella (German Measles) Encephalitis

9.1 Epidemiology, Clinical Presentation, Therapy

The rubella virus is transmitted to foetus via a transplacental route by viraemia. The markedness of the disease depends on gestational age during infection. The fully expressed rubella syndrome develops from infection in the first trimester. Due to the far-reaching immunization of the population, the disease has become rare. Depending on the time point of infection, spontaneous abortion, stillbirths or severe organ damage may occur. Besides encephalitis, malformation of the eye and heart may arise. Deafness is the most important late symptom. The virus disturbs cell division and cell maturation, preferentially of cells of the germinal matrix. Histologically, inflammatory infiltration of the meninges and perivascular spaces is evident.

9.2 Imaging

Microcephaly and parenchymal calcifications, especially in the basal ganglia, are typical.

10 Tick-Borne Meningoencephalitis

10.1 Epidemiology, Clinical Presentation, Therapy

With tick-borne meningoencephalitis (spring–summer meningoencephalitis), the incidence is about 1–2/-100,000 persons per year. Causative agents are arboviruses. Small wild rodents are reservoirs for the virus. The transmission usually occurs by ticks, gnats or mosquitoes. Mostly, the disease occurs from June to July. In Germany the tick species *Ixodes rizinus* predominates. About 0.1 % of the ticks in Germany are infected. Lumbermen and farmers are particularly at risk. In 60 % of the cases human infections pass unnoticed. Of the infected persons, 30 % have influenza complaints within the first 3 weeks.

In only 10 % of the cases does a meningoencephalitis arise, with a latency of 1 week. The typical clinical symptoms of the tick-borne meningoencephalitis are acute onset of high fever and psychosis. Cranial nerve palsies, extrapyramidal motor hyperkinesis, cerebellar signs and pareses may develop. In children, who mostly develop only a benign lymphocytic meningitis, the prognosis is far better than in adults. If vegetative centres of the brain stem are involved, the prognosis is poor. The overall mortality is 1 %. In severe cases the administration of acyclovir is indicated.

10.2 Imaging

In the majority of the cases imaging findings are normal. Occasionally, hyperintensity on T2-weighted images in the thalamus, cerebellum, brain stem and caudate nucleus may be evident.

11 Rabies Encephalitis

11.1 Epidemiology, Clinical Presentation, Therapy

Rabies encephalitis is an acute infection of the CNS involving men and other mammalians. Rabies has a worldwide incidence. Only few countries are free of the disease, among them England, Japan, Australia and New Zealand. The causative agent is a cylindriforme RNA virus of the Rhabdo virus family. Commonly the disease is transmitted to men by bites from infected dogs, cats, foxes, hedgehogs, wolves and vampire bats. Cattle, horses and other vegetarians may be infected, but they are only rarely the transmitter of the disease to humans. After the bite from the infected animal the virus migrates along the axons to the CNS, where the virus multiplies. Usually, the incubation period is 3–10 weeks but may amount to several years. The more the portal of entry (bite) is closed to the CNS, the shorter is the incubation period. From the CNS the virus haematogenously spreads into other organs. About 20–50 % of the bitten persons actually contract rabies. Worldwide the yearly number of deaths from rabies is estimated to at least 40,000–70,000. About 10 million people have to be treated precautionary after contact with an animal suspected of being infected with the rabies virus.

The disease passes in three stages: The *first stage* is characterised by unspecific symptoms such as fever, headache, nausea, vomiting, stomach pain, diarrhoea and cough. Excitability and sensitivity to light, noise and air flow may be additional symptoms in the subsequent course. The fever rises continuously. The second stage, the neurologically acute or excitational stage, is characterised by hyperactivity with twitching muscles, spasms and cramps. Sensations of fear, anxiety and fear of water may be additional symptoms. In 80 % of cases this stage has an encephalitic course, and in 20 % of cases, a paralytic course with palsies is typical. This *second stage* lasts for 2–7 days. Afterward, the patient falls into a coma and dies from paralysis of the respiratory system or from heart or circulation failure. Once the first symptoms are evident, a rabies infection almost always leads to death. The therapy has to be initiated immediately after the bite by an animal suspected of carrying the rabies virus, if possible. After the disease has broken out, the fatal course can only be delayed by the use of intensive medical care. The tissue around the wound should be injected with anti-rabies hyperimmunoglobulin. Furthermore, anti-rabies hyperimmunoglobulin should be applied intramuscularly, possibly in combination with interferon. At first, 1 day later, the administration of a dead vaccine is performed. Prophylactic immunisation is indicated in persons with an increased occupational risk such as hunters, veterinarians, laboratory staff or travellers to Asia or Africa. Histopathologically, axonal necrosis with degeneration of the axons and demyelination are found. In 70 % of rabies cases cytoplasmic inclusion bodies (Negri bodies) can be detected. Mostly, they are found in the pyramidal cells of the hippocampus, the cerebral cortex and the Purkinje cells of the cerebellar cortex.

11.2 Imaging

There are only few reports of rabies in the medical literature. In the initial stage the grey matter is preferentially involved. Diffuse hyperintensity on T2-weighted images in the basal ganglia, pulmonary thalami, periventricular white matter, hippocampus and brain stem can be detected. Signal increase on native T1-weighted images is the correlate for haemorrhage. Also, vasculitis-like lesions with vessel stenoses and ischaemic infarcts are described.

12 Other, Rare Viral Infections of the CNS

In Sweden about 50 % of all cases of encephalitis are caused by the tick-borne virus. Japanese B encephalitis is the most common encephalitis in Asia and is caused by a virus of the St. Louis complex of the flavi virus group. The disease is endemic in China, the northern parts of Southeast Asia, India and Sri Lanka. The virus is transmitted by mosquitoes. Mostly children are involved. Non-immunised adults, who travel into an epidemic area, may suffer a severe encephalitis. The infection may be clinically asymptomatic or may manifest with simple influenza-like symptoms. Encephalitis is accompanied by severe fever, headache, epilepsy and coma. Tremor or other Parkinson-like symptoms may occur. The virus involves the nuclei of the brain stem, basal ganglia and thalamus.

The lymphocytic choriomeningitis virus (group of the arena viruses) is transmitted by domestic mice and hamsters. It can cause meningitis with slight accompanying encephalitis. Encephalitis caused by paramyxoviruses, such as the parainfluenza virus, is rare.

13 Differential Diagnosis

Generally, non-viral inflammations of brain parenchyma have to be included in the differential diagnosis, because they may sometimes resemble viral encephalitis. In patients with relapsing–remitting clinical course, which often occurs in immunocompromised persons, a low–grade glioma has to be considered if only non–enhanced T1-weighted and T2-weighted images were acquired. A change of the contrast enhancement pattern within days in viral encephalitis, absent in haemorrhage in low-grade gliomas and the rapid expansion of the inflammatory changes into limbic structures, as in HSV encephalitis type 1, may be helpful for the differentiation. High-grade glioma and metastases reveal a rrCBV at least twice the normal values. Solid lymphoma and toxoplasmosis, the most important differential diagnoses in AIDS-associated diseases, always show contrast enhancement. For cerebral lymphoma a massive leakage of contrast medium into the interstitial space is typical; therefore, significant blood – brain barrier damage is evident, outweighing the T2* effect by the (only slightly) increased rrCBV in PerfMRI. Acute ischaemic brain

Table 3 Differential diagnostic criteria for the discrimination between infectious (viral) encephalitis and acute disseminated encephalomyelitis (ADEM)

	Infectious (viral) encephalitis	ADEM
MR imaging	Irregular hyperintensity on T2-weighted images; cortex, basal ganglia, brain stem and cerebellum often involved, contrast enhancement possible, if visible, then homogeneous and not circular	Multifocal, round or ovoid hyperintensity on T2-weighted images; typically cerebral white matter, rarely basal ganglia or cortex involved; callososeptal interface typically not involved; ringlike, punctuate or peripheral enhancement; cord involvement possible; cranial nerves may enhance
CSF findings	Lymphozygotic pleocytosis, increased concentration of proteins and glucose	Lymphozygotic pleocytosis, increased concentration of proteins and normal concentration of glucose
	HSV encephalitis: possibly erythrocytes detectable	Acute haemorrhagic encephalomyelitis: possibly erythrocytes detectable
Vaccination days or weeks before	No	Typical
Typical age	No age preference	Children and young adults
Fever	Typical	Possible
Prodromal complaints	Occasionally	Typical
Uni- or bilateral visual loss	Rare	Possible
Cord signs	Rare	Possible

infarction is characterised by a reduced ADC during the first 1–8 days after clinical onset. Signal abnormalities due to ischaemic infarction are oriented to vessel territories and demarcate more rapidly as compared with inflammation. Depending on their stage, the MRI features of ischaemic infarctions are so characteristic that a differentiation between ischaemia and inflammation is possible in the majority of the cases, at the latest after the acquisition and analysis of follow-up examinations. The VZV encephalitis may resemble other forms of cerebral vasculitis. Due to the involvement of basal ganglia, thalamus and brain stem, the imaging pattern of rabies encephalitis may resemble the following diseases: spongiforme encephalopathies; Wilson's disease; Leigh's disease; toxic encephalopathies due to intoxication by carbon monoxide; methanol; and cyanides; or hydrogen sulphide, hypoglycaemia or a haemolytic uraemic syndrome.

The definite identification of the virus is performed by enzyme-linked immunosorbent assay (ELISA) technique. To prove disease in the acute stage, IgM antibodies must be detected.

For the viruses of the herpes group (HSV type 1, HSV type 2, CMV, VZV, EBV), and for increasingly more other viruses, PCR is presently available as a highly sensitive method for early, direct detection at a time when MRI is still the norm. Sometimes it may be difficult to distinguish an acute viral encephalitis from a postinfectious acute demyelinating encephalomyelitis. Differential diagnostic criteria are summarised in Table 3.

Further Reading

Bakshi R (2004) Neuroimaging of HIV and AIDS related illness: a review. Front Biosci 9:632–646

Falcone S, Post MJ (2000) Encephalitis, cerebritis, and brain abscess: pathophysiology and imaging findings. Neuroimag Clin N Am 10(2):333–353

Hähnel S, Storch-Hagenlocher B, Seitz A (2006) Infectious diseases of the brain: imaging and differential diagnosis. Radiologie Up2Date 3:207–234 [in German]

Kennedy PG (2004) Viral encephalitis: causes, differential diagnosis, and management. J Neurol Neurosurg Psychiatry 75(Suppl 1): i10–i15

Roos KL (1999) Encephalitis. Neurol Clin 17(4):813–833

Tan CS, Koralnik IJ (2010) Progressive multifocal leukoencephalopathy and other disorders caused by JC virus: clinical features and pathogenesis. Lancet Neurol. 9(4):425–37

Weber W, Henkes H, Felber S et al (2000) Diagnostic imaging in viral encephalitis. Radiologe 40 (11):998– 010 [in German]

Spongiform Encephalopathies

Horst Urbach and Henriette Tschampa

Contents

Abstract

Sporadic and variant Creutzfeldt–Jakob disease as the most important spongiform encephalopathies are fatal neurodegenerative disorders caused by infectious proteins called prions which aggregate, accumulate and induce neuronal death and spongiform changes of the brain. Definite diagnosis of sporadic CJD (sCJD) requires biopsy. Clinical probable diagnosis is based on typical clinical symptoms associated with a characteristic EEG and/or detection of 14-3-3 protein in CSF and/or bilateral striatal and/or cortical signal hyperintensity on Diffusion-weighted and FLAIR MRI sequences. With a typical clinical picture, this MRI pattern is highly specific. Variant CJD (vCJD) has a different clinical course and MRI pattern. It consists of symmetric bilateral increased signal intensity of the pulvinar thalami (pulvinar sign) in about 80 % of cases, the mediodorsal thalamic nuclei can be additionally affected (hockey stick sign), in contrast to sCJD signal intensity in the thalamus is always higher than in the striate.

1 Epidemiology, Clinical Presentation, Therapy

1.1 Epidemiology

Spongiform encephalopathies are rare and fatal neurodegenerative disorders caused by infectious proteins called prions (proteinaceous infectious particles that lack nucleic acid) that can be transmitted to laboratory animals. According to the prion hypothesis, the normal cellular prion protein (PrP^c, c for cellular) is transformed into an abnormal insoluble form (PrP^{Sc}, Sc for scrapie), which tends to aggregate, accumulate and induce neuronal death and spongiform changes of the brain (Tschampa et al. 2006).

In humans, the most frequent form is Creutzfeldt–Jakob Disease (CJD) with four different types: the sporadic type

H. Urbach (✉) · H. Tschampa
Department of Radiology/Neuroradiology,
Sigmund Freud-Strasse 25,
53105 Bonn, Germany
e-mail: horst.urbach@ukb.uni-bonn.de

S. Hähnel (ed.), *Inflammatory Diseases of the Brain*, Medical Radiology. Diagnostic Imaging,
DOI: 10.1007/174_2012_628, © Springer-Verlag Berlin Heidelberg 2012
Published Online: 22 May 2012

(sCJD) (85 % of cases, incidence 1 per 1–1.5 million persons per year), the genetic type (10–15 % of cases), the iatrogenic type (<5 % of cases), and the variant type (vCJD).

In animals, the most frequent prion diseases are Scrapie, an endemic disease in sheep, and bovine spongiform encephalopathy (BSE), an epidemic disease in cattle. Although the transmission from cattle to human is still under debate, the variant CJD type (vCJD) is strongly associated with the epidemiology of BSE in the United Kingdom (UK): BSE was amplified by feeding cattle meet and bone meal infected with Scrapie and/or BSE, the rendering process changed in the late 1970s. The first verified BSE case occurred in 1986, and a BSE epidemy in the UK in the early 1990s. The first vCJD patient was reported in the UK in March 1996, and until November 2011, the majority of cases ($n = 173$) has been reported in the UK. Four cases occurred in Ireland, 25 in France and 20 in other countries. Seven of 49 persons, who were down with CJD outside the UK, had lived in the UK between 1980 and 1996 for more than 6 months, and the year by year incidence is now declining. For further details see http://www.cjd.ed.ac.uk/vcjdworld.htm. Transmission experiments to macaques and mice indicate that the infectious agent in BSE and vCJD is the same. The pathologic prion protein is detectable in intestinal lymphatic tissue and the tonsils in vCJD, but not in sCJD. A transmission via blood products has been reported for at least three vCJD patients, albeit it has never been considered impossible in sCJD patients (Ironside 2010).

Unfortunately, the proteinaceous agents are resistant to conventional disinfection/sterilization and can be transmitted to humans via contaminated medical instruments and grafts. Before 1980, two iatrogenic CJD cases following depth electrodes implantation, up to four cases transmitted by neurosurgical instruments, 114 dura mater and two corneal grafts transmissions have been known. When CJD is suspected—and MR interpretation plays crucial role either to raise the suspicion or to supersede biopsy—single-use instruments are recommended. Reusable instruments must be decontaminated by immersion in 1N NaOH and autoclaved (121 °C/30 min), cleaned, rinsed and steam sterilized.

1.2 Clinical Presentation

1.2.1 Sporadic CJD

Sporadic CJD patients are predominantly affected between 70 and 79 years of age without a gender predilection. They typically suffer from rapidly progressive dementia and focal neurological signs. These focal signs include ataxia, myoclonus, pyramidal and extrapyramidal disorders and visual disturbances. Clinical deterioration is extremely rapid and leads to a state of akinetic mutism. Mean survival is 6 months with a span ranging from 3 months to 2 years. 14-3-3 protein in CSF is positive in over 95 % of the age groups over 40 years. It is less frequently positive (75 % of cases) in younger CJD patients (Heinemann et al. 2007), and may be also positive in other rapid progressive brain diseases (e.g. Alzheimer's disease, encephalitis).

Table 1 Diagnostic criteria for sporadic CJD (sCJD)

	Diagnostic criteria
Definite CJD	Neuropathological confirmation
Probable CJD	Progressive dementia with at least two of four clinical features: 1. Myoclonus 2. Visual or cerebellar disturbances 3. Pyramidal/extrapyramidal dysfunction 4. akinetic mutism At least one of the following features: periodic sharp and slow wave complexes (PSWCs) in EEG 14-3-3 proteins in CSF and a clinical duration >2 years High DWI and/or FLAIR signal in the striate and at least two cortical regions
Possible CJD	Clinical features as above No PSWCs in EEG No 14-3-3 detection in CSF Duration <2 years

Periodic sharp wave complexes on EEG are rarely found in younger age groups, but continuously increase up to 66 % in the age over 80 years (Heinemann et al. 2007), (Table 1).

In 1999, Parchi et al described molecular subtypes of sCJD (Parchi et al. 1999). They proposed a classification according to the homo or heterozygosity for methionine (M) and valine (V) at the codon 129 of the prion protein gene and the electrophoretic mobility of the protease-resistant fragment of the pathological prion protein (types 1 and 2). Six subtypes (MM1, MV1, VV1, MM2, MV2, VV2) with different clinical profiles were defined, for further details see Table 2.

1.2.2 Variant CJD

Variant CJD predominantly affects young persons (<30 years of age). The disease course is longer than in sCJD and at disease onset, psychiatric and sensory symptoms like dysaesthesiae or sensation of pain predominate. Later, neurologic symptoms like cerebellar signs and involuntary movements (dystonia, chorea, myoclonus) develop. Finally, the patients are immobile and severely dement. EEG is not specific and does not show periodic sharp wave complexes, the 14-3-3 protein in CSF is detected in about 50–60 % of cases. From a clinical point of view, vCJD can be mismatched with the MV2 subtype of sCJD (Table 3).

Table 2 Diagnostic criteria for sporadic CJD (sCJD)

sCJD subtype	%	Clinics	EEG with PSWCs, CSF: 14-3-3-pos	MRI: high signal on T2/FLAIR/DWI
MM1, MV1	60–70	"Classical" form: rapidly progressive dementia and neurological signs including "Heidenhain" form (predominantly visual changes)	75–80, >96 %	Striatum 80 %
MM2 cortical	1–2	Slowly progressive dementia, late myoclonus, pyramidal/extrapyramidal signs. DD: Alzheimer dementia, DLB	50, 100 %	Striatum 0 % Cortex 100 %
MM2 thalamic	1–2	Psychiatric symptoms, autonomic failure, ataxia, dementia	0–20, 20–100 %	Negative
MV2	10	Slow cognitive decline, ataxia, psychiatric symptoms, extrapyramidal signs (88 %) DD: vCJD	0, 30–57 %	Striatum 50–100 %, Thalamus 88 %
VV1	1–2	Young patients, prolonged duration, personality changes, dementia. DD: vCJD	0, 100 %	Striatum 28 %, Cortex 100 %
VV2	10–15	Dementia, ataxia, myoclonus	0, 84 %	Striatum 70, Cortex 100 %

DD Differential diagnosis, *DLB* Dementia with Lewy bodies

1.3 Therapy

There is no causative therapy.

2 Imaging

The imaging hallmark of sCJD has increased signal intensity of the striatum and the cortex on long TR/long TE images (Fig. 1). It occurs in between around 80 % of cases

Table 3 Diagnostic criteria for variant CJD (vCJD)

	Diagnostic criteria
Definite vCJD	Progressive neuropsychiatric disorder + neuropathological confirmation
Probable vCJD	Progressive neuropsychiatric disorder with a duration >6 months + positive tonsil biopsy or Progressive neuropsychiatric disorder with a duration >6 months + four of the five following symptoms: Early psychiatric symptoms, persistent painful sensory symptoms, ataxia, myoclonus or chorea or dystonia, dementia + EEG without PSWC characteristic of sCJD + MRI with bilateral "pulvinar sign"
Possible vCJD	Progressive neuropsychiatric disorder with a duration > 6 months + four of the five following symptoms: Early psychiatric symptoms, persistent painful sensory symptoms, ataxia, myoclonus or chorea or dystonia, dementia + EEG without PSWC characteristic of sCJD

(Zerr et al. 2009; Tschampa et al. 2005). Other grey matter structures like the thalamus are involved to a lesser degree (Figs. 1, 2) (Tschampa et al. 2003). Especially the cortical signal changes are best appreciated on Diffusion-weighted and FLAIR images, while striatal and thalamic high signal intensities are also visible on Proton density and T2-weighted images (Kallenberg et al. 2006). Increased striatal signal intensity is bilateral, but sometimes somehow asymmetric. It starts in the anteroinferior part of the putamen and always involves the caudate head. High cortical signal is always bilateral with preferential involvement of the parasagittal cortex, while the precentral and postcentral gyri are usually spared (Fig. 3), (Tschampa et al. 2007).

T1-weighted images are usually normal and contrast enhancement does not occur.

White matter involvement occurs but whether it represents a distinct entity (panencephalopathic type) or is a nonspecific end stage of sCJD remains a matter of debate (Matsusue et al. 2004). Since white matter changes are unspecific a closer look to the basal ganglia is essential.

Areas of high signal intensity on DW images reflect diffusion impairment with reduced ADC values. Lesser reduced ADC values can also be measured in visually not affected grey matter (Tschampa et al. 2003). Diffusion changes persist over weeks to months but may disappear in the end stage of CJD. At this time, there is usually severe brain atrophy and in many cases extensive white matter hyperintensities in parallel with a clinical picture of akinetic mutism.

In the early phase of sCJD, DWI signal changes may precede those visible on FLAIR images; however, diagnostic certainty is higher, when signal changes are visible on both sequences. Note that the normal cortical signal is

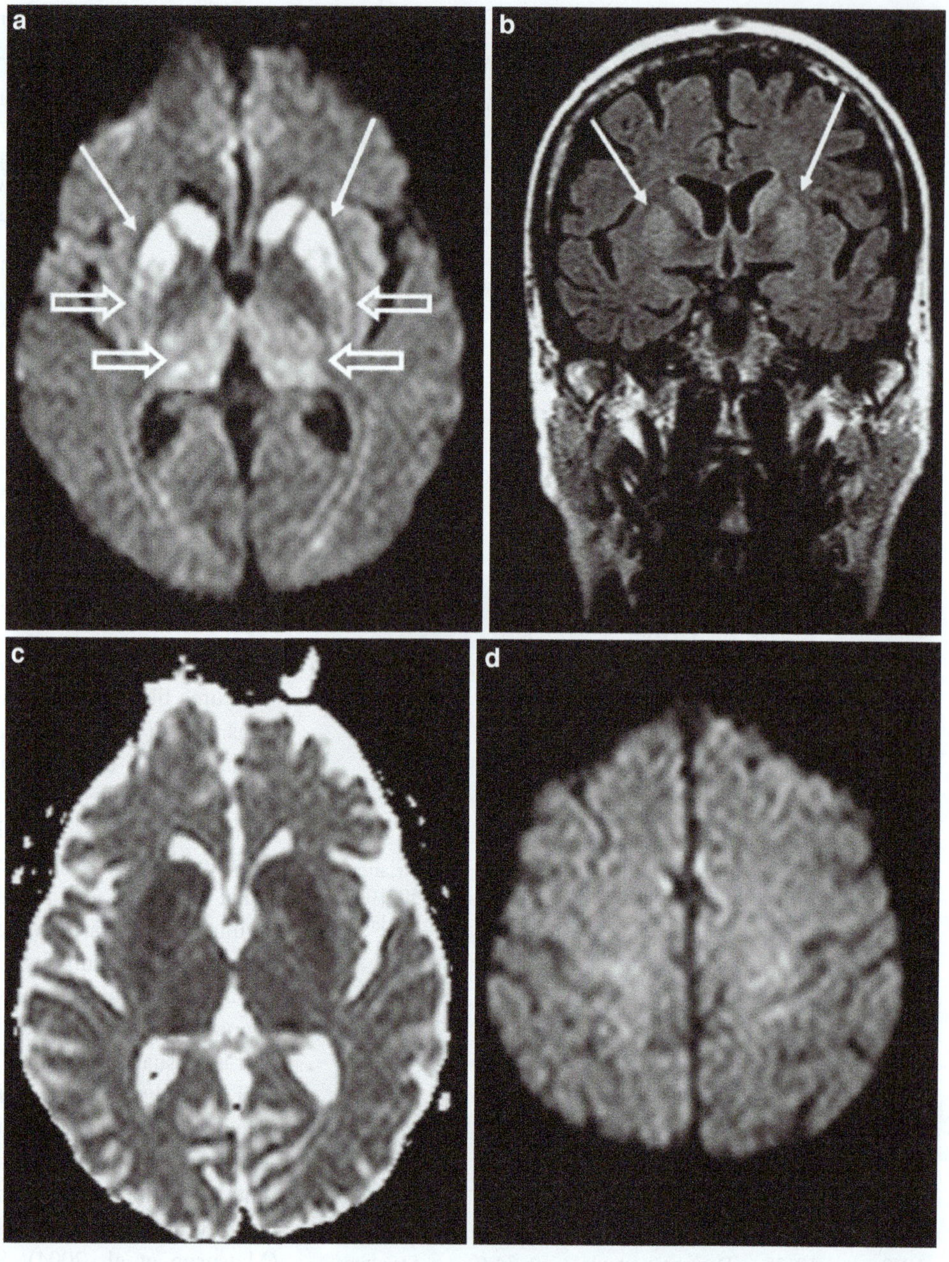

Fig. 1 "Classical" sporadic Creutzfeldt Jakob disease (sCJD). A 66-year-old woman with dementia and myoclonus rapidly progressive over 4 months. Axial Diffusion-weighted at the level of the basal ganglia (**a**) shows markedly increased signal intensity of the anterior putamen and the head of the caudate nucleus on both sides. The posterior part of the putamen as well as the thalami have moderately increased signal intensity. Signal changes are also visible, but not as conspicuous on coronal FLAIR MRI (**b**). Apparent diffusion coefficient (ADC) map proves reduced diffusion of basal ganglia lesions (**c**). The cortex is not involved (**d**) which fits to a molecular MM1 or MV1 subtype

different on FLAIR MRI: it is higher in the limbic structures than in the remaining cortex (Hirai et al. 2000).

There is a correlation between the clinical picture, the distribution of MRI signal changes and the degree of neuropathological changes consisting of pathologic prion protein PrP^{sc} accumulation, neuropil vacuolation (spongiform changes), nerve cell loss and astrogliosis. Increased signal intensity on FLAIR MRI is likely due to astrogliosis (Urbach et al. 1998; Ironside and Head 2004), the pathological substrate of diffusion impairment is not clear yet.

With respect to the molecular sCJD subtypes, MRI is especially helpful in MV2, VV1, and MM2 cortical patients. In MV2 patients, EEG is mostly negative, 14-3-3 is detected in 76 % of patients, whilst about 90 % of patients show increased striatal signal intensity (Krasnianski et al. 2006a). In VV1 patients, EEG is negative whilst 14-3-3 and increased cortical signal intensity has been reported in all patients (Meissner et al. 2005). MM2 cortical patients typically have both, increased cortical signal intensity and high 14-3-3 protein in CSF, PSWCs are found in half of these patients (Krasnianski et al. 2006b).

In vCJD, symmetric bilateral increased signal intensity of the pulvinar thalami is the hallmark of the disease (Fig. 4), (Zeidler et al. 2000). The "pulvinar sign" occurs in between 78 and 90 % of vCJD cases, its specificity is considered to be 100 %. The mediodorsal nuclei of the

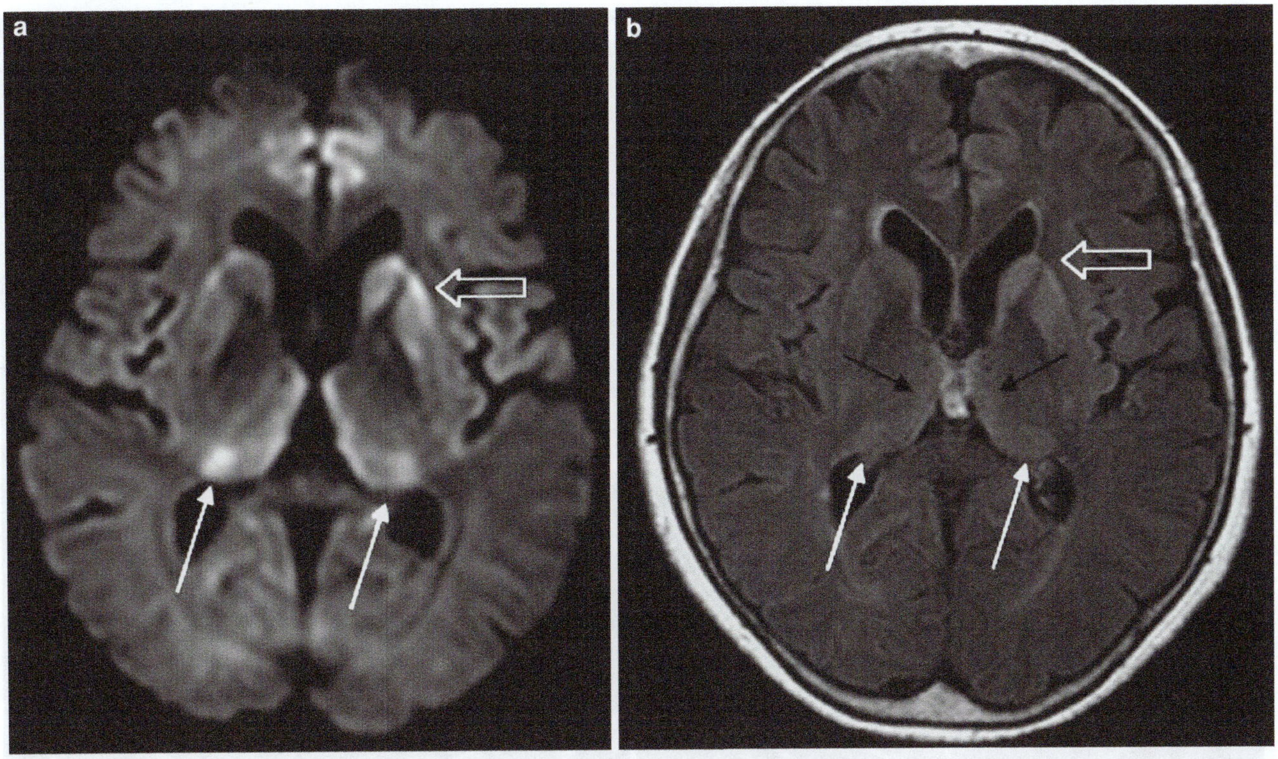

Fig. 2 Sporadic Creutzfeldt Jakob disease (sCJD). A 64-year-old woman with ataxia and cognitive decline since 3 months. Axial Diffusion-weighted (**a**) and FLAIR (**b**) MRI show asymmetrically increased signal intensity of the striate and the thalami. Note the left caudate head and anterior putamen (*open arrow*) have a higher signal than the pulvinar thalami (*white arrows*) and the mediodorsal thalami nuclei (*black arrow*)

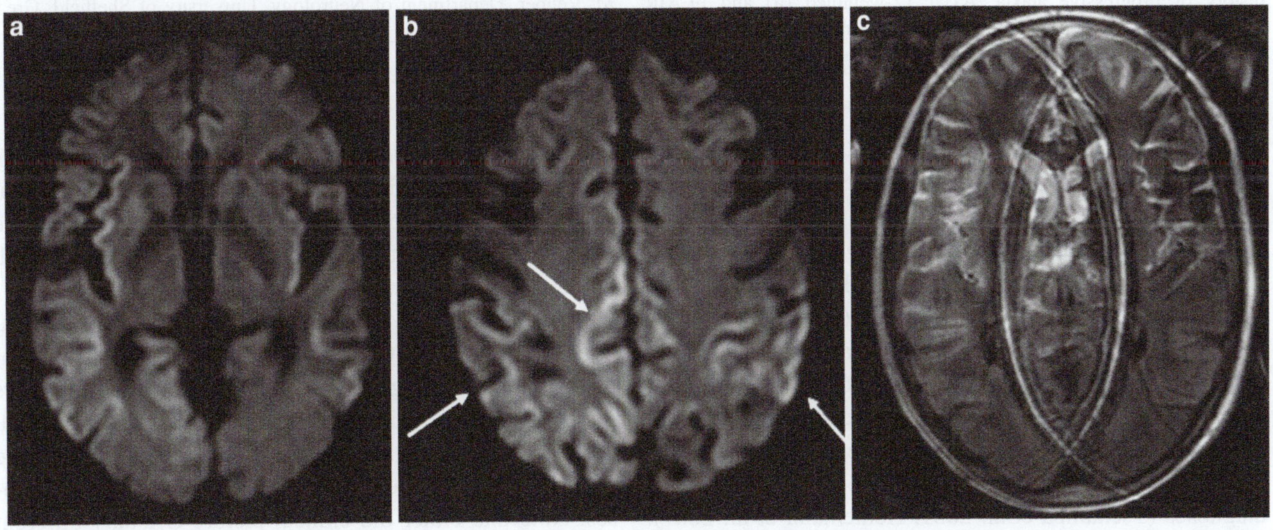

Fig. 3 Sporadic Creutzfeldt Jakob disease (sCJD). A 81-year-old woman with dementia and myoclonus rapidly progressive over 4 months. Axial Diffusion-weighted images (**a**, **b**) show slightly increased signal intensity of the striate whilst the cortex has distinct signal increase. The relatively symmetrical distribution with involvement of the paramedian cortex and sparing of the central region is characteristic for cortical CJD signal changes (**b** *arrows*). One advantage of DWI as compared to FLAIR (**c**) sequences is the shorter acquisition time rendering them insensitive to motion artefacts (Waldman et al. 2003)

thalami are additionally affected in about 56 % of cases, resembling the figure of a hockey stick on axial FLAIR, T2, Proton density or DW images (Collie et al. 2003). Note—in contrast to sCJD—that the signal intensity of the pulvinar thalami is always higher than those of the striate (Linguraru et al. 2006).

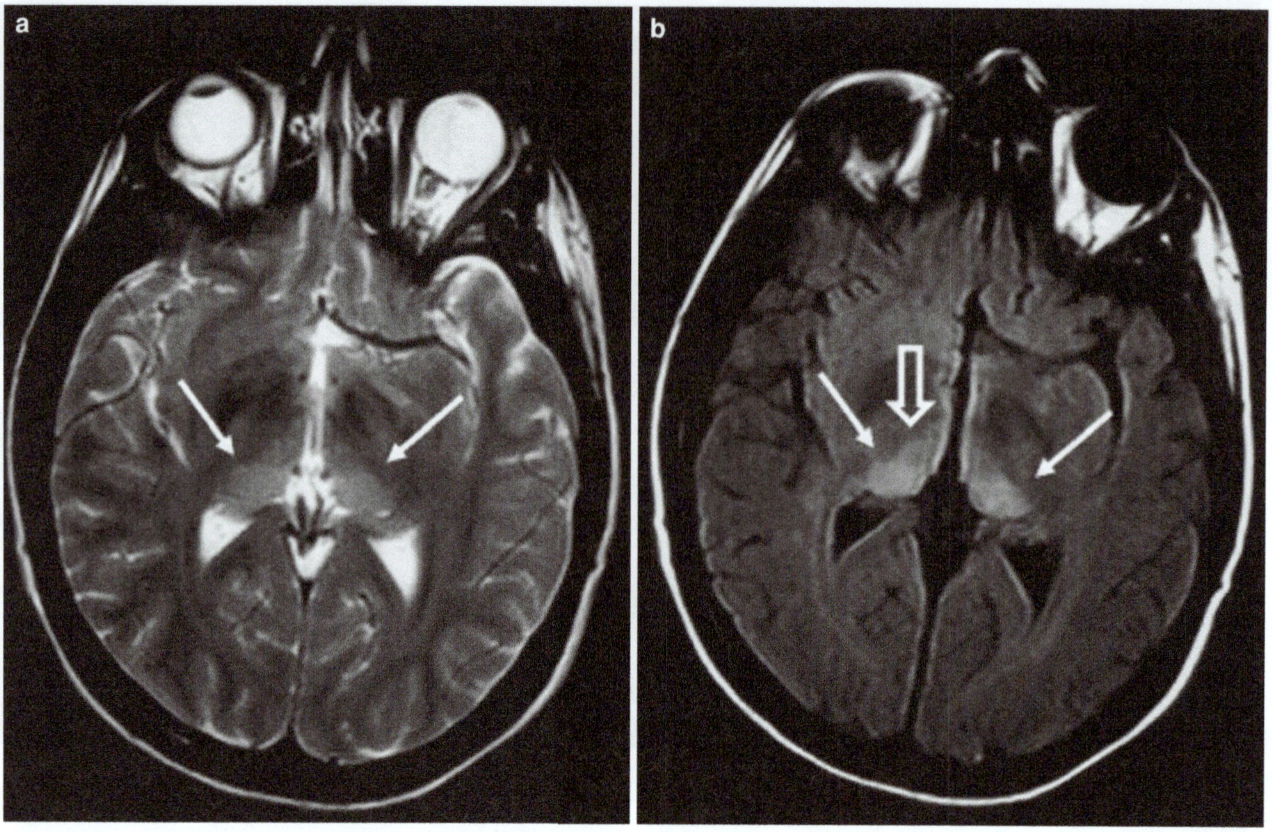

Fig. 4 Variant Creutzfeldt Jakob disease (vCJD). A 38-year-old man with a 9 month history of depression and anxiety and a 3 months history of progressive ataxia. Axial T2-weighted (**a**) and FLAIR (**b**) MRI show symmetrically increased signal intensity of the pulvinar thalami (pulvinar sign). Note subtle signal increase of the dorsomedial thalami (*open arrows*) together resembling a hockey stick. Courtesy of M. Reuber, Department of Neurology, University of Sheffield, Great Britain

3 Differential Diagnosis

From clinical grounds, mainly neurodegenerative disorders are mistaken for CJD. In the German CJD surveillance unit, (rapid progressive) Alzheimer's disease (35 %), Lewy body dementia (9 %), vascular dementia (Urbach et al. 2007) and other vascular diseases (see Fig. 5c) (16 %), multiple system atrophy (3 %), paraneoplastic diseases (see Fig. 5d) (6 %), metabolic disorders (Wernicke encephalopathy, see Fig. 5g–h) and encephalitis were the main differential diagnoses (Tschampa et al. 2001; Heinemann et al. 2007). Note that some progressive disorders like Alzheimer's disease or encephalitis can be accompanied by 14-3-3 detection in CSF which increases the likelihood to falsely diagnose CJD (Burkhard et al. 2001).

From an imaging point of view, there is no other disease that would regularly show high DWI and FLAIR signal in the distribution typical for sCJD. A careful MRI inspection is fundamental in order to avoid misdiagnoses, and the high sensitivity and specificity of MRI in an appropriate clinical context has led to the suggestion to incorporate MRI in the diagnostic WHO criteria (Urbach et al. 2001; Zerr et al. 2009; Chitravas et al. 2011).

For patients with hyperintense basal ganglia, cerebral hypoxia (Fig 5a–b), CO poisoning (Fig 5f), mitochondrial cytopathies including Leigh's disease, metabolic disorders including Wilson's disease and diabetic uraemia (Lee et al. 2007), and encephalitis (Japanese encephalitis, Handique et al. 2006) are frequently mentioned as differential diagnoses. Note that either the clinical picture is totally different (cerebral hypoxia, Leigh's disease) or MRI shows subtle but significant differences: In CO poisoning, bilateral pallidum necrosis occurs whilst the globus pallidus is not affected in CJD. In Wilson's disease, symmetrical T2 hyperintensity, hypointensity or mixed intensity is present in putamina, globi pallidi, caudate nuclei and thalami. Characteristic is (1) a peripheral hyperintense putaminal rim and hypointensity of

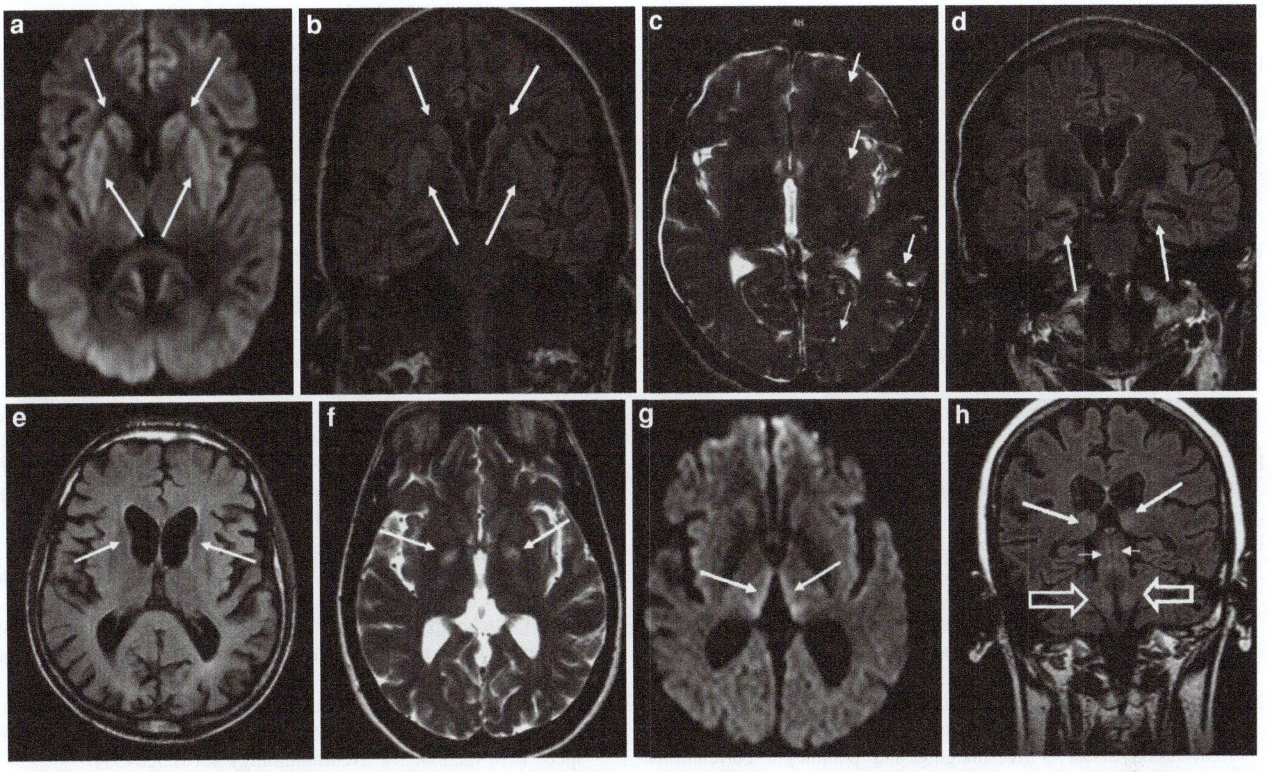

Fig. 5 Differential diagnoses: **a**, **b** Diffuse hypoxia. Moderate signal increase of both putamen and caudate heads (*arrows*) 6 weeks after a 26-year-old woman had been resuscitated following a cardiac arrest. **c** Dural a.v. fistula. Note the serpenginous flow void structures (*arrows*) representing the retrograde venous filling in a 75-year-old male with rapid cognitive decline and progressive aphasia. **d** Paraneoplastic limbic encephalitis in a 64-year-old man who developed complex partial seizures and progressive memory disturbances. MRI shows bilateral hippocampus atrophy (*arrows*), tumor search revealed small cell lung cancer. **e** Huntington's chorea with atrophy of both caudate heads and consecutive dilatation of the frontal horns of the lateral ventricles. **f** CO posioning with bilateral pallidum necrosis. **f–h** Wernicke encephalopathy of a 74-year-old woman. Note the signal changes along the IIIrd ventricle (*arrows*), periaqueductal (*short arrows*), and in the dorsal medulla (*open arrows*)

thc globi pallidi and (2) the "face on the giand panda sign" on axial slices through the midbrain (Sinha et al. 2006). In Wernicke encephalopathy, signal intensity on T2-weighted and Diffusion-weighted sequences is symmetrically increased in the periventricular region of the third ventricle (about 85 % of patients), in the periaqueductal area (65 %), in the mamillary bodies (58 %), in the tectal plate (38 %) and in the dorsal medulla (8 % of patients). Contrast enhancement of the mamillary bodies occurs in about half of patients and is positively correlated with alcohol abuse (Zuccoli et al. 2007).

For patients with hyperintense cortex, postictal changes (non-convulsive status epilepticus), cortical infarcts and posterior reversible encephalopythy syndrome (PRES) could be possible differential diagnoses. The symmetric pattern and the involvement of the anterior putamen and caudate heads should lead to the diagnosis of sCJD.

For patients with vCJD, the most important differential diagnosis is sCJD. Radiological differential diagnoses include post-infectious encephalitis and Alpers syndrome (progressive infantile poliodystrophy, a rare genetically determined mitochondrial cytopathy).

References

Burkhard PR, Sanchez JC, Landis T, Hochstrasser DF (2001) CSF detection of the 14-3-3 protein in unselected patients with dementia. Neurology 56:1528–1533

Chitravas N, Jung RS, Kofskey DM, Blevins JE, Gambetti P, Leigh RJ, Cohen ML (2011 Sep) Treatable neurological disorders misdiagnosed as Creutzfeldt–Jakob disease. Ann Neurol 70(3):437–444

Collie DA, Summers DM, Sellar RJ, Ironside JW, Cooper S, Zeidler M, Knight R, Will RG (2003) Diagnosing variant Creutzfeldt–Jakob disease with the pulvinar sign: MR imaging findings in 86 neuropathologically confirmed cases. AJNR Am J Neuroradiol 24:1560–1569

Handique SK, Das RR, Barman K, Medhi N, Saharia B, Saikia P, Ahmed SA (2006) Temporal lobe involvement in Japanese encephalitis: problems in differential diagnosis. AJNR Am J Neuroradiol 27:1027–1031

Heinemann U, Krasnianski A, Meissner B, Varges D, Kallenberg K, Schulz-Schaeffer WJ, Steinhoff BJ, Grasbon-Frodl EM, Kretzschmar HA, Zerr I (2007) Creutzfeldt–Jakob disease in Germany: a prospective 12-year surveillance. Brain 130:1350–1359

Hirai T, Korogi Y, Yoshizumi Y, Shigematsu Y, Sugahara T, Takahashi M (2000) Limbic lobe of the human brain: evaluation with turbo fluid-attenuated inversion recovery imaging. Radiology 215:470–475

Ironside JW (2010) Variant Creutzfeldt–Jakob disease. Haemophilia 16(Suppl 5):175–180. (Review)

Ironside JW, Head MW (2004) Neuropathology and molecular biology of variant Creutzfeldt–Jakob disease. Curr Top Microbiol Immunol 284:133–159

Kallenberg K, Schulz-Schaeffer WJ, Jastrow U, Poser S, Meissner B, Tschampa HJ, Zerr I, Knauth M (2006) Creutzfeldt–Jakob disease: comparative analysis of MR imaging sequences. AJNR Am J Neuroradiol 27:1459–1462

Krasnianski A, Meissner B, Schulz-Schaeffer W, Kallenberg K, Bartl M, Heinemann U, Varges D, Kretzschmar HA, Zerr I (2006a) Clinical features and diagnosis of the MM2 cortical subtype of sporadic Creutzfeldt–Jakob disease. Arch Neurol 63:876–880

Krasnianski A, Schulz-Schaeffer WJ, Kallenberg K, Meissner B, Collie DA, Roeber S, Bartl M, Heinemann U, Varges D, Kretzschmar HA, Zerr I (2006b) Clinical findings and diagnostic tests in the MV2 subtype of sporadic CJD. Brain 129:2288–2296

Lee EJ, Park JH, Ihn YK, Lee SK, Park CS (2007) Acute bilateral basal ganglia lesions in diabetic uraemia: diffusion-weighted MRI. Neuroradiology 49:1009–1014

Linguraru MG, Ayache N, Bardinet E, Ballester MA, Galanaud D, Haïk S, Faucheux B, Hauw JJ, Cozzone P, Dormont D, Brandel JP (2006) Differentiation of sCJD and vCJD forms by automated analysis of basal ganglia intensity distribution in multisequence MRI of the brain–definition and evaluation of new MRI-based ratios. IEEE Trans Med Imaging 25:1052–1067

Matsusue E, Kinoshita T, Sugihara S, Fujii S, Ogawa T, Ohama E (2004) White mater lesions in panencephalopathic type of Creutzfeldt–Jakob disease: MR imaging and pathologic correlations. AJNR Am J Neuroradiol 25:910–918

Meissner B, Westner IM, Kallenberg K, Krasnianski A, Bartl M, Varges D, Bösenberg C, Kretzschmar HA, Knauth M, Schulz-Schaeffer WJ, Zerr I (2005) Sporadic Creutzfeldt–Jakob disease: clinical and diagnostic characteristics of the rare VV1 type. Neurology 65:1544–1550

Parchi P, Giese A, Capellari S, Brown P, Schulz-Schaeffer W, Windl O, Zerr I, Budka H, Kopp N, Piccardo P, Poser S, Rojiani A, Streichemberger N, Julien J, Vital C, Ghetti B, Gambetti P, Kretzschmar H (1999) Classification of sporadic Creutzfeldt–Jakob disease based on molecular and phenotypic analysis of 300 subjects. Ann Neurol 46:224–233

Sinha S, Taly AB, Ravishankar S, Prashanth LK, Venugopal KS, Arunodaya GR, Vasudev MK (2006 Sep) Swamy HS Wilson's disease: cranial MRI observations and clinical correlation. Neuroradiology 48(9):613–621

Tschampa HJ, Neumann M, Zerr I, Henkel K, Schröter A, Schulz-Schaeffer WJ, Steinhoff BJ, Kretzschmar HA, Poser S (2001) Patients with Alzheimer's disease and dementia with Lewy bodies mistaken for Creutzfeldt–Jakob disease. J Neurol Neurosurg Psychiatry 71:33–39

Tschampa HJ, Mürtz P, Flacke S, Paus S, Schild HH, Urbach H (2003) Thalamic involvement in sporadic Creutzfeldt–Jakob disease: a diffusion weighted MRI study. Am J Neuroradiol AJNR 24:908–915

Tschampa HJ, Kallenberg K, Urbach H, Meissner B, Nicolay C, Kretzschmar HA, Knauth M, Zerr I (2005) MRI in the diagnosis of sporadic Creutzfeldt–Jakob disease: a study on inter-observer agreement. Brain 128:2026–2033

Tschampa HJ, Zerr I, Urbach H (2006) Radiological assessment of Creutzfeldt–Jakob disease. Eur Radiol 17:1200–1211

Tschampa HJ, Kallenberg K, Kretschmar HA, Meissner B, Knauth M, Urbach H, Zerr I (2007) Pattern of cortical changes in sporadic Creutzfeldt–Jakob disease. Am J Neuroradiol AJNR 28:1114–1118

Urbach H, Klisch J, Wolf HK, Brechtelsbauer D, Gass S, Solymosi L (1998) MRI in sporadic Creutzfeldt–Jakob disease: correlation with clinical and neuropathological data. Neuroradiology 40:65–70

Urbach H, Paus S, Tschampa HJ, Keller E, Schild HH (2001) Creutzfeldt–Jakob-Krankheit: Stellenwert der MRT. Fortschr Röntgenstr 173:509–514

Urbach H, Tschampa H, Flacke S, Thal D (2007) MR Imaging of vascular dementia and differential diagnoses or is it really vascular dementia? Clin Neuroradiol 17:88–97

Waldman AD, Jarman P, Merry RT (2003) Rapid echoplanar diffusion imaging in a case of variant Creutzfeldt–Jakob disease; where speed is of the essence. Neuroradiology 45(8):528–531

Zeidler M, Sellar RJ, Collie DA, Knight R, Stewart G, Macleod MA, Ironside JW, Cousens S, Colchester AC, Hadley DM, Will RG (2000) The pulvinar sign on magnetic resonance imaging in variant Creutzfeldt–Jakob disease. Lancet 355:1412–1418

Zerr I, Kallenberg K, Summers DM, Romero C, Taratuto A, Heinemann U, Breithaupt M, Varges D, Meissner B, Ladogana A, Schuur M, Haik S, Collins SJ, Jansen GH, Stokin GB, Pimentel J, Hewer E, Collie D, Smith P, Roberts H, Brandel JP, van Duijn C, Pocchiari M, Begue C, Cras P, Will RG, Sanchez-Juan P (2009 Oct) Updated clinical diagnostic criteria for sporadic Creutzfeldt–Jakob disease. Brain 132(Pt 10):2659–2668

Zuccoli G, Gallucci M, Capellades J, Regnicolo L, Tumiati B, Giadás TC, Bottari W, Mandrioli J, Bertolini M (2007) Wernicke encephalopathy: MR findings at clinical presentation in twenty-six alcoholic and nonalcoholic patients. AJNR Am J Neuroradiol 28:1328–1331

Fungal Infections

Markus Möhlenbruch and Jens Fiehler

Contents

M. Möhlenbruch (✉)
Division of Neuroradiology,
University of Heidelberg Medical Center,
Im Neuenheimer Feld 400, 69120 Heidelberg, Germany
e-mail: Markus.Moehlenbruch@med.uni-heidelberg.de

J. Fiehler
Department of Diagnostic and Interventional Neuroradiology,
Clinic and Policlinic of Neuroradiology,
University of Hamburg-Eppendorf Medical Center,
Martinistrasse 52, 20246 Hamburg, Germany

Abstract

The manifestations of fungal infections result in life-threatening conditions and the major role of the neuroradiologist is to recognize the manifestation and make an educated guess as to the type of pathogen. Magnetic resonance imaging is the imaging modality of choice, and administration of gadolinium contrast is essential to identify areas of enhancement that may be subtle. In principle, fungal CNS infections can lead to meningitis (with secondary hydrocephalus), meningoencephalitis, vasculitis, and formation of abscesses and granulomas. The small yeast forms (*Coccidioides, Histoplasma, Cryptococcus*) usually reach the small arterioles and capillaries. They cause leptomeningitis and subpial ischemic lesions as they have access to the microcirculation from which they seed the subarachnoid space. The large hyphal forms (*Aspergillus and Zygomyces*) obstruct larger arteries and thus cause large infarcts. A ring-enhancing inhomogeneous lesion with irregular walls and projections into the cavity with low apparent diffusion coefficient and without contrast enhancement of these projections carries a high probability of being a fungal abscess. Due to the lack of inflammatory response, neuroradiological findings in fungal infections are often atypical and thus hard to interpret.

1 General Considerations

A fungus is a unique eukaryotic organism that reproduces commonly via spores. For medical purposes fungi may be differentiated into hyphae and yeasts. Hyphae are multicellular colonies of long, branching filamentous cells that reproduce by forming spores or by budding. In contrast, yeasts are colonies of unicellular organisms. Some genera of fungi are dimorphic–hyphae and yeast coexist.

S. Hähnel (ed.), *Inflammatory Diseases of the Brain*, Medical Radiology. Diagnostic Imaging,
DOI: 10.1007/174_2012_638, © Springer-Verlag Berlin Heidelberg 2012
Published Online: 15 June 2012

Table 1 Fungal infections and immunostatus

Immunocompromised only	Immunocompetent and immunocompromised
Aspergillus	*Cryptococcus*
Candida	*Coccidioides*
Mucor	*Histoplasma*

Occurring worldwide, most fungi are largely invisible to the eye, living for the most part in soil and dead matter and as symbionts of plants or animals. Several fungi are an integral part of the gastrointestinal tract, the lung, and the surface of the body, and usually do no harm. The occurrence of fungal infections depends on the environment, the climatic conditions, and the socioeconomic status of the human hosts, on their habits and, inevitably, on genetic factors. Atypical forms of fungal infections originating from other regions of the world emerge in local hosts as a result of global travel and migration. With the exception of *Candida albicans*, which is a normal inhabitant of the intestinal tract, most fungi enter the body by inhalation or via skin abrasions.

Generally, fungal infections of the central nervous system (CNS) have been recognized and diagnosed for decades but usually still represent a clinical surprise since they are still very rare in the general population. In most cases, fungal infections present without specific characteristics. They are frequently mistaken for other infections such as tuberculosis, pyogenic abscess, or even brain tumors like lymphoma.

Normally, fungal infections are of low virulence and confined to local infections. In immunocompromised states, the same fungus tends to produce invasive infection with devastating consequences. The increase in frequency that has been observed over the past two decades results from the increasing number of people with longstanding diabetes and immunocompromised patients who are surviving longer periods because of either widespread use of immunosuppressive drugs, a larger aging population, increased number of malignancies, spread of AIDS, and numerous less frequent reasons. Nevertheless, immunocompetent hosts may also suffer from some types of fungal infections (Table 1).

Although almost any fungus may cause encephalitis, cryptococcal meningoencephalitis is most frequently seen, followed by aspergillosis, and more rarely by candidiasis. Patients with AIDS appear to be prone to infections by *Candida*, *Cryptococcus*, and *Histoplasma*, whereas aspergillosis is uncommon in those patients. Aspergillosis is usually observed in patients with hematological malignancies, with autoimmune disorders with prolonged steroid therapy, or in patients who had undergone transplantation of solid organs.

The manifestations of fungal infections often result in life-threatening conditions. The major role of the neuroradiologist is to recognize the manifestation and make an educated guess as to the type of the pathogen based on the combination of patient history and imaging appearance. Fungal infection should always be considered in patients at risk since untreated fungal CNS infections have extremely high mortality rates. On the other hand, the suspected diagnosis should be based on careful consideration since fungal therapy often has serious side effects (Dubey et al. 2005).

Magnetic resonance imaging is the modality of choice, and contrast administration is essential to identify areas of enhancement that may be subtle in these patients. In principle, fungal CNS infections can lead to meningitis with the possible consequence of hydrocephalus, meningoencephalitis, vasculitis, and formation of abscesses and granulomas. Due to the lack of inflammatory response, neuroradiological findings are often atypical and thus difficult to interpret. Especially immunocompromised patients with AIDS and those who had undergone bone marrow transplantation often do not show any enhancement or perifocal edema.

Knowledge about the morphology and size of the pathogenic organism helps to understand the implications of this sort of aggression against the CNS and dictate the development, location, and appearance of CNS lesions. The small yeast forms (*Coccidioides*, *Histoplasma*, *Cryptococcus*) usually reach the small arterioles and capillaries. They cause leptomeningitis and subpial ischemic lesions as they have access to the microcirculation from which they may seed the subarachnoid space (Table 2). In contrast, the large hyphal forms (*Aspergillus* and *Zygomyces*) have no such access to the microvasculature. Hyphae form mycelian colonies instead, which invade and obstruct larger arteries and occasionally veins. By doing so they cause large infarcts or form colonies that retrogradely disseminate along larger vessels.

Routine histology, special stains, and morphological characteristics indicate the type of fungus, but assignment to a certain species needs culturing and biochemical characterization; however, the final diagnosis must be based on epidemiological, clinical, laboratory, and imaging knowledge. The most important specific fungal infections are discussed in the following section.

Table 2 Differential diagnosis

	Affected persons	Disease spread	CNS manifestation	Typical imaging appearance features
Cryptococcus neoformans	AIDS patients	Yeast cells	Leptomeningitis, cryptococcomas in plexus and parenchyma	Imaging often negative, leptomeningeal enhancement with minimal inflammatory reaction, mucoid matter in Virchow-Robin spaces (soap-bubble pattern)
Coccidiodes	Immunocompromised in southwestern U.S., Central and South America	Yeast cells	Leptomeningitis	Marked meningeal enhancement, vasculitic infarcts, communicating hydrocephalus
Histoplasma capsulatum		Yeast cells	Leptomeningitis, rarely parenchymal granulomas (histoplasmomas)	Nodular or annular foci of hematogenous distribution with variable edema
Candida albicans	AIDS patients and microbial selection by medication	Pseudohyphae	Scattered brain microabscesses	Multiple hypointense lesions on T1-weighted, ring enhancement after gadolinium application, and intermediate-signal lesions within surrounding high signal on T2-weighted
Mucor	Diabetes mellitus, with diabetic ketoacidosis	Hyphae	Massive rhinocerebral spread	Confluent regions of T2-weighted hyperintense signal in the basal portions of the frontal and temporal lobes, hemorrhages
Aspergillus fumiginatus	Hematological malignancies, solid organ transplantation, prolonged steroid therapy	Hyphae	Maxillary sinusitis with direct infiltration into the basal bones, invasion of the vascular wall of arteries and veins, infarcts, hemorrhage	Hemorrhagic lesions, solid enhancing lesions in frontal and temporal lobes, cortical and subcortical infarction, pseudoaneurysms

2 Cryptococcus

2.1 Epidemiology, Clinical Presentation, Therapy

2.1.1 The Fungus

Cryptococcus neoformans is an encapsulated yeast-like fungus that can live in both plants and animals. It usually grows as yeast (unicellular) and replicates by budding. When grown as a yeast, *Cryptococcus neoformans* has a prominent capsule composed mostly of polysaccharides, which protects it from host inflammatory response. Microscopically, the India ink stain is used for easy visualization of the capsule. The particles of ink pigment do not enter the capsule that surrounds the spherical yeast cell, resulting in a zone of clearance or "halo" around the cells. Infection with *Cryptococcus neoformans* is termed cryptococcosis.

2.1.2 Epidemiology

In general, *Cryptococcus neoformans* is considered the most frequent cause of fungal leptomeningitis and considered among the two most frequent CNS fungal infections. The fungus is most frequently isolated from mammal and bird feces, particularly pigeon droppings, but also from soil, wood, and trees. *Cryptococcus* is mostly limited to tropical and subtropical regions but is usually a saprophyte in the human skin and mucous membrane. It seems to be very robust: Recent studies made on the Chernobyl Nuclear Power Plant have shown that colonies of *Cryptococcus neoformans* were even developing on the ruins of the melted-down reactor. Cryptococcosis is reported worldwide with male predominance. This has been explained partly by the fact that estrogen inhibits its growth. It may cause infection both in immunocompromised and immunocompetent individuals. More than half of the patients with disseminated disease are immunocompromised. Transmission from person to person has not been reported. Approximately 5–10 % of HIV-infected patients develop cryptococcal meningitis as an AIDS-defining illness and in about 40 %, this represents the initial clinical manifestation. While *Cryptococcus neoformans* causes the most common CNS fungal infection in patients with AIDS, its relative frequency ranks third after HIV encephalitis and cerebral toxoplasmosis among all CNS infections in AIDS.

2.1.3 Manifestation and Disease Spread

Cryptococcosis is a deep visceral, systemic cutaneous mycosis. Because of presence of soluble anticryptococcal factors in serum and absence in cerebrospinal fluid (CSF) the CNS is the preferred site for cryptococcal infection. Through inhalation the lung is believed to be the major entry site for these fungi. They then spread hematogenously and involve the walls of meningeal vessels and thence Virchow-Robin's spaceVirchow-Robin's perivascular spaces and the CSF-producing meningitis. Meningitis is the most common manifestation of hematogenous dissemination of *Cryptococcus* infection. The CSF flow in complement and immunoglobulins facilitates establishment of infection in the basal meninges and choroid plexus.

Cryptococcal meningitis is seen in immunocompromised patients. Intracranial colonies within the Virchow-Robin's perivascular spaces lead to the accumulation of mucoid matter with gelatinous pseudocysts forming later that enlarge the local spaces to give them a "soap-bubble" pattern. Due to stability of the BBB and to the absence of local inflammatory response, no significant enhancement is seen in this disease pattern. Cryptococcosis typically produces a chronic basal meningitis or meningoencephalitis with minimal inflammatory reaction. Rarely, *cryptococcomas*, as localized granulomatous masses, ventriculitis, and inflammation of the choroid plexus, are observed. Occasionally, space-occupying lesions at the choroid plexus have been described. *Cryptococcus neoformans* infection, though, has significant affinity for CNS, and rarely results in infarction. Extraneural cryptococcosis (mainly in lung, skin, and genitourinary tract) may accompany CNS disease. The systemic infection of *Cryptococcus* from the primary pulmonary and cutaneous focus is essentially hematogenous.

2.1.4 Clinical Presentation

The disease may manifest subacutely with headache and signs of meningeal irritation, or may even present as an acute fulminating, rapidly fatal form. *Cryptococcus neoformans* causes minimal inflammation in patients with AIDS, accounting for the frequent absence of meningeal signs. Fever and neck stiffness may be slight or absent. Symptoms are often mild and nonspecific and may present in an acute or, more commonly, indolent form dating from 2 to 4 weeks earlier. The most common clinical manifestations are fever and headache (75–90 % of patients), nausea and vomiting (40 % of patients), meningismus (30–45 % of patients), photophobia and visual disturbances (20–30 % of patients), behavioral changes (20–30 % of patients), lethargy, altered mental status, personality changes and memory loss (11–30 % of patients), and seizures (10 % of patients). Elevated intracranial pressure, a very important sign that has prognostic value, is observed in 50–75 % of patients.

2.2 Serologic Tests, Therapy, and Prognosis

The CSF analysis is an effective complementary method of diagnosis that enables measurement of exit pressure and CSF studies. The detection of cryptococcal capsular polysaccharide antigen in the serum and CSF is highly sensitive and specific for cryptococcosis, which corresponds to the severity of illness. India ink stains of the CSF are also very helpful because they often confirm the presence of the characteristically round encapsulated forms of cryptococci. Even with intensive antifungal treatment (i.e. amphotericin B), outcome is often poor and mortality as high as 70 %.

2.3 Imaging

In the majority of cases with cryptococcosis the MRI is normal ("cryptic" disease), particularly in AIDS patients. A mild atrophy has been described; thus, in individuals with suspected fungal infection, above all those with AIDS, it is of utmost importance to analyze the CSF.

The following four distinct patterns may be differentiated only rarely:

1. Fungal leptomeningitis with mild enlargement of the ventricles and rarely nodular enhancement of the leptomeninges (Fig. 1).
2. Dilated Virchow-Robin spaces appearing as symmetric non-enhancing gelatinous pseudocysts in basal ganglia and thalami. Those preformed spaces are filled with fungi and mucoid material in variable relative amounts without invasion of the surrounding brain.
3. Cryptococcomas consisting of fungi, mucoid material, and inflammatory cells that form solid or ring-enhancing masses preferentially in the choroid plexus (Table 2).
4. A mixed pattern.

Signs of leptomeningitis are often missing in immunocompromised patients. If visible, basal meningitis is hard to distinguish from *Mycobacterium tuberculosis*, with T1 shortening of CSF in the basal cisterns and enhancement of loculated collections after contrast administration (Erly et al. 1999). On the other hand, patients with cryptococcomas are found in patients who are not immunocompromised. In CT studies, these lesions are usually hypoattenuating, and their specific location within the perivascular spaces, as well as their expanding aspect, help prevent them being mistaken for vascular lesions as sequelae.

Magnetic resonance is the most effective imaging method for demonstrating small focal perivascular space enlargements in the basal ganglia, thalami, substantia nigra,

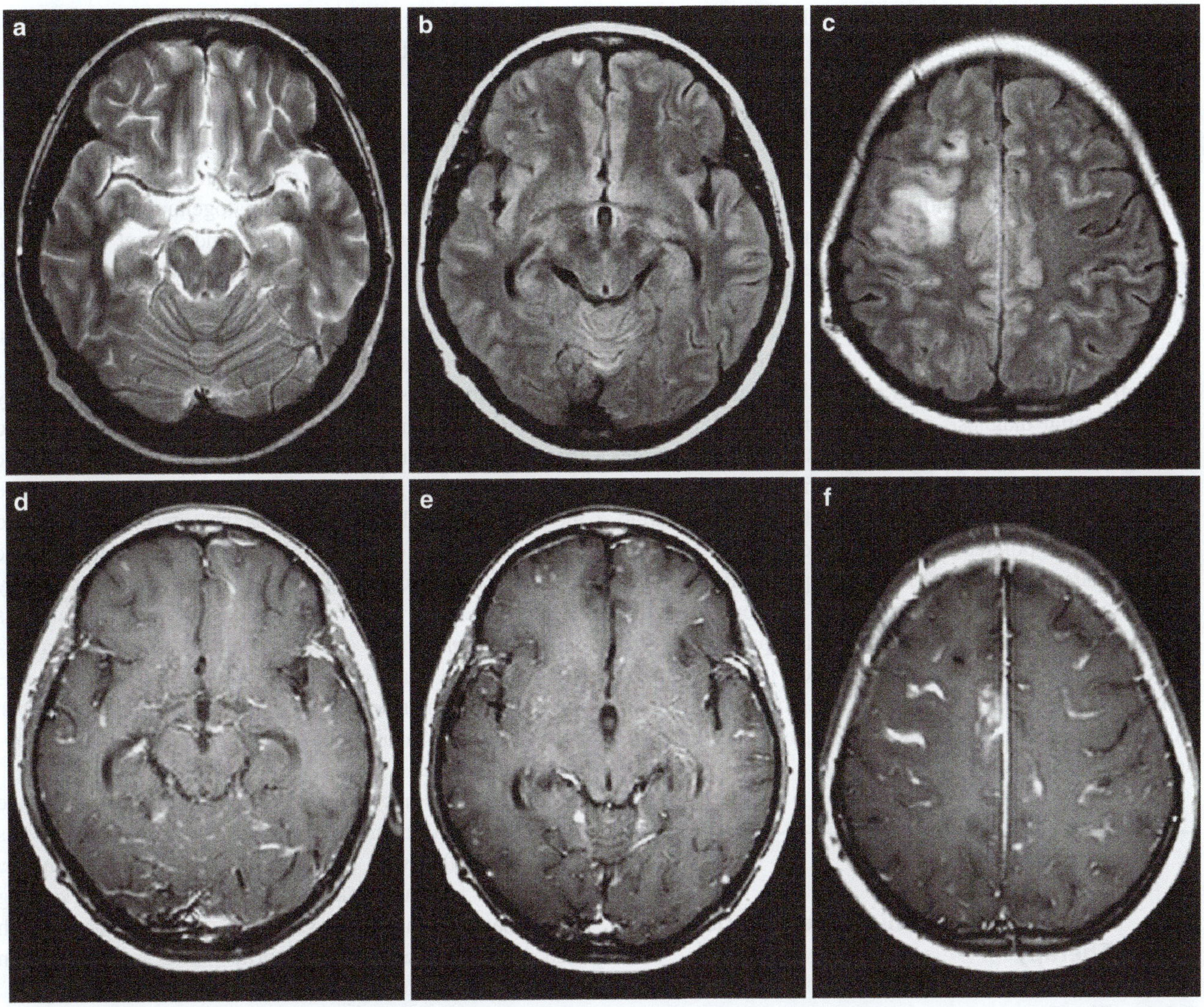

Fig. 1 Cryptococcocal leptomeningitis. **a** Axial T2-weighted image. **b** Axial FLAIR images. **c** Axial FLAIR images. **d, e** Axial T1-weighted images after contrast administration. The parenchymal reaction may be absent in the basal sections of T2-weighted images (**a**) but is usually seen on FLAIR images (**b**, **c**). There is marked parenchymal edema frontally in FLAIR (**b**, **c**) and continuous or mild nodular enhancement of the leptomeninges in the related meninges on T1-weighted images (**d–f**). (Courtesy of S. Geibprasert-Krings)

periventricular regions, and also in choroid plexus. These lesions constitute a "soap-bubble appearance." This pattern allows a quick provisional diagnosis that leads to rapid antifungal treatment. These lesions usually have a similar signal to CSF on T1- and T2-weighted images but may be hyperintense on FLAIR images. Perilesional edema and enhancement can occur but are usually minimal or absent in individuals who have not yet undergone specific treatment. In immunocompetent patients or in patients with AIDS under highly active antiretroviral treatment who develop an immune reconstitution syndrome, the lesions can become ring enhancing. Enlargement of the enhancement and the edema areas may be an indicator for a favorable response to treatment.

Small parenchymal lesions can be demonstrated best by the use of contrast-enhanced MR images. These small lesions result from parenchymal dissemination of the disease from the involved deep small vessels. These foci will have a nodular or annular aspect, depending on their size, and stem from the formation of parenchymal granulomas. These small foci may grow through the multiplication of fungi leading to local accumulation of gelatinous matter, which gives them a cystic aspect, associated with the presence of inflammatory cells, perilesional edema, and rupture of the blood–brain barrier with focal enhancement.

Focal involvement of the choroid plexus has been well demonstrated due to the presence of large local perivascular spaces. Intraventricular granulomas have been described with a very peculiar imaging pattern with a signal isointense to CSF on T1- and T2-weighted images but hyperintense to CSF on DWI mimicking intraventricular epidermoid tumor. It is believed that this may reflect inorganic structures of cryptococcal granuloma in an active state. Incidence of large granulomas by intraventricular *cryptococcus* is very rare.

In immunocompetent individuals the most common form of presentation for cerebral involvement is the formation of cryptococcomas, which might enhance as a result of an immunologic reaction by the host. Only approximately 5 % of individuals with immunodeficiencies will present isolated cryptococcomas. This form shows on DWI hypointensity in the central cavity and thus is a major diagnostic challenge. The differential diagnosis must be carried out for several types of infectious and even tumoral lesions. H-1 MR spectroscopy demonstrates marked increase in lactate along with decrease in N-acetyl aspartate (NAA), choline, and creatine.

It should be pointed out that the demonstration of the imaging patterns mentioned is highly specific for the diagnosis of cryptococcosis, particularly in the form of gelatinous pseudocysts inside deep perivascular spaces; however, the sensitivity of the imaging methods is compromised owing to the occurrence of forms of cryptococcosis without enlargement of the perivascular spaces, but only with colonization of the CSF.

3 Aspergillosis

3.1 Epidemiology, Clinical Presentation, Therapy

3.1.1 The Fungus

Aspergillus spp. was first cataloged by an Italian priest and biologist who was reminded of the shape of a holy-water sprinkler (aspergillum). *Aspergillus* spp. are highly aerobic and are found in starchy food, decaying vegetation, and organic debris matter. *Aspergillus fumigatus* is the most common human pathogen; however, *A. flavus*, *A. niger*, and *A. oxyzae* are also frequently seen. It consists of branching septate hyphae varying from 4 to 12 mm in width, producing numerous spores. The asexually produced conidia are the infective form of the organism that is inhaled through the respiratory route. Tissue destruction and disease are caused by filamentous forms after germination.

3.1.2 Epidemiology

Aspergillosis has a worldwide distribution. Although essentially an opportunistic disease, it is surprisingly rare in the CNS of individuals with AIDS. In contrast, it is usually related to immunosuppression such as neutropenia and long-term corticosteroid use. As a patient cohort, CNS aspergillosis is most often seen in cardiac, renal, and other organ transplantation patients—most frequently after bone marrow transplantation.

3.1.3 Disease Spread and Pathobiology

Intracranial infection can affect the parenchyma or the meninges via two principal routes. First, cerebral manifestations are a typical site for hematogenous spread from a primary pulmonary infection. Second, direct inoculation into the CNS may occur during surgical procedures or spread from the paranasal sinuses, and the mastoid and middle ear as *Aspergillus* fungal spores are commensal in the respiratory tract and external auditory canal.

Maxillary sinusitis is the most common site of primary *Aspergillus* infection, where direct infiltration (Fig. 2) into the basal bones may lead to osteomyelitis. The chronic indolent form of paranasal sinus aspergillosis may invade the orbit, the skull base as well as the anterior, middle, and posterior cranial fossae, and the parasellar regions with the formation of intracranial granulomas. This pattern is usually termed the sinocranial or rhinocerebral form. An abscess caused by *Aspergillus* contains a central necrosis area surrounded by a wall of hemorrhagic necrosis with acute inflammation interspersed with numerous hyphal elements. A spectrum of manifestations with more than one pathological process can be present at any given time.

Aspergillosis has an angiotropic predilection to invade the vascular wall of arteries and veins, with microorganisms growing in the wall and lumen of vessels, leading to thrombosis and subsequent aseptic infarcts. The evolving hemorrhagic infarcts convert into septic infarcts with associated abscesses and cerebritis since infarcted brain tissue is an excellent environment for culture.

The ability of *Aspergillus* to produce elastase, which degrades the vessel wall, may lead to cerebral hemorrhage or, rarely, to the formation of true mycotic aneurysms. In contrast to aneurysm-based bacterial infection, aneurysms in aspergillosis tend to be more fusiform and involve longer and more proximal segments of intracranial vessels such as basilar, middle, and posterior cerebral arteries. Less commonly, aneurysms follow after meningitis or aneurysm clipping.

3.1.4 Clinical Presentation and Prognosis

Aspergillosis should be considered in cases of acute focal neurological deficits resulting from a suspected vascular or space-occupying lesion in immunocompromised hosts and has a predilection for the frontal lobes (Dubey et al. 2005), basal ganglia, thalami, and corpus callosum, which, however, is rather unspecific. Granuloma formation has been reported to be most common with *Aspergillus*. According to the site and nature of lesion, the patient may present with signs of meningitis, focal neurological deficits, or raised intracranial pressure.

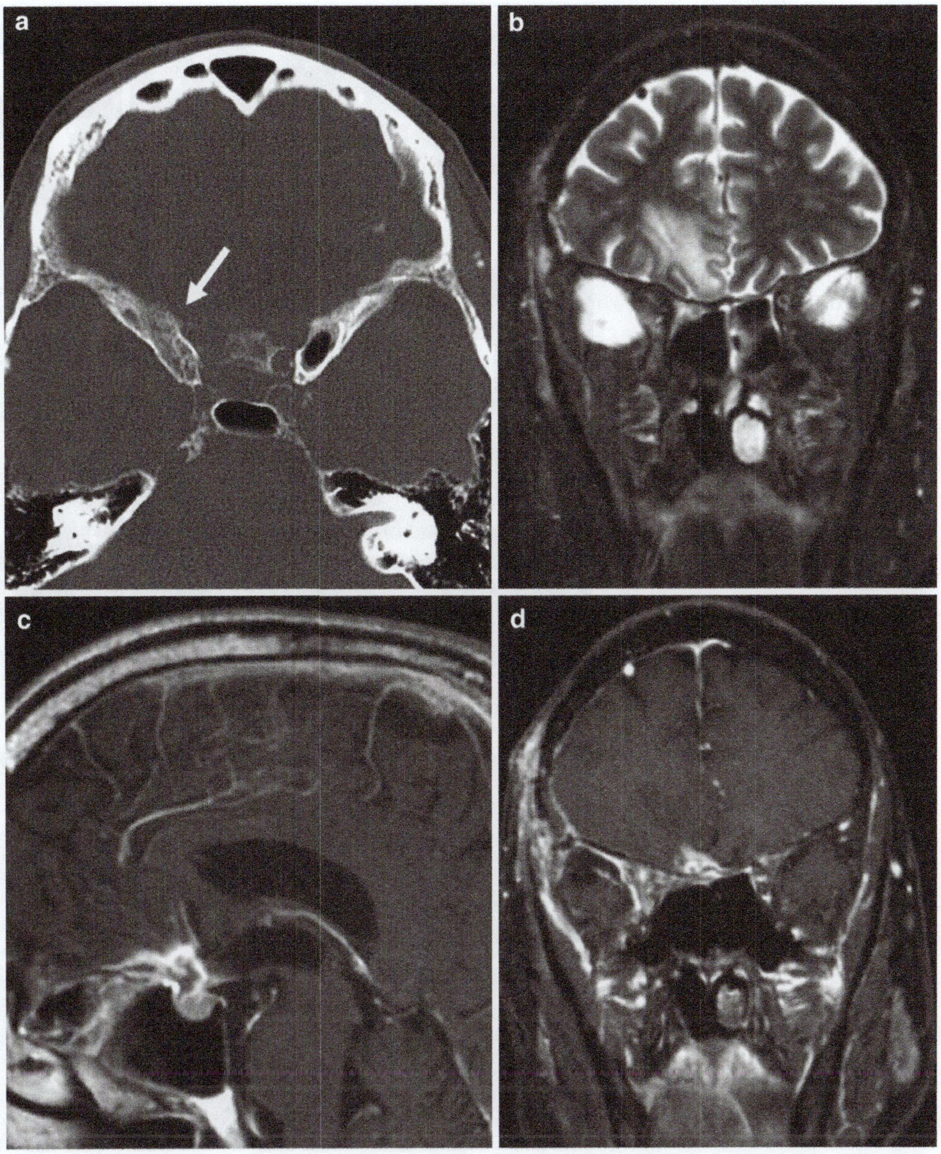

Fig. 2 Invasive aspergillosis. **a** Axial computed tomogram. **b** Coronal T2-weighted image. **c** Sagittal T1-weighted image after contrast administration. **d** Coronal T1-weighted image after contrast administration. Signs of bone erosion on the right sphenoid wing (**a**, *arrow*). In the adjacent frontal lobe there is considerable reactive edema (**b**) originating from the contrast-enhancing infiltrations through the orifices of the skull base into the basal cisterns (**c**) and into brain tissue itself (**d**)

Usually, the patients are afebrile or have only low-grade fever. In patients with paranasal sinus spread, orbital extension with proptosis, ocular palsies, and chemosis may occur. Mycotic aneurysms may get symptomatic with subarachnoid hemorrhage and thereby typical sequelae.

The disease is usually slowly progressive and symptoms may persist for months; however, if brain-stem or cerebellar signs are the presenting features, rapid neurological deterioration and death may occur. Nevertheless, the prognosis for CNS aspergillosis is poor, with by far the most reported cases being fatal. An aggressive surgical approach in non-immunocompromised patients may reduce the mortality.

3.1.5 Serologic Tests and Therapy

Serial serologic tests may be helpful, but laboratory findings do not always confirm the diagnosis of fungal infection so that neuroimaging is crucial. Mortality is high in aspergillosis patients, and early diagnosis is mandatory if survival is to be achieved. Fungostatic therapy, i.e., voriconazole and amphotericin B, and treatment of the source of infection represent the cornerstones of the management. Even lobectomy in patients with a single abscess is considered an acceptable surgical option when non-eloquent areas of the brain are involved. High awareness of the possibilities of *Aspergillus* infection on the basis of imaging findings may help to avoid such drastic measures.

3.2 Imaging

Imaging patterns of cerebral aspergillosis are heterogeneous: meningeal enhancement; edematous lesions; hemorrhagic

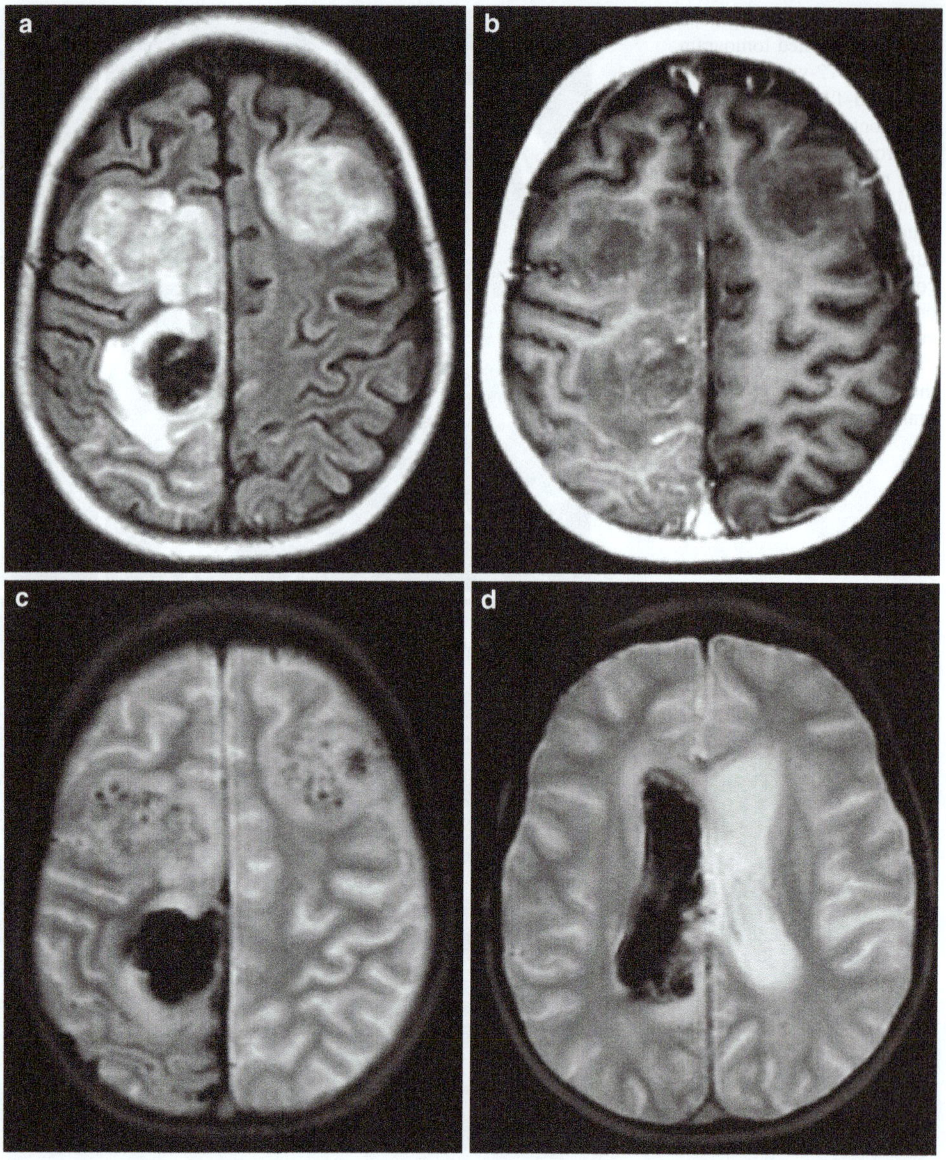

Fig. 3 Multiple aspergillomas. **a** Axial FLAIR image. **b** Axial T1-weighted image after contrast administration. **c, d** Axial T2*-weighted images. Space-occupying lesions with marked surrounding edema (**a**). Contrast enhancement is faint (**b**). Due to the vasodestructive propensities of *Aspergillus*, the masses display hemorrhagic transformation, best visualized on T2*-weighted images (**c**, **d**). Also intraventricular hemorrhage is evident (**d**)

lesions (Fig. 3); solid enhancing lesions referred to as aspergilloma or "tumoral form"; abscess-like ring-like enhancing lesions; infarct lesions; and mycotic aneurysms. Meningeal enhancement is usually seen in lesions adjacent to infected paranasal sinuses. The immunological state of the patient dictates both the type of clinical manifestation and disease severity and thus the imaging appearance. Patients with AIDS and other severely immunocompromised patients often do not show any enhancement or perifocal edema. In cases of hematogenous dissemination, multiple lesions are observed involving the middle or anterior cerebral arterial territory with acute necrotizing and purulent lesions (cerebrovascular aspergillosis). After local spread from contiguous anatomical structures, chronic granulomas eliciting dense fibrosis often with osseus destruction are observed on CT and MRI.

In the paranasal sinuses fungal involvement appears on CT as a hypodense mass lesion with calcification and separation from the wall of sinuses and hypointense on T2-weighted images with more or less solid contrast enhancement on T1-weighted images (Fig. 2). Beginning with colonization of the paranasal sinuses, imaging changes may extend directly to the orbits and brain, particularly affecting the cavernous sinuses and adjacent parenchyma to form abscesses and areas of ischemia by vascular lesions.

Brain abscesses caused by *Aspergillus* resemble those of other infectious agents, and are usually multiple with a circular enhancement pattern, and with perilesional vasogenic edema. In most *Aspergillus* abscesses a mass effect is observed. Diagnosis of such intracranial mass with intermediate signal and surrounding edema is best confirmed with a CT or MRI scan after contrast administration.

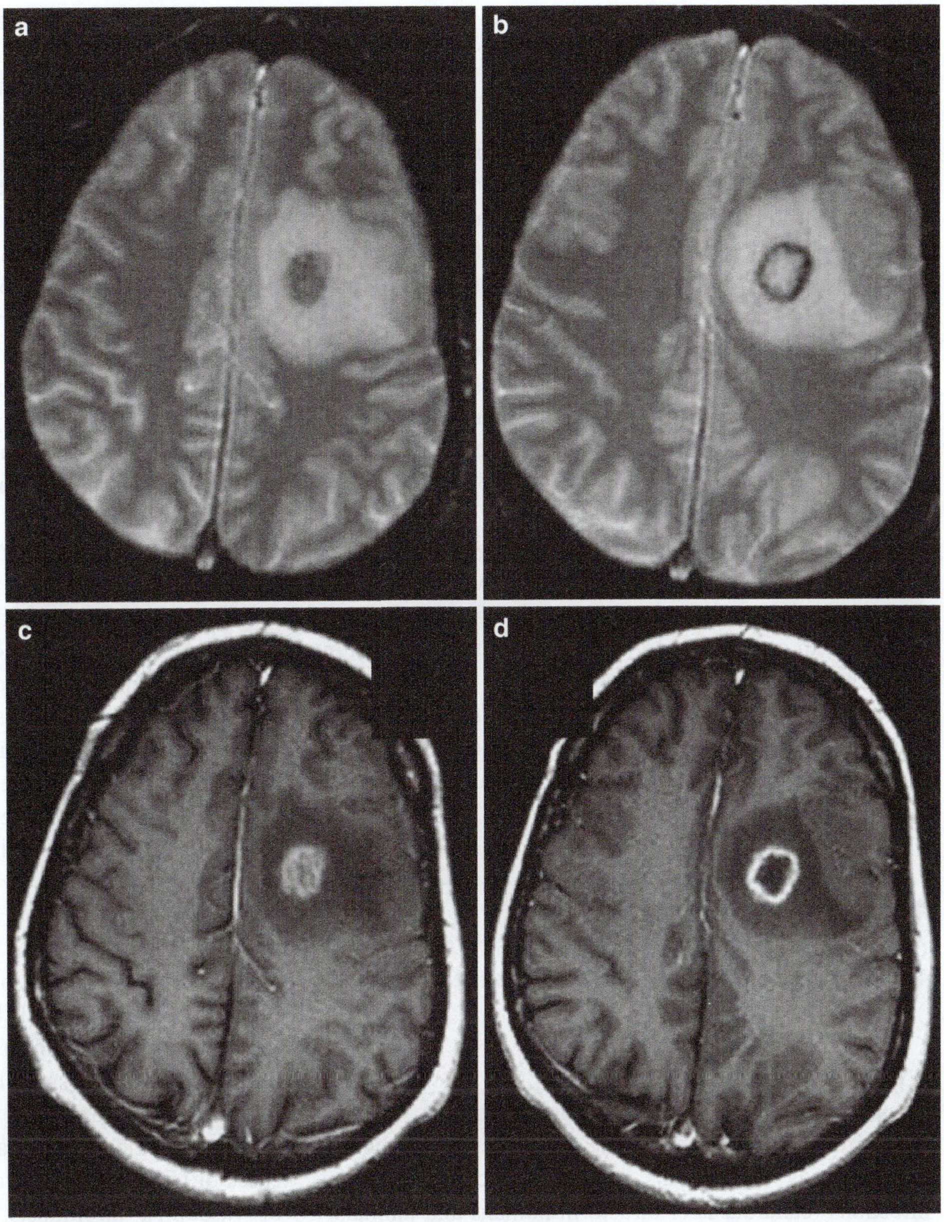

Fig. 4 Development of an intraparenchymal aspergilloma over 6 months. **a** Initial examination. **b** Follow-up after 6 months. **a**, **b** Axial T2-weighted images. **c** Initial examination. **d** Follow-up after 6 months. **c**,**d** Axial T1-weighted images after contrast administration. Solidly hypointense structure (**a**) with compact enhancement (**c**) at the initial examination. Centrally necrotic mass with high signal in the center on T2-weighted image (**b**) and ring enhancement at follow-up after 6 months (**d**)

Sometimes hemorrhagic transformation occurs. On CT, the corresponding abnormalities are usually subtle, with varying densities and minimal mass effect, and poor contrast enhancement, but usually without ring formation. Magnetic resonance imaging is more sensitive for detecting small lesions and can demonstrate a typical aspect of hypointense signal on T2-weighted images in the walls of abscesses. Especially on T2*-weighted images or SWI the walls of hemorrhagic necrosis can be demonstrated easily (Fig. 4). Aside from blood-breakdown products, this pattern has been related to fungal hypha-containing paramagnetic elements primarily. Enhancement in larger chronic abscesses is mostly ring-like, whereas homogeneous enhancement is unusual in larger lesions. Diffusion-weighted imaging has been proven to be useful in diagnosing fungal abscess, including multiple lesions due to *Aspergillus* dissemination. They demonstrate hyperintensity on DWI, probably reflecting a high proteinaceous fluid and cellular infiltration with the consequence of ADC reduction. It is sometimes difficult to differentiate with certainty between parenchymal *Aspergillus* lesions and ischemic vascular lesions. On MR spectroscopy the identification of multiple signals seen between 3.6 and 3.8 ppm assigned to trehalose sugars may further add to the diagnostic confidence (Luthra et al. 2007).

Intracerebral solitary granuloma formation is most common in the frontal and temporal lobes. They present as space-occupying lesions that do not reveal any contiguous extension from paranasal sinuses. Those granulomas are located at the basifrontal or basitemporal regions and are frequently misinterpreted as meningioma or tuberculoma on MRI and even at surgery.

Cerebrovascular aspergillosis denotes a well-recognized syndrome of cerebral infarction and necrosis and/or hemorrhage without suppuration resulting from vascular invasion and thrombosis secondary to endovascular infection from a septic embolus or direct invasion of the vessel wall causing vasculitis. Inflammatory response is usually scarce, with lesions occurring within the territory of affected vessels essentially in the cerebral cortex, subcortical regions, and less commonly the brain stem, cerebellum, and spinal cord. This form is most frequent in immunocompromised patients with hematopoietic stem cell or solid organ transplants and occasionally following corticosteroid therapy. Cortical and subcortical infarction with or without hemorrhage is a common finding in *Aspergillus* infection explained by fungal infiltration of the vessel wall and thrombosis. Recognition of these radiological patterns in patients with cerebral aspergillosis is helpful in establishing an early diagnosis.

Isolated meningitis due to *Aspergillus* infection is extremely unusual, being more often a complication of other *Aspergillus*-related lesions. Spinal cord involvement has been reported very rarely.

4 Candida Albicans

4.1 Epidemiology, Clinical Presentation, Therapy

4.1.1 The Fungus

Candida is a diploid fungus that grows both as yeast and filamentous cells. Clinically, the most relevant member of the genus is *C. albicans*, which can cause numerous infections (candidiasis or thrush) in humans and animals.

4.1.2 Epidemiology

C. albicans is part of the flora of mucous membranes and the gastrointestinal tract in 80 % of healthy individuals. The gastrointestinal tract is the gateway for systemic infection in individuals with some predisposing condition such as diabetes, lymphoproliferative disease, intravenous drug abuse, and those in whom the use of broadspectrum antibiotics leads to microbial selection through impairment of the competitive inhibition of the normal flora. Although mucocutaneous candidiasis is probably one of the commonest disease manifestations of HIV positive status with an incidence of about 50–100 % the occurrence of generalized candidiasis in individuals with AIDS is rare.

4.1.3 Manifestation and Disease Spread

Candida meningitis may manifest spontaneously after iatrogenic inoculation—most often catheter related. A variety of further conditions, such as prolonged antibiotics, steroids, immunosuppressive agents, chemotherapeutic treatment, indwelling catheters, parenteral nutrition, abdominal surgery, burns, malignancies, neutropenia, and AIDS, may promote the hematogenous spread. The severity of disease is dictated by the dose of inoculum. Phagocytosis is the principal non-specific mechanism protecting the host against *Candida albicans* infection. The hyphal form of *Candida* can resist digestion by both polymorphs and macrophages; thus, the highest incidence of candidiasis is seen in neutropenic patients (chemotherapy) and defects in neutrophil/macrophage function (long-term steroid therapy). There are two main CNS manifestations of candidiasis: meningitis and abscesses.

Candida meningitis is the most frequent clinical manifestation of CNS candidiasis. It is most common in neonates, where it usually shows an acute progression. In the more rare manifestation, in adults, the picture usually has a chronic and indolent course. About 50 % of adult patients dying from invasive candidiasis had evidence of CNS involvement, but meningeal disease was observed in only 10–15 % of the adult cases with CNS affection.

Scattered brain microabscesses with little or no meningeal involvement (Fig. 5) have been consistently found in about half of the patients dying from invasive candidiasis with, in turn, candidiasis being the second most common agent causing this sort of brain microabscess. With the occlusion of small vessels by the pseudohyphae, colonies of yeast enmeshed in fibrin and acute polymorph reaction primarily present as small hemorrhagic infarcts, progressing to microabscess and later granulomatous abscess reaction. Histopathological confirmations of vascular involvement in cases of CNS candidiasis are well described with evidence of vasculitis, thrombosis, intraluminal proliferation, and small-vessel invasion. Several case reports of cerebrovascular complications are related to *Candida meningitis*. Clinical presentations include basilar artery thrombosis and subarachnoid hemorrhages resulting from rupture of true mycotic aneurysm or arteritis with vascular invasion.

4.1.4 Serologic Tests, Clinical Presentation, Therapy

Difficulties in growing *Candida* from the CSF have been reported; thus, a large-volume CSF needs to be collected from patients with chronic meningitis that might be fungal. The Gram stain is positive in only 30 % of cases. Patients with CNS microabscesses develop a progressive encephalopathy associated with waxing and waning signs and symptoms.

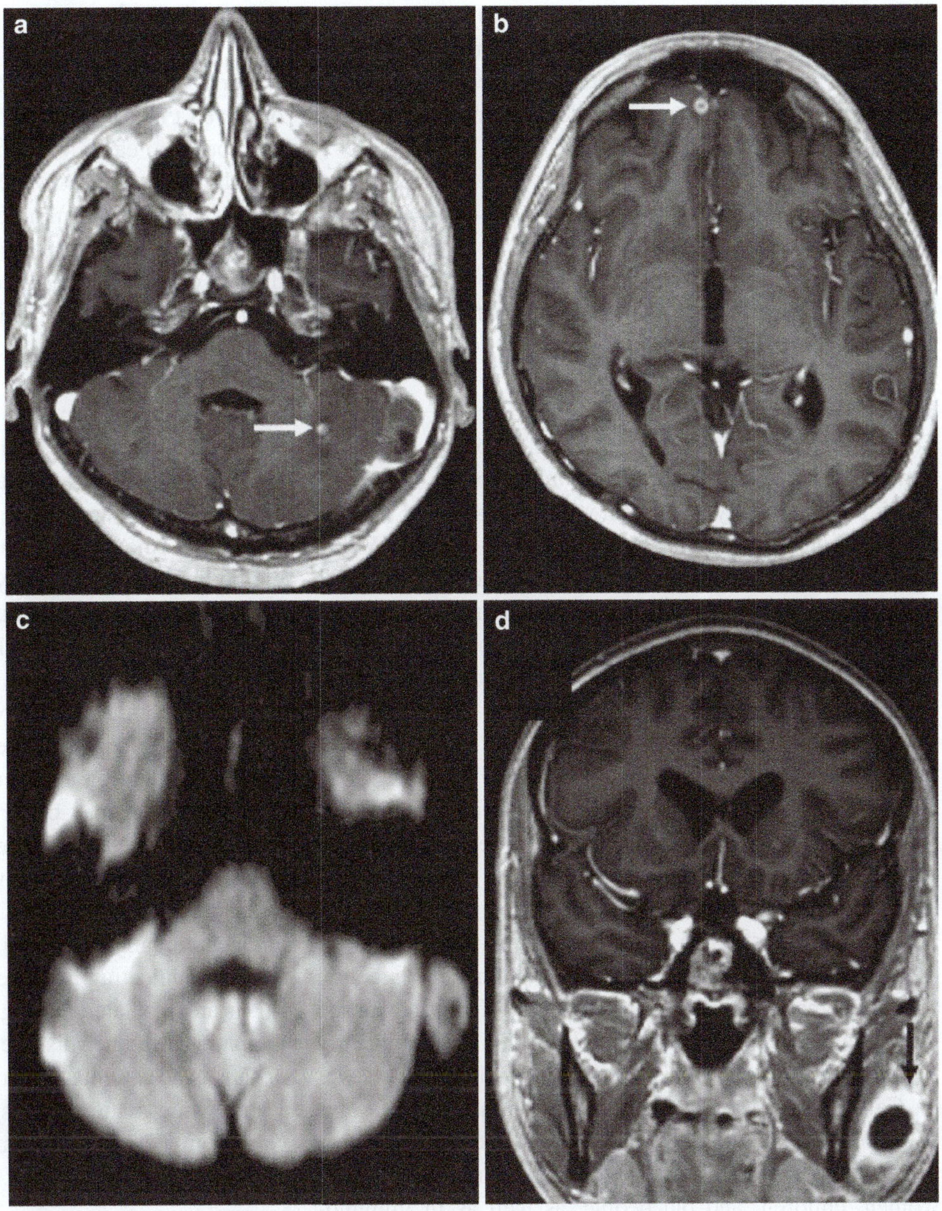

Fig. 5 *Candida* infection with cerebral microabscesses. **a**, **b** Axial T1-weighted images after contrast administration. **c** Axial DWI. **d** Coronal T1-weighted image after contrast administration. Typical scattered pattern after contrast enhancement (*arrows* in **a**, **b**). Lesions are not necessarily detectable on DWI (**c**). Moreover, this patient showed a cervical abscess (**d**, *arrow*). Complete resolution after treatment in further course (Courtesy of J. Spreer)

Multiple microabscesses are not infrequent but usually unrecognized and should be considered in the differential diagnosis of encephalopathy in hospitalized patients with chronic disease, immunosuppression, and sepsis. Intravenous or intraventricular administration of antifungal agents (i.e., amphotericin B, caspofungin, or fluconazole) is suggested. Duration of treatment should be decided on a case-by-case modality, based on results of serial CSF cultures.

4.2 Imaging

Usually, MR images show multiple hypointense lesions on T1-weighted images, ring enhancement after gadolinium administration, and intermediate-signal lesions within surrounding high signal on T2-weighted images. However, in immunocompromised patients, abscesses appear as patchy or punctate T2 hyperintense lesions with frequently absent enhancement. Such diminutive nodular or annular lesions in the transition from white matter to gray matter, and in the basal nuclei, are compatible with microabscesses or non-caseous granulomas. Usually the microabscesses are observed in the territory of the anterior and middle cerebral arteries, which might be explained simply by the relative extension of the vascular supply of these territories; however, cerebellar involvement also has been reported. Given the history of chronic disease or immunosuppression, this pattern should alarm the neuroradiologist who should suggest *Candida* abscesses among the differential diagnoses. Even on histology, unless suspected and looked for, the *Candida* organisms may be overlooked. In immunocompetent patients, candidiasis may manifest as solid or abscess-like lesions giving rise to the differential diagnosis of a pyogenic abscess. These findings alone do not allow a specific diagnosis, so that treatment decisions must be based on clinical parameters and CSF findings.

5 Coccidiomycosis

5.1 Epidemiology, Clinical Presentation, Therapy

5.1.1 The Fungus

Coccidioidomycosis is a systemic infection caused by a dimorphous fungus *Coccidioides immitis* or *C. posadasii*, which exist in the mycelial form within the soil and become infective when the airborne arthrospores are inhaled. Within the host, the arthrospore develops into a globular structure (spherule). This spherule is 20–100 mm in diameter and later develops hundreds of endospores within a thick-walled capsule. When the spherule ruptures, the tiny endospores are released continuing the infection cycle.

5.1.2 Epidemiology

Coccidioides are fungi predominantly endemic in the southwestern United States as well as in Central and South America.

5.1.3 Manifestation

After inhalation of fungus from dust, a pulmonary infection spreads hematogenously. Approximately 40 % of exposed individuals develop a flu-like picture with predominantly self-limited pulmonary symptoms, the so-called valley fever or California fever. The rate of disseminated disease is about 5 % of symptomatic patients, and meningitis occurs in about half of those cases with increased risk in pregnant women, children, and old people, as well as in immunocompromised patients.

5.1.4 Serologic Tests, Therapy, and Prognosis

The fungal infection can be demonstrated by microscopic detection of diagnostic cells in body fluids, by PCR or by serologic analysis detecting fungal antigen or host antibody. Disseminated disease is associated with high morbidity and mortality. Generally, the involvement of the CNS is considered a late, and not infrequently a terminal, event. Without intravenous antifungal therapy (i.e. fluconazole), the clinical course of coccidioidal meningitis is almost always fatal. Although the disease may be controlled with chronic antifungal therapy, relapse after withdrawal of therapy is common.

5.2 Imaging

Generally, findings on MRI are much more frequently observed than on CT. The initial head CT is usually negative, but also early MRI studies are inconspicuous in about one-third of the cases. With ongoing disease, however, almost all MRI examinations will show marked meningeal enhancement. Meningeal enhancement may be primarily diffuse or nodular enhancement in the basal cisterns and may later progress to confluent diffuse enhancement patterns that represent focal collections of the organism with surrounding inflammation. In areas of meningeal enhancement the corresponding regions on the non-enhanced T1-weighted images are isointense with brain and isointense to slightly hypointense relative to brain on the T2-weighted images. The low signal on the T2-weighted images is thought to represent ferromagnetic material within the fungus or simply reflect a dense cellularity of the focal lesion. A typical but facultative CT finding is the poor visualization of basal and sylvian cisterns secondary to hyperdense exudates, and hydrocephalus. Cisternal involvement may lead to vasculitis and thus territorial infarcts in the dependent territories supplied by perforating vessels. In addition to vasculitis, it has also been speculated that vasospasm may occur as a result of the inflammatory process or direct invasion of the vessel by the fungus. Typically, those infarcts involve the brain stem, cerebellum, thalamus, or basal ganglia. Cortical infarction seems to be an exceptionally rare manifestation.

Communicating hydrocephalus with or without ventriculitis is an associated finding that is observed in up to 90 % of the patients in later disease stages. True mass lesions, hemorrhage, and calcification are seen less frequently. Multifocal vague white matter lesions have also been described. Coccidioidomycotic parenchymal abscesses are exceptional.

6 Zygomycosis

6.1 Epidemiology, Clinical Presentation, Therapy

6.1.1 The Fungus

Zygomycosis (mucormycosis) is caused by several genera belonging to the family *Mucorace*. *Rhizopus oryzae* is the most common cause of infection. Mucorales grow profusely on decaying vegetables, seeds, fruits, and animal excrement. The fungi can usually be cultivated from the oral cavity, nasal fossa, and pharynx of healthy individuals. In immunodeficiency they multiply and the spores germinate, forming hyphae, which become invasive and can spread.

6.1.2 Epidemiology

Zygomycosis is a worldwide polymorphic disease and is closely linked to the occurrence of diabetes mellitus in about 75 % of the patients especially in diabetic ketoacidosis. Other predisposing conditions include hematological malignancies, neutropenia, immunosuppressive medication, renal failure, organ transplantation, septicemia, trauma, burns, starvation, and others—a feature common to the majority of these is possible ketoacidosis.

6.1.3 Disease Spread and Manifestation

The manifestations of zygomycosis can be classified into several forms with rhinocerebral mucormycosis being a typical one. After colonization of the nasal and paranasal sinuses, where a spread occurs to the orbits, the disease spreads to the cavernous sinuses and brain parenchyma, particularly in the frontal lobes. Occluded vessels with thrombosis, vasculitis, mycotic aneurysms, and parenchymal infarcts are the hallmarks of disease similar to an *Aspergillus* infection.

6.1.4 Therapy and Prognosis

Orbital extension from the ethmoid sinuses produces proptosis, chemosis, superior ophthalmic vein thrombosis with extension, and subsequent thrombosis of the cavernous sinus. Resulting clinical symptoms are facial pain, bloody nasal discharge, chemosis, exophthalmos, and cranial nerve palsy, progressing rapidly to stroke, encephalitis, and death. The progression of infection is often so rapid that imaging does not offer much beyond demonstrating the extent of involvement. While most reports suggest intracranial involvement to be almost invariably fatal, a relatively high survival rate of 70 % has been reported after timely medical or surgical intervention.

6.2 Imaging

Imaging shows a similar pattern to aspergillosis, but usually with even greater extent of damage to the cerebral parenchyma particularly in the basal nuclei and frontal lobes. Typically, confluent regions of hyperintense signal on T2-weighted images in the basal portions of the frontal and temporal lobes with mild mass effect are visible that result from vasogenic edema. Foci of annular contrast enhancement can be visible. Usually those lesions are associated with vascular involvement, including obstruction of the cavernous sinuses and even of the carotid arteries, revealing thrombosis or wall enhancement, probably due to local inflammatory involvement. CT imaging may reveal soft tissue surroundings along the walls of the paranasal sinuses. On MRI, low intensity of the sinuses may be present on T1- and T2-weighted images. Proton MRS may show a profile similar to that of bacterial abscess. Resonances of the amino acids valine, leucine, and isoleucine may be evident both in pyogenic and fungal abscesses.

7 Histoplasma Capsulatum

7.1 Epidemiology, Clinical Presentation, Therapy

Histoplasma capsulatum is a fungus found in several regions of the world, above all in some regions of North America, especially in the Ohio and Mississippi River valleys. The fungi are abundant in the droppings of birds and bats and are released into the air as spores that can be inhaled, causing pulmonary involvement. In the environment, it grows as a brownish mycelium, whereas after inoculation at body temperature it morphs into a yeast. The inoculum once inhaled germinates and then transforms into budding yeast cells. Histoplasmosis, also known as Darling's disease, is caused by the fungus *H. capsulatum*. Its symptoms vary greatly, but the disease is usually restricted to the lungs and rarely presents systemic dissemination in immunocompetent individuals. Exposure to *H. capsulatum* is very common in this region and usually follows a benign clinical course.

7.2 Imaging

On chest CT, calcification of the mediastinal adenopathy is common and is seen in up to 85 % of cases. CNS involvement may accompany hematogenous dissemination of the disease and may be characterized by cisternal meningitis or, more rarely, by the occurrence of parenchymal granulomas (histoplasmomas) that may mimic neoplasms. Histoplasmomas may present as single ring-enhancing lesions in brain parenchyma enlarging over a period of months. The MRI appearance is unspecific. Usually it consists of nodular or annular foci of hematogenous distribution with variable edema, characterized by hypointense signal on T1- and hyperintense signal on T2-weighted images, as has also been shown with other fungal lesions.

8 Differential Diagnosis

The microscopic verification of the causative agent and analysis of the CSF are decisive in fungal infections of the CNS. In the neuroradiological differential diagnosis other granulomatous diseases, such as neurotuberculosis, neurosarcoidosis, and parasitic infections, and also multifocally growing brain tumors, such as gliomas and brain metastasis, should be included. In cases of dural involvement also meningiomas and dural metastases should be considered. The wall of a fungal abscess usually shows decreased diffusion on DWI, whereas the inner core of the fungal abscess shows lesser restriction of diffusion. This is in contrast to pyogenic and tubercular abscesses where restricted diffusion is observed in the lesion center; however, heterogeneity of diffusion in fungal infection has been described (Mueller-Mang et al. 2007) with both increased and decreased diffusion in fungal abscesses in the cerebritis stage and the early capsular stage. The presence of multiple signals seen between 3.6 and 3.8 ppm in the wall of abscesses of aspergillosis, cryptococcosis, and zygomycosis assigned to the disaccharide trehalose may add further to the diagnostic confidence (Luthra et al. 2007).

References

Dubey A, Patwardhan RV, Sampth S, Santosh V, Kolluri S, Nanda A (2005) Intracranial fungal granuloma: analysis of 40 patients and review of the literature. Surg Neurol 63:254–260

Erly WK, Bellon RJ, Seeger JF, Carmody RF (1999) MR imaging of acute coccidioidal meningitis. Am J Neuroradiol 20:509–514

Luthra G, Parihar A, Nath K, Jaiswal S, Prasad KN, Husain N, Husain M, Singh S, Behari S, Gupta RK (2007) Comparative evaluation of fungal, tubercular, and pyogenic brain abscesses with conventional and diffusion MR imaging and proton MR spectroscopy. Am J Neuroradiol 28:1332–1338

Mueller-Mang C, Castillo M, Mang TG, Cartes-Zumelzu F, Weber M, Thurnher MM (2007) Fungal versus bacterial brain abscesses: is diffusion-weighted MR imaging a useful tool in the differential diagnosis? Neuroradiology 49:651–657

Parasitic Infections

Christoph Stippich

Contents

Abstract

The wording "parasite" originates from the ancient greek "parasitos" (*pará* = besides, *sítos* = eating). Parasites are organisms living in (endoparasites, intracellular parasites) or on (ectoparasites) other species (host). The host provides nutrients for the parasite and is injured by the parasite. The relationship between host and parasite is "antagonistic" in favor of the parasite. Detrimental effects to the host include malnutrition, organ injury, inflammation, toxicity, mass effects, and others. Typically, the host is undermined but not killed. Parasitism has been extremely successful during evolution. It has been suggested that approximately 50 % of all organisms are parasitic permanently or have a parasitic period in life. This is supported by the fact that nearly all animals host a number of different parasites, each specifically adapted to their host. Stationary parasites are in permanent contact with the host, whereas temporary parasites attack the host only for feeding (e.g., mosquitoes). The cycle of life of most parasites is very complex including changes between different hosts (intermediate and definite) as well as sexual and non-sexual reproduction. There are different ways of parasite transmission leading to infection of the host: direct surface contact; active percutaneous; oral; feco-oral; cyclic-alimentary (e.g., malaria: while feeding the anopheles mosquitoes transmit parasites between individuals); sexual and diaplacental (e.g., in fetal toxoplasmosis). This chapter addresses the most relevant CNS manifestations of human pathogen parasites including imaging features and differential diagnoses. These are the protozoans *Toxoplasma gondii* (toxoplasmosis), *Plasmodium* sp. (malaria), and *Entameba histolytica* (amebiasis), as well as the *Helminthes* (worms), *Taenia solium* (neurocysticercosis), *Echinococcus granulosus* and *Alveolaris* (echinococcosis), *Trichinella spiralis* (trichinosis), and *Schistosoma sp.* (schistosomiasis). In general, MRI is superior to CT in diagnostic neuroimaging of parasitic CNS infections.

C. Stippich (✉)
Universitätsspital Basel, Klinik für Radiologie,
Neuroradiologie und Nuklearmedizin, Petersgraben 4,
4031 Basel, Switzerland
e-mail: CStippich@uhbs.ch

S. Hähnel (ed.), *Inflammatory Diseases of the Brain*, Medical Radiology. Diagnostic Imaging,
DOI: 10.1007/174_2012_654, © Springer-Verlag Berlin Heidelberg 2012
Published Online: 02 September 2012

1 Toxoplasmosis

1.1 Epidemiology, Clinical Presentation, Therapy

1.1.1 Epidemiology

Approximately 1.5 billion people worldwide are infected with the obligate intracellular protozoan *Toxoplasma gondii*, representing the most common human parasite. Toxoplasmosis is also the most common opportunistic CNS infection in patients with AIDS. Typically, the oocytes are ingested with infected meat, raw milk, or through cat feces. Cats may be definite or intermediate hosts, whereas all other mammals, including humans and birds, are intermediate hosts. The evolution of *Toxoplasma gondii* continues over various stages in the host intestine and the parasites enter different organs including the CNS actively after hematogenous spreading. Infections through contaminated needles, transfusion, or organ transplantation have also been reported. Diaplacental infection of the fetus is possible. Inside the organ parenchyma *Toxoplasma gondii* forms cysts—preferentially in the brain, heart, and peripheral muscles—where the parasites may persist infectious over several years.

1.1.2 Clinical Presentation

In immunocompetent individuals toxoplasmosis is usually a subclinical, self-limiting disease that may present with initial fever and lymph node swelling. The prevalence in adults ranges from 15 to 85 % and increases with age. In immunodeficient patients toxoplasma cysts may be reactivated in the brain. The parasites then invade the surrounding tissue resulting in local inflammation, vascular leakage, or thrombosis with concomitant infarctions and necrosis. A first infection during pregnancy has a 50 % risk for affecting the embryo and here mainly the CNS. Severity is inversely related to the duration of pregnancy.

1.1.3 Therapy

Medication includes sulfadiazine, pyrimethamine, and clindamycin.

1.2 Imaging

Overall neuroimaging and pathology findings correlate well. On MRI toxoplasmosis appears with T1-hypointense and T2-hyperintense lesions—typically 1–3 cm in diameter—with surrounding edema. Isointense lesions may also be present. Contrast enhancement is common and often spares the necrotic center (ring enhancement). Small lesions may show nodular enhancement. Calcifications in regressing lesions appear as (punctate) signal loss and are better depicted on CT. Here, the lesions are hypo- to isodense, ring enhancing, and surrounded by edema. Infarctions associated with toxoplasmosis are typically linked to vascular territories and show the classic changes over time on DWI, ADC, and CT. Common findings in congenital toxoplasmosis include: intracranial calcifications with a preference for basal ganglia and cortex; hydrocephalus due to aqueductal stenosis after ependymitis; and chorioretinitis (Figs. 1, 2, 3, 4).

1.3 Differential Diagnosis

In immunocompromised patients the differential diagnosis includes lymphoma, tuberculoma, TBC, cryptococcosis, and bacterial abscess.

2 Malaria

2.1 Epidemiology, Clinical Presentation, Therapy

2.1.1 Epidemiology

Malaria is a life-threatening disease endemic in many tropical and subtropical countries. It has been estimated that approximately one billion people are infected with an infection rate over 300 million per year including 10,000–30,000 international travelers. Each year more than one million patients die from the disease, mainly children in Africa. The sporocoids of the four different human pathogen plasmodium species (*P. falciparum*, *P. malariae*, *P. ovale*, and *P. vivax*) are transmitted via blood through the biting female anopheles mosquito, breeding in warm water (lakes, swamps, etc.). Once inside the host liver they mature to merocoids and then enter the erythrocytes for further reproduction leading to recurrent ruptures of the infected red blood cells (schizogony). The released parasites re-enter other erythrocytes, resulting in cyclical schizogony of 48 or 72 h in duration, which is strictly synchronized for plasmodium vivax, ovale, and malariae. Blood-smear microscopy is diagnostic and reveals deformed erythrocytes containing parasites in different characteristic states.

2.1.2 Clinical Presentation

Acute relapsing fever after an incubation time of 1 week or longer is characteristic. *Plasmodium falciparum* causes the most severe form of malaria which may be fatal within 24 h, if untreated. Other non-specific symptoms include chills, headache, weakness, muscular and abdominal pain, vomiting, diarrhea, or cough. Generalized convulsions as well as organ and circulatory failure may occur followed by coma and death. The three other *Plasmodium* species cause a high morbidity but are rarely fatal.

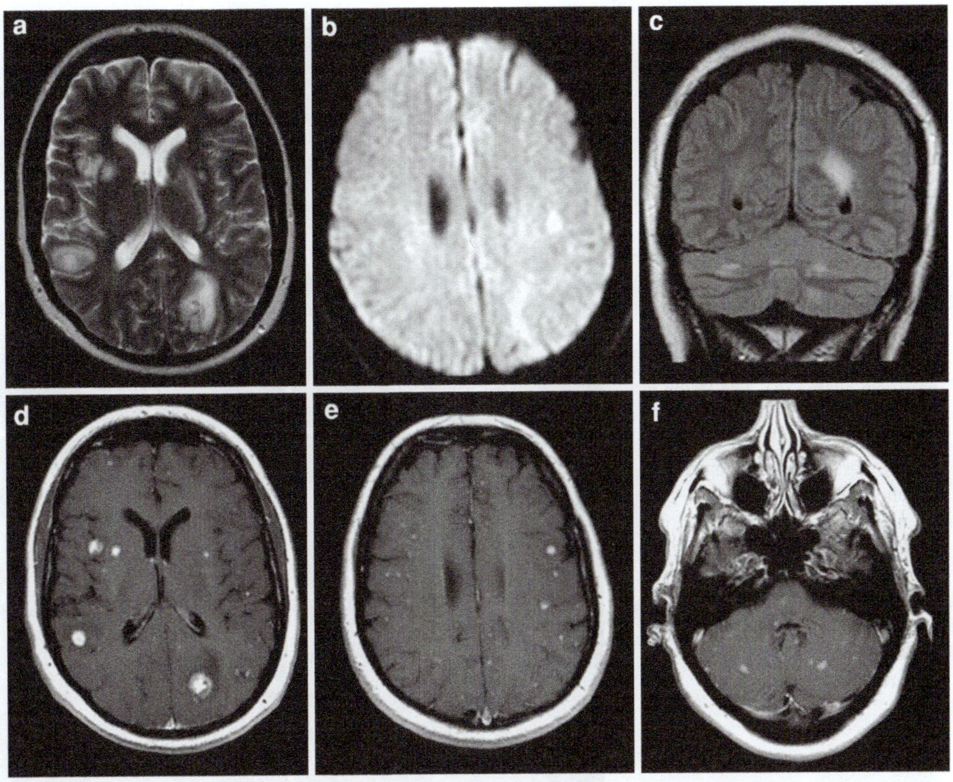

Fig. 1 Cerebral toxoplasmosis in an immunocompetent 49-year-old woman. **a** Axial T2-weighted image. **b** Axial DWI. **c** Coronal FLAIR image. **d** Axial T1-weighted images after contrast administration. Multiple supra- and infratentorial lesions with hyperintense signal on T2-weighted images, DWI, and FLAIR images (**a**, **c**), and strong punctate or circular contrast enhancement (**d–f**)

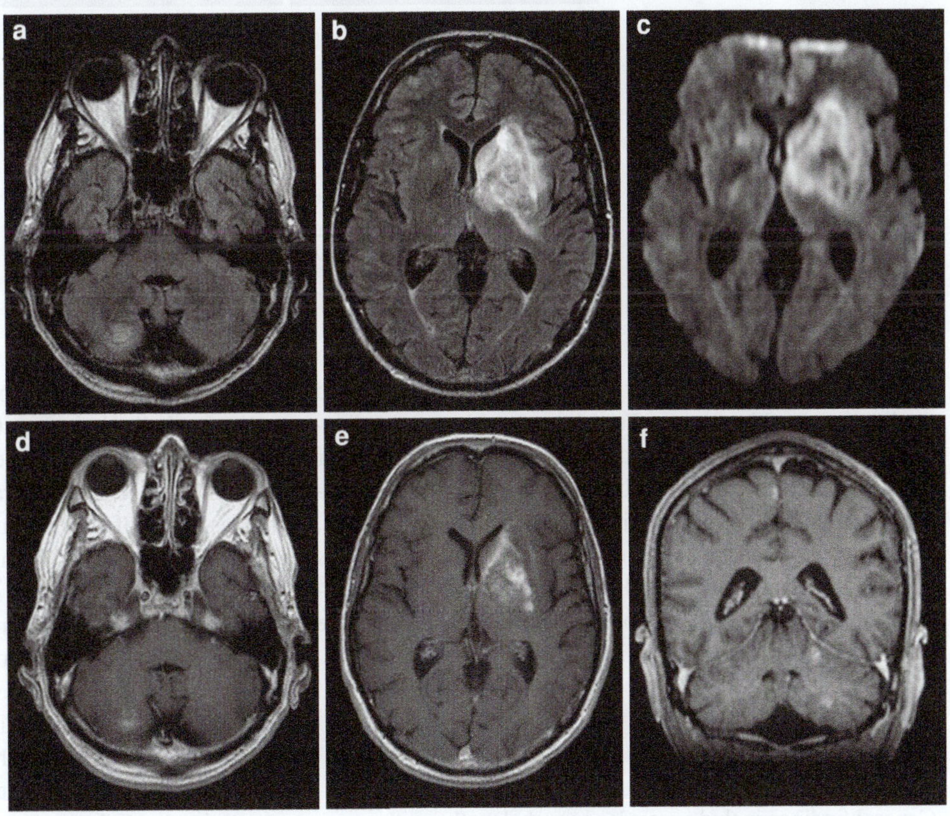

Fig. 2 Cerebral toxoplasmosis in an immunocompromised 56-year-old man. **a**, **b** Axial FLAIR images. **c** Axial DWI; **d, e** Axial T1-weighted images after contrast administration; f Coronal T1-weighted image after contrast administration. Multifocal supra- and infratentorial contrast-enhancing lesions. Note the association with an ischemic infarct in the territory of the left middle cerebral artery including the basal ganglia (**b, c**). The toxoplasmosis lesions and the ischemic infarct reveal contrast enhancement (**d–f**)

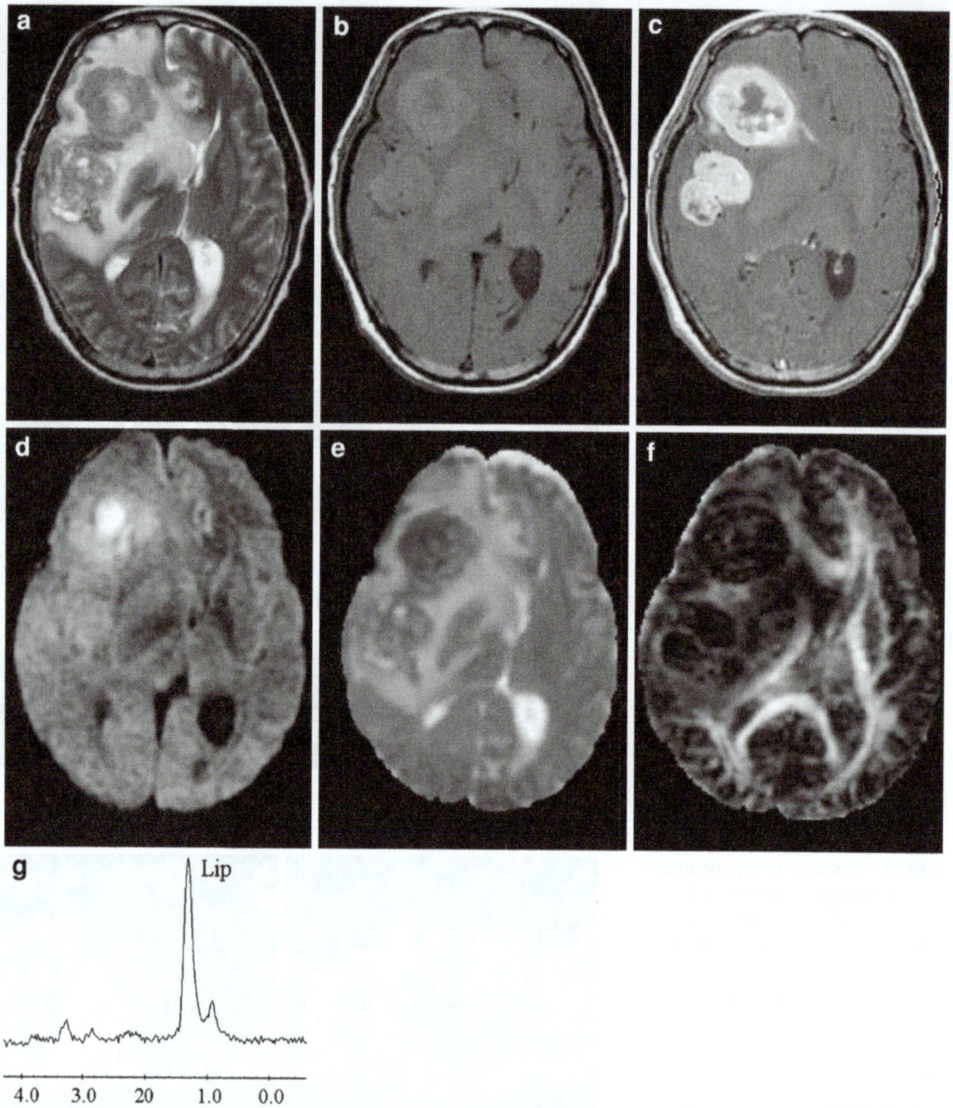

Fig. 3 Toxoplasmosis in a 40-year-old man with headache, fever, and vomiting. **a** T2-weighted image. **b** T1-weighted image before contrast administration. **c** T1-weighted image after contrast administration. **d** Axial DWI. **e** Axial ADC map. **f** FA map. **g** In vivo proton MRS. right frontal and fronto-parietal lesion; T2-weighted image shows peripheral hypointensity with central hyperintensity and perifocal edema (**a**). The lesion is iso- to slightly hyperintense on T1-weighted image (**b**) and shows marked inhomogeneous enhancement (**c**). Vasogenic edema with diffusion restriction on DWI and on the ADC map (**c**, **d**). The FA map shows no anisotropy in the cavity (**f**). Resonance of lipid peak (1.30 ppm) on proton MRS. (Courtesy of R.K Gupta)

2.1.3 Therapy

Mosquito-bite protection is a general precaution. Standard medication is chloroquine. Travelers should start medication 1 week before arrival and continue until 4 weeks after the last possible exposition. Long-term medication is possible but carries significant risks and adverse side effects. *P. falciparum* is increasingly resistant to antimalarial drugs making the combination of different pharmaceuticals necessary, e.g., proguanil, mefloquine, doxycycline, etc. We refer the reader to the specialist literature for details.

2.2 Imaging

General findings include vascular encephalopathy with punctate or ring hemorrhages, infarctions, and edema. The predilections are cortex and basal ganglia. On CT four different patterns can be identified: (1) normal; (2) diffuse edema; (3) infarctions with or without hemorrhages; and (4) thalamic and/or cerebellar hypodensity. On MR general brain swelling may be seen due to increased cerebral blood flow caused by vasodilatation and sequestration of infected erythrocytes as well as signs of venous and arterial thrombosis. Typically infarctions appear as T1-hypointense and T2-hyperintense lesions. Blood–brain barrier disruption may be present leading to lesional contrast enhancement. The signal characteristics of hemorrhages change from acute to chronic stages on T1-weighted and T2-weighted images and finally induce signal loss. White matter ischemia or toxic edema cause diffuse hyperintensities on T2-weighted, PD-, and FLAIR images, and show characteristic changes on DWI. White matter lesions may regress in part under treatment. Central pontine myelinolysis, myelinolysis of the upper medulla, and cerebellar infarctions have been described as other CNS manifestations of malaria.

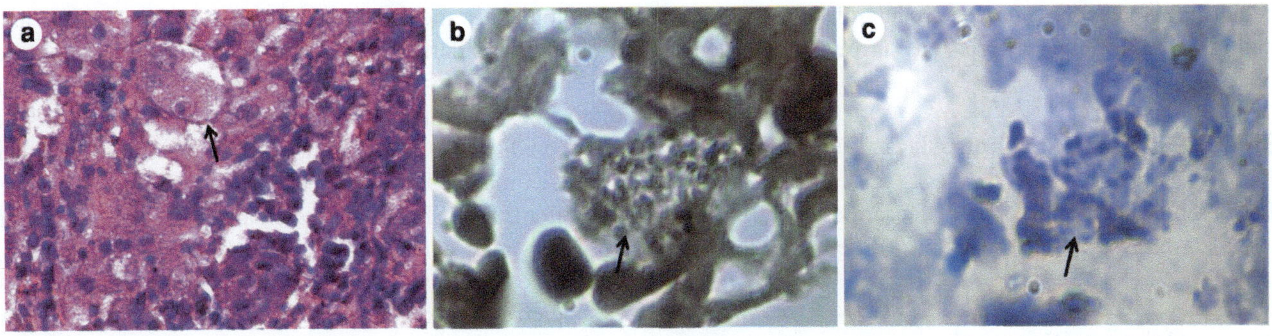

Fig. 4 Toxoplasmosis: hematoxylin–eosin stain (**a**) shows oval cytoplasmic parasites (*arrow*). Gomori methenamine silver stain (**b**) shows clusters of small oval intracytoplasmic parasites (*arrow*). Giemsa stain (**c**) of squash smear shows oval intracytoplasmic parasites with dot-like red nuclei and blue cytoplasm (*arrow*) (courtesy of R. K. Gupta)

3 Amebiasis

3.1 Epidemiology, Clinical Presentation, Therapy

3.1.1 Epidemiology

Entameba histolytica has a worldwide distribution but is endemic in South and Middle America, Southeast Asia, and Africa. Probably 10 % of the world's population is infected, and up to 100,000 patients die from amebiasis each year. The typical route of entry is feco-oral through contaminated food and water. Cysts of *E. histolytica* can also be transmitted with dust via the respiratory tract. The cysts remain infectious for several weeks, are highly resistant to heat, and survive even in chlorinated water. The majority of patients have intestinal manifestations with a subclinical course. Severe colitis and—after hematogenous spreading—multiple abscesses in different organs (liver, lung, skin, etc.) characterize the aggressive form. Cerebral amebiasis is extremely rare but represents a severe illness with a high mortality. The diagnosis may be delayed, as the cerebral manifestation often occurs several months after the intestinal symptoms. *Entameba histolytica* actively attacks the cells of the organs with proteolytic agents and induces a local invasion of neutrophil granulocytes. The neutrophils get killed by the protozoans and release additional aggressive agents into the parenchyma accelerating the lytic and necrotic processes. This results in large fluid-filled cavities in the affected organs (amebic abscesses) that can progress rapidly. Other amebic parasites are *Naegleria fowleri*, a facultatively human pathogen parasite, with a worldwide distribution, endemic to the United States and Australia. Infections are typically acquired when swimming in pools, lakes, and polluted industrial waters. The trophocoids enter the CNS via the nasal cavity and follow the olfactory tract into the brain where they cause the fatal primary amoebic meningoencephalitis (PAME). Infections with *acanthameba* usually affect immunocompromised individuals causing a fatal granulomatous encephalitis. Routes of entry are the olfactory tract and the respiratory tract followed by hematogenous spread.

3.1.2 Clinical Presentation

Amebiasis usually has a subclinical course with self-limiting diarrhea. Asymptomatic patients may remain infectious for several years and expel amebic cysts with their feces. The aggressive form is characterized by colitis with abdominal pain, severe diarrhea containing blood, and slime. Only one-third of patients have fever. Amebic abscesses can be giant (>1 l) and exhibit considerable mass effects on the affected organs. Together with the ongoing parenchymal destruction, this results in organ failure and finally death. Cerebral manifestations may be complicated by hydrocephalus. During a chronic course seizures are frequently found. PAME typically affects children and adolescents. Symptoms of this lethal disease are similar to bacterial meningitis.

3.1.3 Therapy

Metronidazole is the antiparasitic medication of choice. Biopsy and CSF testing are the primary diagnostic tools. Neuroimaging is supportive.

3.2 Imaging

Cerebral amebiasis is characterized by single or multiple nodular or ring-enhancing masses with a preference for the frontal lobes and basal ganglia. Signs of meningoencephalitis may be present with diffuse edema and parenchymal contrast enhancement seen on CT and MRI. Amebic abscesses are well delineated, with a hypodense core on CT. On MR T1 hypointensity, T2 hyperintensity, and marked heterogeneous ring enhancement are typical. The lesion rim (capsule) may be isointense to hypointense on T2-weighted images and hemorrhages may be present. Nodular lesions appear as multiple punctate enhancing lesions surrounded by edema.

3.3 Differential Diagnosis

Besides other cerebral parasites, nocardiosis, tuberculosis, and metastases represent the primary differential diagnoses.

4 Neurocysticercosis

4.1 Epidemiology, Clinical Presentation, Therapy

4.1.1 Epidemiology

Taenia solium has a worldwide distribution and is the most common human helminthosis. More than 80 million people are infected. Cysticercosis is endemic in areas with a combination of high human population and low hygienic standards. For example, it has been suggested that approximately 1 % of the habitants in Mexico city are infected and neurocysticercosis accounts for approximately 25 % of "brain tumors." The adult tapeworm is up to 4 m long and lives in the intestine of pigs (definite host). Humans are intermediate hosts. The infection is acquired from contaminated pork, water, or feco-orally (eggs). The oncospheres (embryos) hatch in the intestinal tract where they invade vessels and distribute to different organs, mainly the CNS (60–90 %) and the muscles. There they transform into the larval state (cysticercus). Depending on the localization of the cysticerci in the CNS parenchymal, leptomeningeal, intraventricular, or spinal manifestations can be distinguished, which also occur in combination. *Parenchymal* manifestations are most frequent. Four different pathological stages of parasite evolution can be identified:

1. In the vesicular stage the fully grown cysticerci present as fluid-filled round cysts of 1–2 cm in diameter with a mural nodule (scolex).
2. The colloid–vesicular stage is characterized by larval degeneration leading to turbid fluid in the cysts, thickening of the capsule, and host inflammatory response.
3. During the granular nodular stage the larvae retract, fluid filling gets absorbed, and the capsule thickens considerably.
4. Finally, the lesions shrink and calcify (nodular calcified stage).

The evolution of the different cisticerci is not synchronized and varies considerably in duration. As a consequence, multiple lesions of different stages are seen in the same patient. Cisternal cysticercosis may be caused by cysticercus cellulosae (cyst with scolex) or by cysticercus racemosus (grape-cluster-like larva without scolex), the latter preferring the basal cisterns, sylvian fissure, or ventricles. Chronic granulomatous meningitis, associated hydrocephalus and proliferative endarteritis causing infarctions, may complicate the clinical course of cisternal cysticercosis. Intraventricular cysticercosis accounts for 7–20 % of neurocysticercosis. The site of predilection is the fourth ventricle. The intraventricular cyst itself may be hard to detect when the fluid content does not differ from CSF, but the scolex and subependymal tissue retraction may guide to the correct diagnosis. Aqueductal stenosis or obliteration is a common complication. Spinal cysticercosis is extremely rare and typically involves the subarachnoid space (intradural extramedullary cyst, arachnitis), less often the spinal cord (intramedullary cyst with or without scolex), or epidural space.

4.1.2 Clinical Presentation

Clinical symptoms are not specific. Seizures occur in 50–80 % of patients with parenchymal neurocysticercosis but are rarely present in the other manifestations. About 20–30 % of patients develop a symptomatic hydrocephalus. Mass effects may induce focal neurological deficits. Ischemic infarctions may complicate neurocysticercosis with a subarachnoid manifestation more likely than with pure parenchymal manifestation, whereas endarteritis may cause deep lacunar infarcts. Children and adolescents may present with acute encephalitis induced by a massive inflammatory response to the parasites. Compression of the spinal cord or cauda equina is extremely rare and occurs in less than 1 % of the spinal manifestations. Spinal neurocysticercosis most likely affects the subarachnoid space rather than the medulla itself. Serological testing and neuroimaging are diagnostic. Eggs may be detectable in stool.

4.1.3 Therapy

Antiparasitic medication includes niclosamide, praziquantel, and mebendazole over several months. Cortisone can be applied in addition to reduce edema and inflammation. The encephalitic form represents a contraindication for antiparasitic agents. Solitary parenchymal and intraventricular lesions may be removed or drained surgically.

4.2 Imaging

Neurocysticercosishas a predilection for the subarachnoid space over the convexities but may also involve the basal cisterns, brain parenchyma—typically at the gray/white matter junction—and the ventricles with a preference for the fourth ventricle. Rare manifestations affect the spine, orbits, and sella. The size of cysticercus cysts is highly variable between several millimeters up to 10 cm. A mural nodule of a few millimeters in diameter (scolex) is a characteristic feature of neurocysticercosis as well as the presence of different evolutionary stages in multiple cysticerci. Solitary or

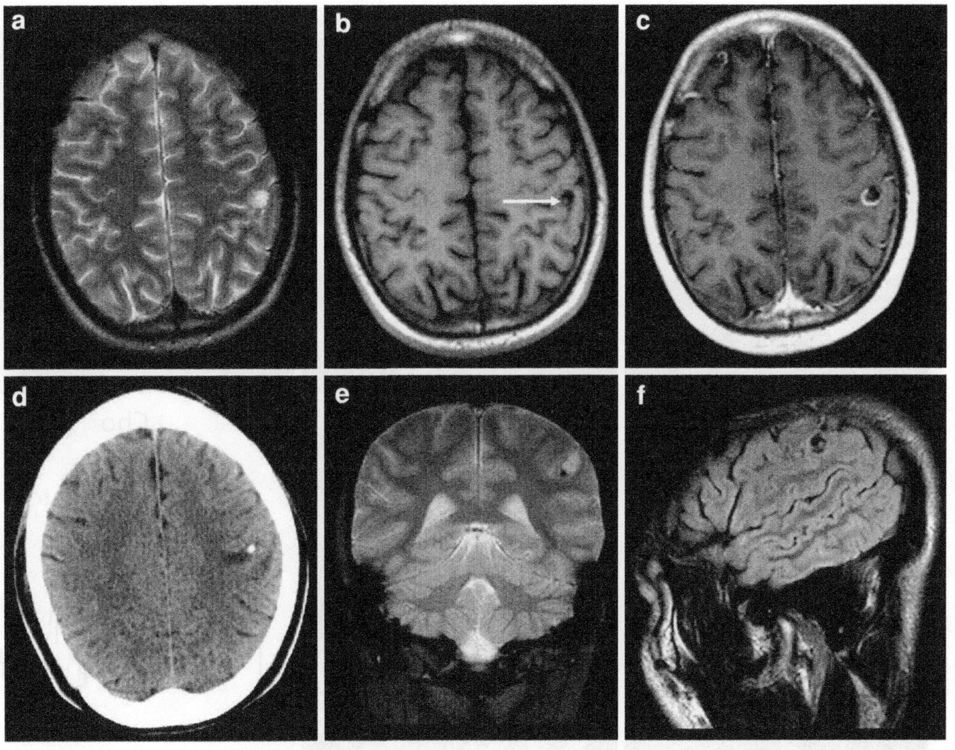

Fig. 5 Neurocysticercosis in a 22-year-old man. **a** Axial T2-weighted image. **b** Axial T1-weighted image before contrast administration. **c** Axial T1-weighted image after contrast administration. d Axial CT. **e** Coronal T2*-weighted image. **f** Sagittal FLAIR image. The solitary cysticercus has a classical localization in the subarachnoid space over the convexity, in this case the left postcentral sulcus. The lesion is fluid-filled resembling CSF, and appears hyperintense on T2-weighted images, hypointense on T1-weighted images, and shows circular contrast enhancement, but nearly no peripheral edema. The scolex can be visualized on the T1-weighted image before contrast administration (**b**, *arrow*). CT and T2*-weighted sequence shows mural calcification

multiple lesions are common, and a true miliary dissemination is uncommon. The vesicular stage is characterized by smooth, thin-walled cysts without peripheral edema and often without contrast enhancement that are filled with fluid resembling CSF on CT (hypodense) and MRI (T1 hypointense, T2 hyperintense). During the colloid vesicular stage the cyst fluid gets hyperdense compared with CSF on CT and hyperintense on T1-weighted and PD-weighted MRI reflecting high protein content. Fluid–fluid levels may be visible. Cyst wall and scolex remain isodense/isointense to brain parenchyma. The ongoing inflammation induces peripheral edema and (ring) enhancement which may progress under treatment. The diffuse encephalitic form in young individuals is characterized by severe brain swelling. During the granular nodular stage the thick-walled retracting lesions appear isointense on T1-weighted and T2-weighted MRI with or without T2 hyperintense center. Contrast enhancement is solid or ring shaped. Surrounding edema may be present or not. Finally, the shrunken and calcified lesions of the nodular calcified stage appear hyperdense on CT and iso- to hypointense on T1-weighted and T2-weighted MRI, typically without contrast enhancement and surrounding edema. T2*-weighted MRI is useful to detect calcifications. FLAIR sequences are helpful to better assess the extent of edema and for identifying hyperintense intraventricular cysts. Magnetic resonance imaging is the imaging modality of choice. Calcifications can be depicted best on GRE sequences and CT (Figs. 5, 6, 7).

4.3 Differential Diagnosis

Neurocysticercosis may be differentiated from brain abscess using T2-weighted and diffusion-weighted MRI. Brain abscesses typically have T2 hypointense rims, high signal on DWI, and low ADC values in the cavity. Tuberculomas are usually solid enhancing lesions often accompanied by meningitis. Primary CNS neoplasms and metastases typically present with more irregular, strongly enhancing margins and signs of tissue infiltration. A primary may be known. In solitary lesions differentiation from pilocytic astrocytoma or hemangioblastoma may be difficult without having additional diagnostic information at hand (serological testing, etc.). Arachnoid cysts do not enhance, follow CSF signal on all MR sequences, and have no "mural nodule." The same holds true for enlarged perivascular spaces.

According to Del Brutto et al. (2001) diagnostic criteria for neurocysticercosis based on objective clinical, imaging, immunological, and epidemiological data have been defined. Four categories of criteria stratified on the basis of their diagnostic strength, including the following, have been set up: (1) absolute—histological demonstration of the parasite from brain or spinal cord lesion biopsy, cystic lesions with visualization of the scolex on CT or MRI, and direct visualization of subretinal parasites by funduscopic examination; (2) major—lesions highly suggestive of neurocysticercosis on neuroimaging studies, positive serum enzyme-linked immunoelectrotransfer plot for the detection

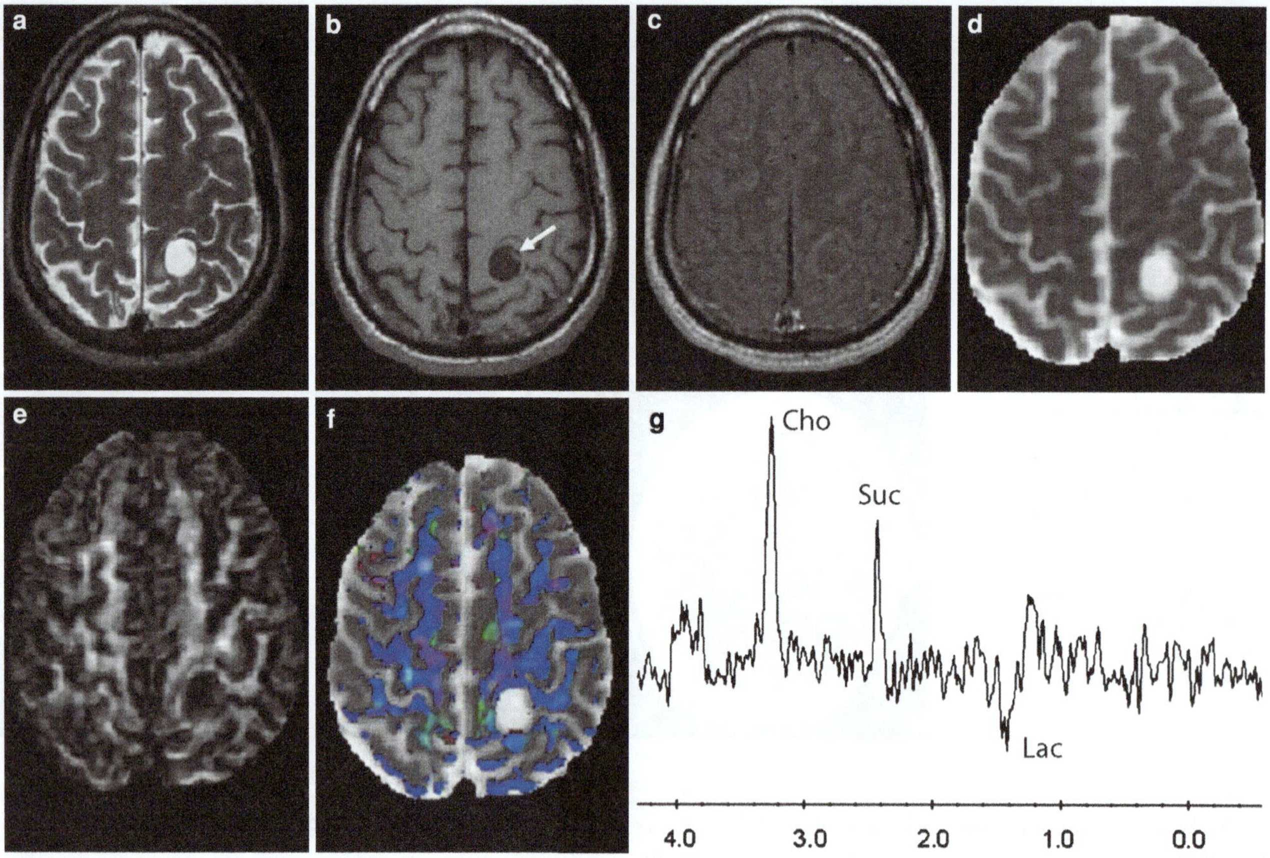

Fig. 6 Neurocysticercosis in a 40-year-old man who presented with headache. **a** Axial T2-weighted image. **b** Axial T1-weighted image before contrast administration. **c** Axial T1-weighted image after contrast administration with MT contrast. **d** Axial ADC map. **e** FA map. **f** Color-modulated FA map. **g** Proton MRS. Hyperintense cyst on the left side with eccentrically placed hypointense scolex on T2-weighted image. The lesion appears hypointense with isointense scolex on non-enhanced T1-weighted image (**b**, *arrow*) and shows minimal rim enhancement (**c**). Elevated ADC (**d**) and absent anisotropy in the cyst (**e**). Color-modulated FA map (**f**) shows no orientation in the cavity. In vivo proton MRS. **g** Demonstrates resonances of lactate (1.33 ppm), succinate (2.4 ppm), and choline (3.22 ppm) (courtesy of R.K. Gupta)

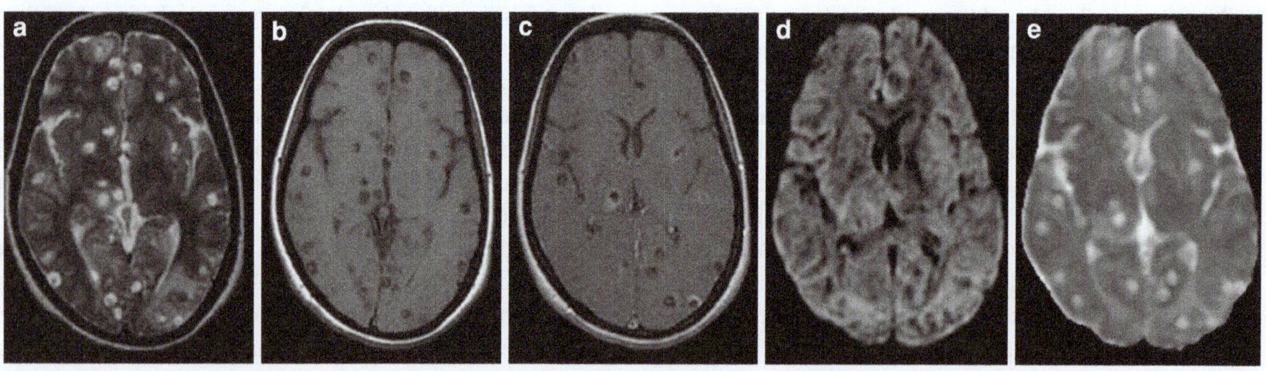

Fig. 7 Multiple neurocysticercosis cysts in a 25-year-old man with headache, nausea, and vomiting. **a** Axial T2-weighted image. **b** Axial T1-weighted image before contrast administration. **c** Axial T1-weighted image after contrast administration. **d** Axial DWI. **e** Axial ADC map. Multiple cysts with eccentrically placed hypointense scolex (**a**). The lesions appear hypointense with isointense scolex on T1-weighted images (**b**) and show minimal rim enhancement (**c**). Diffusion is not restricted (**d, e**) (courtesy of R.K. Gupta)

of anticysticercal antibodies, resolution of intracranial cystic lesions after therapy with albendazole or praziquantel, and spontaneous resolution of small single contrast-enhancing lesions; (3) minor—lesions compatible with neurocysticercosis on neuroimaging studies, clinical manifestations suggestive of neurocysticercosis, positive CSF enzyme-linked immunosorbent assay for detection of anticysticercal antibodies or cysticercal antigens, and cysticercosis outside the CNS; and (4) epidemiological—evidence of a household contact with *Taenia solium* infection, persons coming from or living in an endemic area, and history of frequent travel to endemic areas. From these criteria two degrees of diagnostic certainty may derived: (1) definitive diagnosis, in patients who have one absolute criterion or in those who have two major plus one minor and one epidemiological criterion; and (2) probable diagnosis in patients who have one major plus two minor criteria, in those who have one major plus one minor and one epidemiological criterion, and in those who have three minor plus one epidemiological criterion.

5 Echinococcosis

5.1 Epidemiology, Clinical Presentation, Therapy

5.1.1 Epidemiology

Echinococcus granulosus (main definite host: dog) has a worldwide distribution, whereas *Echinococcus multilocularis* (main definite host: fox) is endemic in the northern hemisphere in zones with intermediate climate (Central Eurasia, North America). The larval form is pathogenic to humans who represent an erroneous intermediate host. Adult tapeworms live in the intestine of their definite hosts and expel their eggs through feces. After oral ingestion (contact or smear infection) or indirect infection through contaminated water or food, the parasites are released in the human intestine and penetrate the mucosa, enter the venous (and/or lymphatic) system, and distribute to different organs, mainly into liver (50–70 %) and lung (15–30 %), seldom into spleen, kidneys, and brain. The CNS manifestations have a prevalence of approximately 2–6 % in infected individuals. Inside the organs *E. granulosus* develops large solitary cysts that contain scolices, broad capsules, and often daughter cysts embedded in a thick pericyst with nutritive vessels. Clinical symptoms are mainly due to mass effects. Mortality is low with 2–4 % (Germany, Switzerland). *E. multilocularis* forms an alveolar network of communicating cysts that grows by external budding of the germinal membrane, progressively infiltrates the surrounding tissue, and finally destructs the affected organ. Necrosis and calcifications are common. After a long chronic course, alveolar echinococcosis is often fatal—even under treatment—with a 10-year mortality rate of up to 90 %.

5.1.2 Clinical Presentation

The incubation time is highly variable ranging from months to several years. Children and adults can be infected. The majority of patients are in their third to fifth decade of life. Clinical presentation is typically unspecific. In later stages, the disease symptoms of vascular or biliary compression (including icterus) may occur due to significant mass effects as well as ascites, abdominal and pulmonary symptoms, and pain. Spontaneous rupture of *Echinococcus* cysts leads to parasitic spread and may induce severe allergic reactions. Vessel erosion may cause unlimited bleeding. Patients with cerebral echinococcosis may present with headaches, focal neurological deficits, seizures, and hydrocephalus. Serological tests and neuroimaging are diagnostic. ELISA enables an early diagnosis and differentiation between *E. granulosus* and *E. alveolaris*.

5.1.3 Therapy

Prophylaxis includes anti-helminthic medication of pets (dogs, cats) and proper hygiene. Treatment is multidisciplinary. Surgery is the treatment of choice in *E. granulosus*, typically in combination with perioperative chemotherapy. In punctate lesions PAIR (puncture, aspiration, injection, reaspiration) is an option, with installation of alcohol to neutralize the parasites before surgery. Resection of the pericyst usually enables a safe removal of the hydatid. Rupture or incidental surgical opening of the cyst is a severe complication, however, with uncontrollable spread of parasites. In non- or incompletely resectable hydatids long-term medication with mebendazole and albendazole is required. In contrast, surgical treatment is rarely an option in *E. multilocularis*. Organ invasion and destruction often makes a complete removal of the conglomerated alveolar cysts impossible. Lifelong parasitostatic medication with benzimidazoles is the only therapeutic option but is not a curative approach.

5.2 Imaging

Cerebral hydatids have a predilection for the hemispheres, in particular the parietal lobe and the vascular territory of the middle cerebral artery. The lesions appear as solitary or multiple thin-walled spherical cysts that show no contrast enhancement and no peripheral edema. Magnetic resonance imaging may show particulate substrate within the cyst that represents daughter scolices and hydatid sand (aggregates of scolices). Their content resembles CSF on CT and MRI. Calcification is rare. Cerebral alveolar echinococcosis appears as multilocular solid, semisolid, or cystic lesions with definite margins and without scolex. Calcification is common. Peripheral edema and contrast enhancement are typically found in the inflammation zone around the cysts (Figs. 8, 9).

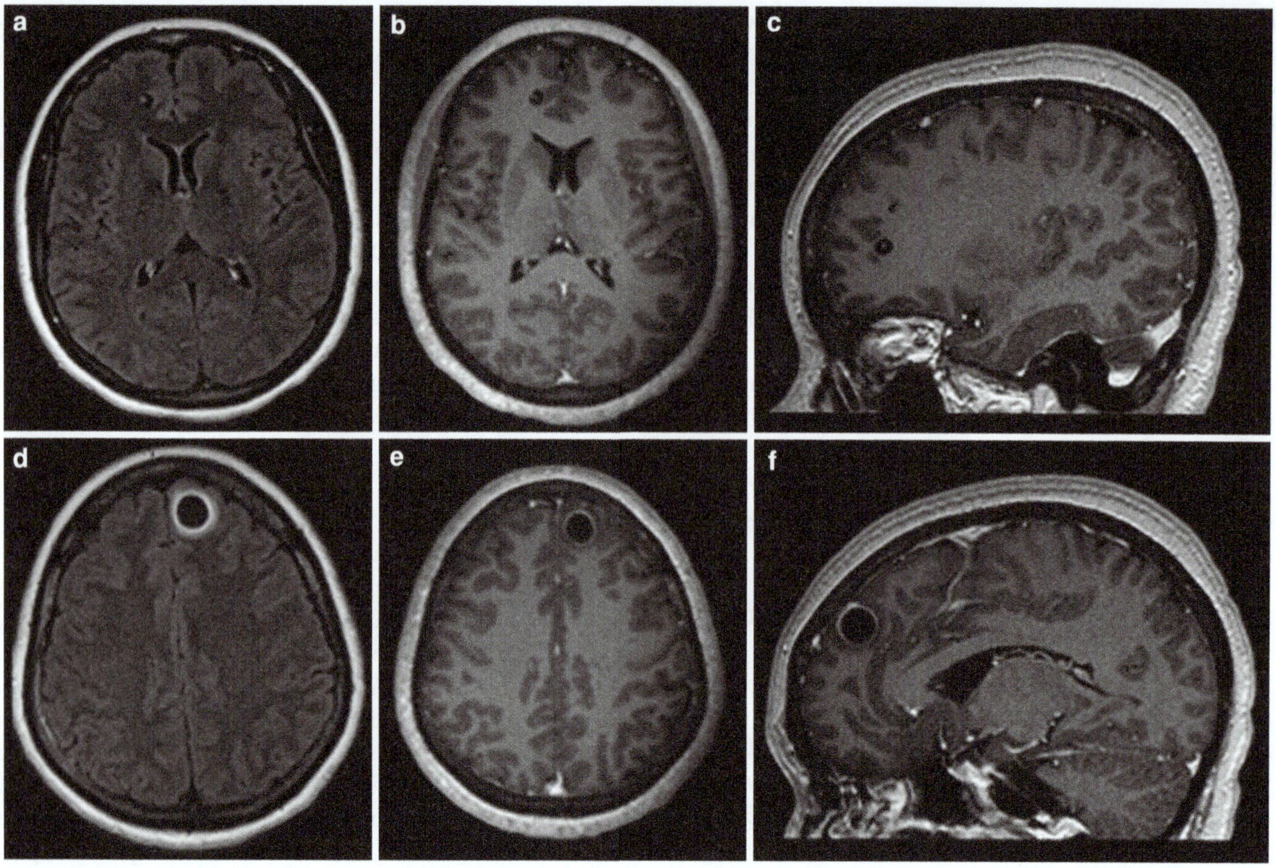

Fig. 8 Different evolutionary stages of neurocysticercosis in a 24-year-old immunocompetent woman; upper row vesicular stage with a scolex, lower row degenerating colloidal vesicular stage. **a, d** axial T2-FLAIR images, **b, e** axial contrast enhanced T1-weighted images, **c, e** sagittal contrast enhanced T1-weighted images

5.3 Differential Diagnosis

The main differential diagnoses for the cystic form (*E. granulosus*) include brain abscess, cystic tumors, and metastases (these lesions typically enhance and are associated with surrounding edema!), arachnoid cyst, or porencephalic cyst. Gliomas, metastases, tuberculomas, and fungal infections are the most important differentials for the alveolar form (*E. multilocularis*).

6 Trichinosis

6.1 Epidemiology, Clinical Presentation, Therapy

6.1.1 Epidemiology

Trichinella spiralis is a human pathogen nematode with a worldwide distribution. After nearly complete elimination of the disease in Europe during the late nineteenth century, the rate of infections is actually increasing with more than 20,000 cases in the past decade. A speciality of *Trichinella* is that each infected animal or human is a definite host and also becomes an intermediate host during the course of the disease. The adult worms live in the intestine (definite host), the larvae in the peripheral muscles (intermediate host). Contaminated meat is the main source of infection containing encapsulated larvae. After oral ingestion, the larvae penetrate the intestinal mucosa where they mature to adult worms that copulate and finally breed living larvae. The larvae actively enter the blood or lymphatic system, from where they distribute to the peripheral muscles. Here the larvae enter muscle cells, encapsulate, and persist infectiously over many years. More than 1 mm-large capsules containing dead larvae calcify and are visible during butchery.

6.1.2 Clinical Presentation

Trichinosis is a biphasic disease. The adult worms are responsible for the enteric period which is characterized by abdominal pain, vomiting, diarrhea, and nausea. The larvae

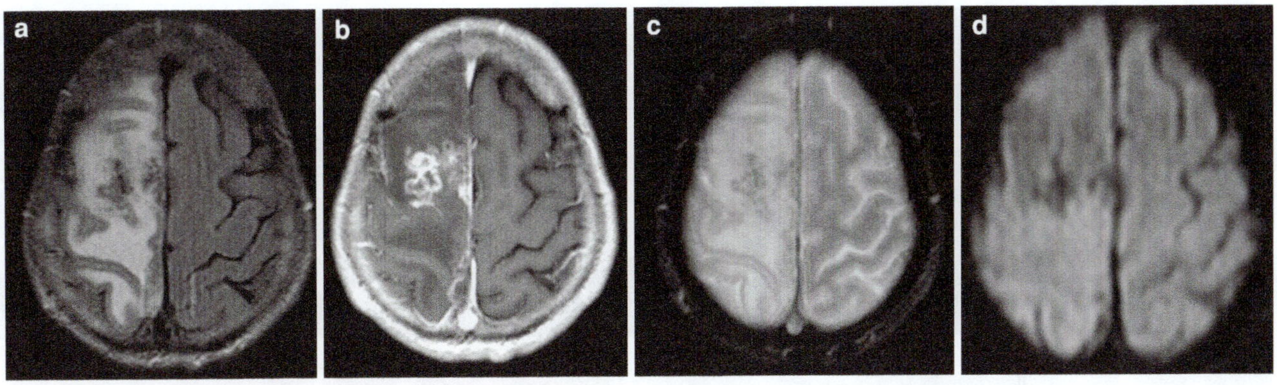

Fig. 9 Cerebral alveolar echinococcosis . **a** Axial FLAIR image. **b** Axial T1-weighted image after contrast administration. **c** Axial T2*-weighted image. **d** Axial DWI. The right frontal lesion is space occupying and appears inhomogeneous on T2-weighted images (**a**) with a mixture of hyperintense and hypointense areas, the latter correlating mainly to calcifications as confirmed on T2*-weighted images (**c**). Marked peripheral edema is present (**a**). Contrast enhancement appears irregularly with diffuse and ring-enhancing parts around necrotic zones underlining the destructive character of the disease (**b**) (courtesy of J. Fiehler)

are responsible for the parenteric period. Initial symptoms include eyelid and ankle swelling due to allergic host reactions, followed by muscular pain, fever, weakness, and dyspnea. Usually, the disease follows a mild to moderate clinical course. Severe illness occurs in 5–10 % of cases which may be complicated by myocarditis and CNS dysfunction mainly due to acute meningoencephalitis and (thrombo-)ischemic events. Neurotrichinosis seems to be related to marked hypereosinophilia and shares similarities with the hy pereosinophilic syndrome. Muscle biopsy is often diagnostic. Additional information on CNS manifestations is provided by CT, MRI, CSF testing (eosinophilia), and serological tests (increased muscle enzymes).

6.1.3 Therapy

Antiparasitic medication includes thiabendazole, alternatively mebendazole or flubendazole. It is noteworthy that the synchronicity of potentially life-threatening neurological and cardiac events in trichinosis makes a complete diagnostic workup necessary when first symptoms occur as a basis for effective treatment.

6.2 Imaging

Cerebral trichinosis is characterized by eosinophilic meningoencephalitis, vascular (arteriolar) thrombosis, and small white and gray matter infarctions. On CT multifocal hypodense small white matter and cortical lesions have been described along with cortical infarctions. After contrast administration, ring enhancement is typical. Diffuse white matter hypodensity of the centrum semiovale may also be present. Literature data about trichinosis are rare: In a case report MRI findings in neurotrichinosis were attributed mainly to multiple microinfarctions at the border zones of major vascular territories, in the periventricular white matter, and the corpus callosum. The lesions appeared hyperintense on T2-weighted and FLAIR images with reduced ADC and showed no contrast enhancement. Most lesions regressed over time (3 weeks and months follow-up). In another case report focal lesional contrast enhancement has been described and bilateral diffuse T2 hyperintensities in the centrum semiovale representing further possible MRI findings. Representative reports with larger numbers of patients addressing specific MR findings in neurotrichinosis and addressing the differential diagnosis are, however, lacking.

7 Schistosomiasis

7.1 Epidemiology, Clinical Presentation,Therapy

7.1.1 Epidemiology

Schistosomiasisis endemic in Asia, Africa, and South America. Approximately 250–300 million people are infected and a further 600 million are at risk for future infections. There are different species of schistosoma that are pathogenic to humans: *S. haematobium* mainly infesting the urogenital tract and *S. mansoni*, *S. intercalatum*, *S. japonicum*, and *S. mekongi* primarily infesting the intestine. Watersnails (*Biomphalaria* sp., *Bulinus* sp.) are the intermediate hosts, man is the definite host. The entry for the schistosoma cercaria is active percutaneous. After mating in the portal vein, male and female blood flukes build lifelong pairs (permanent copula) colonizing the human venous system of the target organ. The adult parasites are harmless, but their fertilized eggs are highly

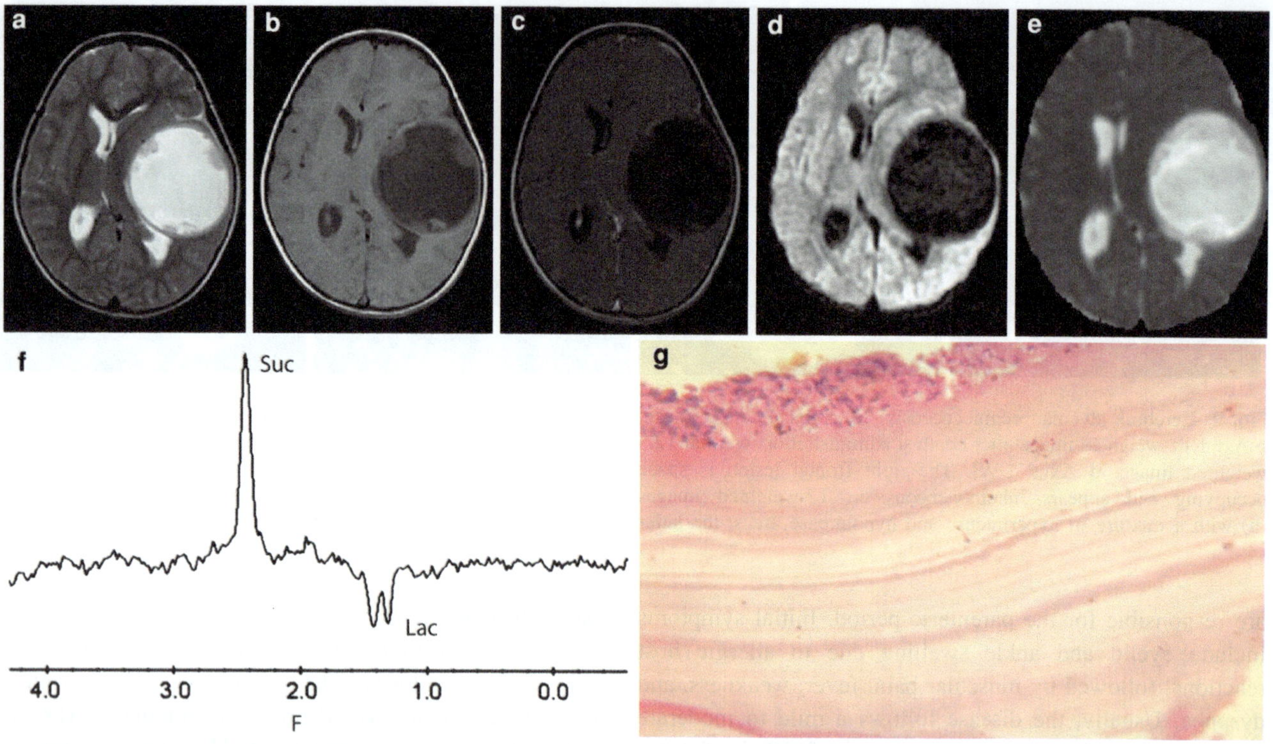

Fig. 10 Hydatid cyst (echinococcosis) in a 12-year-old girl who presented with signs of raised intracranial tension. **a** Axial T2-weighted image. **b** Axial T1-weighted image before contrast administration. **c** Axial T1-weighted image after contrast administration. **d** Axial DWI. **e** Axial ADC map. **f** Proton MRS. **g** Photomicrograph (HE stain). Large, well-defined rounded hyperintense area with hypointense rim on T2-weighted image (**a**). The lesion appears hypointense on non-enhanced T1-weighted image (b) and shows minimal rim enhancement (**c**). Particulate wall-adherent substrate within the cyst that probably represents daughter scolices and hydatid sand (**a–c**). Non-restricted diffusion in the cyst (**d**, **e**). Proton MRS (**f**) demonstrates resonances of lactate (1.33 ppm) and succinate (2.4 ppm). Photomicrograph shows a cellular amorphous laminated layer on HE stain (courtesy of R.K. Gupta)

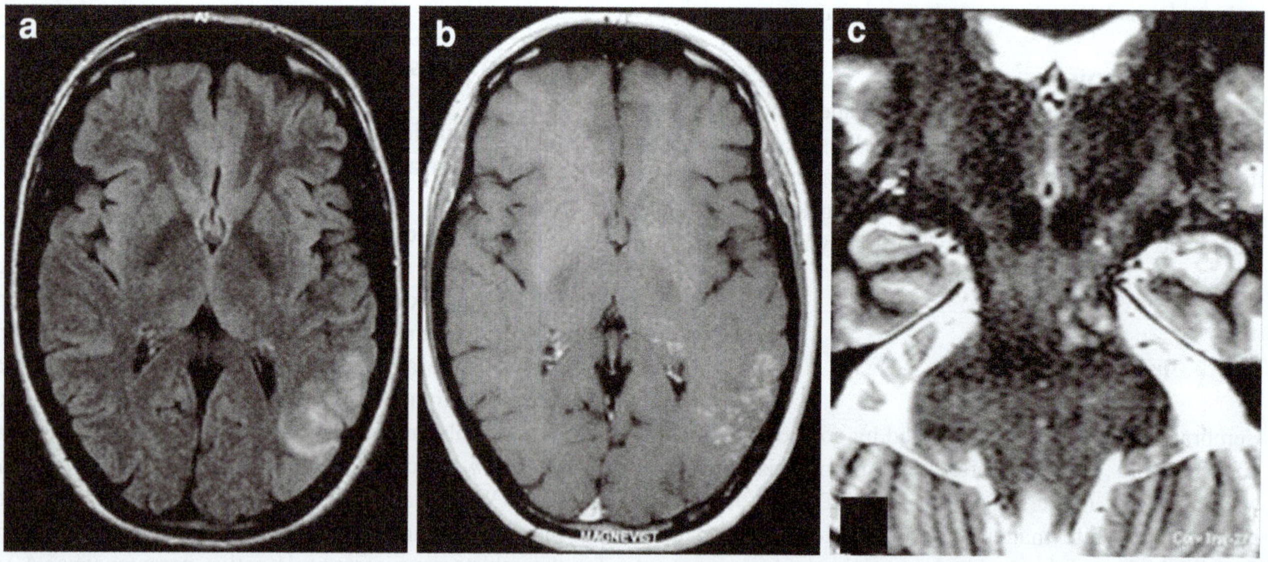

Fig. 11 Cerebral schistosomiasis in a 38-year-old woman. **a** Axial FLAIR image. **b** Axial T1-weighted image after contrast administration. **c** Coronal T2-weighted image. Supratentorial (**a**, **b**) and brainstem manifestations (**c**). The left parietal lesion shows punctate contrast enhancement (**b**) surrounded by edema as vizualized best on FLAIR imaging (**a**). The left-sided brain-stem lesion appears partially cystic and inhomogeneously hyperintense on T2-weighted images (**c**)

pathogenic. The eggs are released into the venous system from where they drift to different organs including the CNS.

7.1.2 Clinical Presentation

The percutaneous invasion of the larvae is accompanied by itching and local cutaneous hyperemia. Clinical symptoms are often delayed and may occur even years after infection. The eggs induce characteristic intravascular granulomas that occlude intrahepatic veins leading to portal hypertension, hepatosplenomegaly, and ascites. The CNS infections in childhood go along with physical, mental, and sexual retardation. Schistosomiasis is associated with an increased risk for cancer of the target organs (bladder, colon, rectum). The acute form has been termed "Katayama fever" and is characterized by fever, chills, cough, headaches, acute hepatosplenomegaly, and lymph node swelling. Usually, the illness regresses over several weeks, but the outcome may also be fatal.

7.1.3 Therapy

The antiparasitic agent is praziquantel. Oxidiazoles represent an alternative. *Phytolacca dodecandra* (plant) is useful for prophylaxis. In endemic areas the availability of uncontaminated water and better sanitary facilities are important.

7.2 Imaging

Cerebral schistosomiasis causes a non-specific granulomatous inflammation with surrounding edema on CT and MRI. Brain and spinal cord can be affected. Computed tomography reveals single or multiple hyperdense masses with surrounding edema. On MRI the lesions are T2 hyperintense and show a characteristic pattern of contrast enhancement on T1-weighted sequences, which is a centrally linear enhancement surrounded by multiple punctate nodules (Figs. 10, 11).

Acknowledgments I would like to thank Professor Rakesch K. Gupta and Dr. Jens Fiehler for providing image material and Dr. Leonie Jestedt for her support in Literature Search.

References

Del Brutto OH, Rajshekhar V, White AC Jr, Tsang VC, Nash TE, Takayanagui OM, Schantz PM, Evans CA, Flisser A, Correa D, Botero D, Allan JC, Sarti E, Gonzalez AE, Gilman RH, García HH (2001) Proposed diagnostic criteria for neurocysticercosis. Neurology 57:177–183

Further Reading

Bükte Y, Kemanoglu S, Nazaroglu H, Özkan Ü, Ceviz A, Simsek M (2004) Cerebral hydatid disease: CT and MR imaging findings. Swiss Med Wkly 134:459–467

Chang KH, Han MH (1998) MRI of CNS parasitic diseases. J Magn Reson Imaging 8:297–307

Cordoliani YS, Sarrazin JL, Felten D, Caumes E, Léveque C, Fisch A (1998) MR of cerebral malaria. Am J Neuroradiol 19:871–874

Feydy A, Touze E, Miaux Y, Bolgert F, Martin-Duverneuil N, Laplane D, Chiras J (1996) MRI in a case of neurotrichinosis. Neuroradiology 38:80–82

Fourestie V, Douceron H, Brugieres P, Ancelle T, Lejonc LJ, Gherardi RK (1993) Neurotrichinosis. Brain 116:603–616

Gelal F, Kumral E, Dirim Vidinli B, Erdogan D, Yucel K, Erdogan N (2005) Diffusion-weighted and conventional MR imaging in neurotrichinosis. Acta Radiol 46(2):196–199

Lucius R, Loos-Frank B (2008) Biology of parasites. Springer, Heidelberg

Newton RJC, Warrel DA (1998) Neurological manifestations of falciparum malaria. Ann Neurol 43:695–702

Osborn AG (1994) Diagnostic neuroradiology. Mosby, St. Louis

Osborn AG (2004) Diagnostic imaging brain. Amirsys, Salt Lake City

Part II

Meninges

Inflammatory Diseases of the Meninges

Stefan Rohde

Contents

S. Rohde (✉)
Division of Neuroradiology,
Heidelberg University Medical Center,
Im Neuenheimer Feld 400, 69120 Heidelberg, Germany
e-mail: Stefan.Rohde@med.uni-heidelberg.de

Abstract

Neuroimaging is of major importance in all cases of suspected infectious meningitis in order to get quick information about the extent of the disease, typical lesion patterns, and potential complications, such as hydrocephalus, involvement of the underlying brain parenchyma, or vasculitis. In bacterial meningitis, abnormal and asymmetrical enhancement of the leptomeninges and the subarachnoid space is typical. Initial neuroimaging has to rule out infectious foci of the skull base such as purulent sinusitis or mastoiditis. In patients with focal deficits or seizures, MRI is the tool of choice to diagnose vascular or septic complications. Neoplastic, viral, or fungal infections of the CNS may present with similar changes of the meninges; however, fungal meningitis normally causes a thicker and more nodular enhancement. In case of basal accentuation of the leptomeningeal contrast enhancement and conspicuous signal changes in the basal cisterns, one has to consider tuberculous meningitis for differential diagnosis, especially in patients with HIV infection. Non-infectious causes of meningeal enhancement comprise several primary and secondary tumors (e.g., CNS lymphoma, medulloblastoma, or breast cancer), granulomatous diseases, intracranial hypotension, and post-operative changes.

1 Introduction

Inflammation of the protective membranes covering the brain and spinal cord, known collectively as the meninges, may develop in response to a number of causes, most prominently bacteria and viruses, but also fungi, parasites, radiation, or neoplasm. Moreover, a number of systemic diseases, such as sarcoidosis or vasculitis, may involve the meninges.

S. Hähnel (ed.), *Inflammatory Diseases of the Brain*, Medical Radiology. Diagnostic Imaging,
DOI: 10.1007/174_2012_633,
Published Online: 21 June 2012

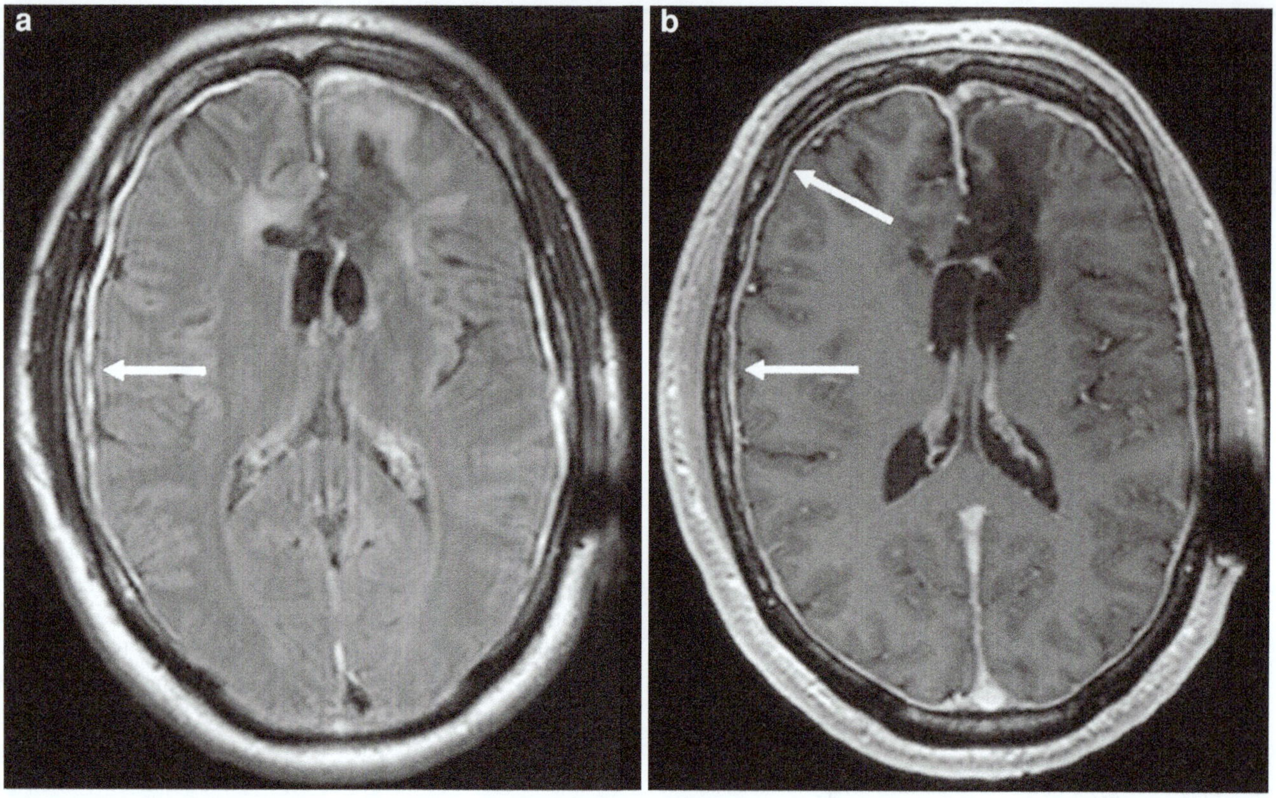

Fig. 1 Intracranial hypotension. A 44-year-old patient who had been surgically treated for an oligodendroglioma of the left frontal lobe. Early post-operative MRI (3 T). **a** Axial FLAIR image. **b** Axial T1-weighted image after contrast administration. Thickening and increased contrast enhancement of the pachymeninges with effusion into the subdural space (*arrows* in **a, b**), representing transient reactions of the dura-arachnoid complex due to intra-operative intracranial hypotension

In cases of acute infectious meningitis, rapid diagnosis and identification of the probable pathogen is mandatory, as early effective antimicrobial treatment is of major importance. While examination of the CSF, laboratory analysis, and biopsy remain the gold standard to identify the infectious agent, neuroimaging plays an important role in visualizing typical lesion patterns, the extent of the disease, and the potential involvement of deeper brain structures. In addition, imaging may help to identify sources of infection, such as fractures of the skull base, infection of the temporal bone or mastoid, and to rule out other, non-infectious causes of inflammatory disease of the meninges, such as granulomatous or neoplastic processes.

2 General Pathophysiological Considerations

Anatomically, the meninges consist of three layers: the dura mater; the arachnoid mater; and the pia mater. However, for a better understanding of meningeal inflammation in neuroimaging, it is helpful to use the anatomic—functional classification of lepto- and pachymeninges (Smirniotopoulos et al. 2007).

The leptomeninges (skinny meninges) comprise the membranes of the arachnoidea and the pia mater; the latter one follows the surface of the brain. The space between the arachnoid mater and the pia mater is the subarachnoid space (SAS). The vessels within the leptomeninges have a blood–brain barrier (BBB) that inhibits leakage of endogenous and exogenous serum compounds under physiological conditions. Infections of the leptomeninges and the SAS cause multiple pathophysiological changes in brain homeostasis. The SAS is infiltrated with inflammatory cells, which release glycoproteins and toxins that affect the tight junctions of the vascular endothelium, leading to a breakdown of the BBB. Serum fluid, proteins, and cells leak into the SAS and the adjacent cortex and cause interstitial and parenchymal edema. The breakdown of the BBB also allows contrast material to leak from the vessels into the CSF. The typical pattern of leptomeningeal enhancement follows the surface of the brain and fills the SAS of the sulci

Table 1 Probable causes of predominant leptomeningeal contrast enhancement in neuroimaging

Etiology	Type of enhancement	Remarks
Bacterial meningitis	Asymmetrical, thin, linear enhancement of the leptomeninges and the SAS, typically affects convexities	Tuberculous meningitis predominantly affects the basal meninges and cisterns, often cranial nerve involvement
Viral meningitis	Thin, linear enhancement	Often no enhancement
Fungal meningitis	Thick, lumpy, or nodular enhancement	May also cause pachymeningeal enhancement
Neoplastic ("carcinomatous") meningitis	Wide range from thin and linear to thick, lumpy, or nodular enhancement; may also involve dural structures	May also involve underlying cortex or pachymeningeal structures; most often in CNS lymphoma, breast cancer, medulloblastoma, and ependymoma
Neurosarcoidosis	Wide spectrum of leptomeningeal (and pachymeningeal) enhancement, especially in basal cisterns, often cranial nerve involvement	–

Table 2 Probable causes of predominant pachymeningeal contrast enhancement in neuroimaging

Etiology	Type of enhancement	Remarks
Intracranial hypotension, e.g., after surgery, lumbar puncture	Linear enhancement of the dura and falx cerebri with global homogeneous thickening	Additional findings: enlargement of the pituitary gland; low cerebellar tonsils; subdural effusions/hemorrhage
Meningioma	Curvilinear enhancement adjacent to the bulky tumor ("dural tail")	–
Metastases	Thick, nodular irregular enhancement	Most often from breast cancer and prostatic cancer
Granulomatous diseases, e.g., sarcoidosis, Wegener's granulomatosis	Wide spectrum of pachymeningeal and leptomeningeal, often irregular enhancement, typically affecting basilar meninges and the cranial nerves	–

and cisterns. While bacterial and viral meningitis are supposed to exhibit enhancement that is thin and linear, fungal meningitis and neoplastic infiltration of the leptomeninges may produce thicker, lumpy, or nodular enhancement in the SAS. A list of the potential causes of leptomeningeal enhancement is given in Table 1.

The pachymeninges (thick meninges) consist of the dura mater and the outer layer of the arachnoid mater; they follow the dural flections of the inner table of the skull, the falx cerebri, tentorium cerebelli, and the venous sinus. The vessels within the dura mater do not produce a BBB; thus, serum compounds, such as albumin, fibrinogen, or contrast agent, can leak into the dura mater. Therefore, the pachymeninges can be seen on contrast-enhanced CT or T1-weighted MR images as a thin, linear, and sometimes discontinuous enhancement, following the inner table of the skull, the falx, and the tentorium cerebelli. Typically, irritation and inflammation of the pachymeninges may arise from various benign or malignant processes, including transient post-operative changes, intracranial hypotension, meningioma, metastases, lymphoma, and granulomatous disease that lead to vasocongestion and interstitial edema of the dura mater (Table 2). Classical imaging features of isolated inflammation of the pachymeninges include thickening and increased enhancement of the dura-arachnoid complex *without* enhancement of the sulci or brain surface (Fig. 1).

3 Bacterial Meningitis

3.1 Epidemiology, Clinical Presentation, Therapy

Bacterial meningitis is the purulent infection of the cerebral and spinal leptomeninges. The incidence in the U.S. and Western Europe is about 5–10/100,000 persons. Meningitis is the most common form of CNS infection in children. Mortality ranges between 20 and 30 %, and neurological sequelae occur in 15–40 % of surviving patients. Infection may arise from hematogenous spread during systemic infection, from a chronic suppurative focus, or per continuitatem during acute or chronic infections of the paranasal sinus, the middle or inner ear, or the mastoid. Another path of infection is brain injury with open or covered disruption of the dura mater, especially when the paranasal sinus or the air-filled cavities of the temporal bone are involved in the fracture.

The type of microorganism responsible for meningitis depends on the age of the patient and the way of infection: while in neonates the most common pathogens are *group-B*

Streptococcus and *Escherichia coli*, in infants it is *Haemophilus influenzae*, *Streptococcus pneumoniae*, and *Neisseria meningitidis*. In adolescents and adults *Streptococcus pneumoniae* and *Neisseria meningitidis* are found most often. In a study on the epidemiology of 696 episodes of community-acquired meningitis in adults, *S. pneumoniae* was determined to be the responsible pathogen in 51 %, *N. meningitides* in 37 %, and *Listeria monocytogenes* in 4 % of cases (van de Beek et al. 2004); however, due to vaccination against *H. influenzae* and *S. pneumoniae*, epidemiology of bacterial meningitis changes constantly.

In patients with ENT infections or after splenectomy, *S. pneumoniae* are the most common causative species in bacterial meningitis. After neurosurgery and in patients with open brain injury or with dural fistulae, *S. aureus* and *Pseudomonas aeroginosa* are found frequently beside *S. pneumoniae* and *H. influenzae*. Immunocompression and alcoholism are associated with *Listeria monocytogenes*, different types of *Enterococcus*, *S. aureus*, and *S. pneumoniae*.

In most of the cases meningitis starts with unspecific prodromes such as abnormal fatigue growing pains that may last for several hours or days before the onset of meningeal symptoms. On admission more than 90 % of patients with bacterial meningitis present with at least two of the following four symptoms: fever; neck stiffness; changes in mental status—the "classical triad" and headache. Headache is the most common symptom in meningitis and is found in more than 80 % of the patients. Further symptoms indicating irritation of the leptomeninges are nausea, conjunctivitis, hyperesthesia, and hyperacusis. Approximately one fourth of the patients develop petechial rash, with *N. meningitidis* as the most frequent causative pathogen. One third of the patients have focal neurological deficits such as cranial nerve palsy, aphasia, hemiparesis, or seizures. These symptoms are associated with a lower level of consciousness and indicate a more severe course of the disease; they are more frequent in pneumococcal than in meningococcal meningitis (van de Beek et al. 2004). Bacterial meningitis may be complicated by cortical and subcortical infarctions due to septic vasculitis of the cerebral arteries, hydrocephalus, brain edema, empyema, or pyogenic abscess. Systemic complications result from bacteremia and comprise the Waterhouse–Friderichsen syndrome (e.g., meningococcal sepsis with disseminated intravasal coagulation and petechial bleeding), the adult respiratory distress syndrome (ARDS), and septic emboli into the lung or peripheral vessels.

Empirical antimicrobial treatment has to be started immediately after lumbar puncture and sampling blood cultures. Therapeutic regimens comprise antibiotic combinations from the penicillin, rifamycine, cephalosporin, and aminoglycoside groups. Antiedematous treatment with dexamethasone before or with the first dose of antimicrobial therapy has been proven to reduce the risk of unfavorable outcome, including mortality and neurological complications (Weisfelt et al. 2006). In cases of transmitted bacterial meningitis from infections of the sinus, mastoid, or middle ear, surgical removal of the focus is mandatory.

3.2 Imaging

In uncomplicated cases and the initial phase of the disease, neuroimaging might reveal normal findings of the brain and meninges; however, a CT exam should be performed in all patients with suspected bacterial meningitis prior to lumbar puncture to rule out brain edema and potential herniation. As a sign of beginning disturbance of the CSF circulation, CT might reveal mild enlargement of the ventricles and the SAS; the basal cisterns can be effaced. After administration of contrast medium, CT might demonstrate linear leptomeningeal enhancement in the sulci and cisterns that might increase during the course of the disease, especially if antibiotic treatment is not started or is started with delay (Kastrup et al. 2005). Parenchymal lesions are often difficult to distinguish; however, CT is a simple and fast tool for monitoring critically ill patients and to rule out severe complications of bacterial meningitis, such as resorptive hydrocephalus, swelling, venous thrombosis, or infarction. Besides cerebral structures, CT provides important information about probable pathologies of the skull base, the temporal bone, and the nasal sinus, such as fractures, purulent sinusitis, otitis media, or mastoiditis; therefore, CT of patients with bacterial meningitis should always include a reconstruction of the skull base in the "bony window".

Although not specific for a certain type of meningitis or a causative pathogen, contrast-enhanced T1-weighted images have been proven to be more effective in demonstrating meningeal enhancement than contrast-enhanced CT (Chang et al. 1990). Abnormal enhancement of the leptomeninges is usually asymmetrical and extends into the basal cisterns. Besides the importance of contrast-enhanced T1-weighted images, MRI may reveal an increased signal of the SAS on T2-weighted and FLAIR images, indicating leakage of the BBB with hypercellularity or increased proportions of proteins in the CSF (Fig. 2). When patients with bacterial meningitis develop focal neurological symptoms or seizures, MRI is the tool of choice to diagnose vascular or septic complications (Fig. 3). Diffusion-weighted imaging (DWI) is highly sensitive in depicting small cortical or deep white matter infarctions that are hardly seen with conventional MRI, whereas vascular changes can be visualized directly with MRA. Moreover, bacterial meningitis may cause subarachnoid hyperintensity on DWI, predominantly around the frontal lobe, a finding that is often associated with poor prognosis (Kawaguchi et al. 2012). In cases of severe stenosis, vasospasm, or vessel occlusion due to septic vasculitis, PerfMRI may help to get functional information about potential collaterals and the "tissue at risk," which is clinically helpful in deciding whether or not to use high-dose steroid therapy.

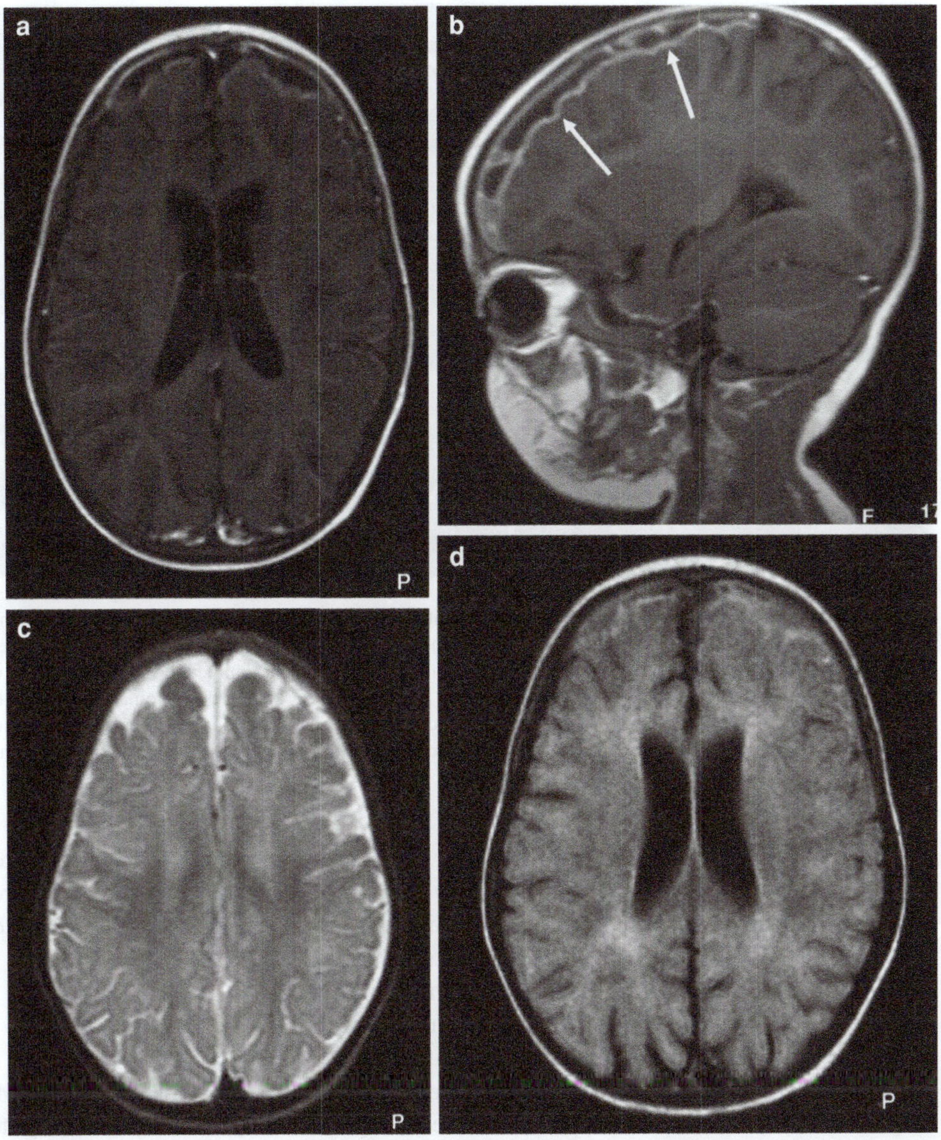

Fig. 2 Pneumococcal meningitis in a 5-year-old child. **a** Axial T1-weighted image after contrast administration. **b** Sagittal T1-weighted image after contrast administration. Pneumococcal meningitis in a 5-year-old child. **c** Axial T2-weighted image. **d** Axial FLAIR image. Bifrontal subdural exudates (**c, d**) with relatively high signal compared with the CSF (**d**), indicating an elevated content of proteins

Subdural or epidural empyemas are slightly hyperintense relative to CSF and hypointense to white matter on T1-weighted images and hyperintense relative to CSF and white matter on T2-weighted images (Fig. 4). They are often associated with edema and mass effect. On DWI subdural empyema usually show high signal, whereas epidural empyema tend to be of low or mixed signal intensity (Kastrup et al. 2005).

3.3 Differential Diagnosis

Isolated enhancement of the leptomeninges is not specific for bacterial infection. Viral or fungal meningitis may present with similar changes of the meninges and the SAS, however, fungal meningitis normally causes a thicker, lumpy, or nodular enhancement in the SAS. Subarachnoid hemorrhage (SAH), acute stroke, high inspired oxygen, or imaging artifacts may cause an increased FLAIR signal in CSF that can be mistaken for infectious exudates in the SAS. Additionally, several primary and secondary tumors, e.g., medulloblastoma, breast cancer, or CNS lymphoma, may cause leptomeningeal enhancement as well, known as "carcinomatous meningitis." In the majority of cases, clinical presentation, medical history, and analysis of the CSF will provide the clue for differential diagnosis.

4 Tuberculous Meningitis

4.1 Epidemiology, Clinical Presentation, Therapy

In Central Europe tuberculous meningitis (TBM) has become relatively rare; however, due to socio-economic changes and the increasing number of HIV infections, the

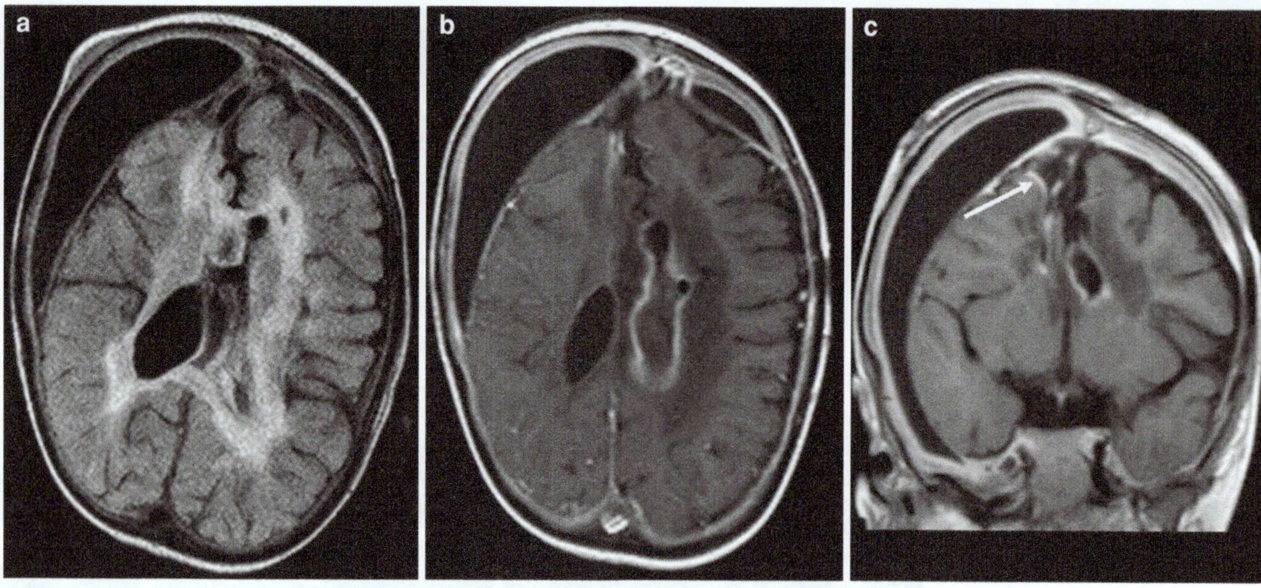

Fig. 3 Ventriculitis after complicated bacterial meningitis. A 3-year-old boy with medical history of premature birth, SAH, and hydrocephalus occlusus. The child developed a pneumococcal meningitis due to shunt infection that was complicated by ventriculitis. **a** Axial FLAIR image. **b** Axial T1-weighted image after contrast administration. **c** Coronal T1-weighted image after contrast administration. Hyperintensity of the ependyma and the subependymal white matter (**a**). The fluid in the left ventricle shows a higher signal than normal CSF (**a**), indicating a higher level of proteins and cell detritus. Chronic subdural hygroma on the right. **c** Coronal T1-weighted image after contrast administration. Thin linear enhancement of the ependyma of the ventricles (**b, c**) and in the channel of the ventricular drainage (**c**, *arrow*)

incidence of TBM is rising again. Worldwide, more than 8 million patients come down with TB annually. The TBM is the most frequent manifestation of CNS TB and is more common in children. The meninges are affected secondarily through hematogenous spread in patients with miliary tuberculosis or from ruptured tuberculous granulomata. In adults, the primary focus often cannot be identified.

Clinically, TBM starts with unspecific symptoms such as fatigue, ill humor, diminished appetite, elevated temperature, and headache that may last for several weeks. Signs of meningeal affection often begin slowly and without disturbances of consciousness. Because of the predominant affection of the basal parts of the meninges, TBM frequently causes cranial nerve palsy, primarily of the abducent nerve, the oculomotor nerve, and the facial nerve. In severe cases TBM may affect also caudal cranial nerves and spinal nerves. Hydrocephalus and secondary vasculitis are main complications. Mortality is still 10–20 %; it is even higher in underdeveloped countries and after delayed diagnosis.

Treatment has to be started as soon as possible, even without direct proof of the causative pathogenic agent, when clinical presentation and liquor results (e.g., moderate pleocytosis of 100–200 cells, strong positive lactate and protein, low glucose) suggest the diagnosis of TBM. Modern regimens comprise an antituberculostatic combination with Isoniazid, Rifampicin, Pyracinamid, or Ethambutol for at least 2 months or longer, when CSF is still positive for tuberculosis. In complicated cases intrathecal injection of streptomycin has been proposed as adjunctive treatment. Steroids should be given to prevent secondary vasculitis.

4.2 Imaging

As the prognosis of TBM depends on starting treatment early, and confirmatory tests take longer time (culture, PCR), imaging of TBM is crucial for immediate diagnosis. The typical imaging feature of TBM is enhancement of the basal cisterns and the corresponding leptomeninges caused by dense fibrinous exudate in the SAS (Fig. 5). Basal meningeal enhancement is found in approximately 60 % of TBM cases. Interestingly, several studies have demonstrated that tuberculous meningitis is not only seen on contrast-enhanced T1-weighted images, but also on non-enhanced T1-weighted MT images, showing the inflamed meninges as distinct basal periparenchymal hyperintensity (Kamra et al. 2004). This phenomenon is reported to be missing in patients with meningitis of other etiology; thus, visibility of the meninges on non-enhanced T1-weighted MT images has to be considered highly suggestive of tuberculous meningitis. Yet, one has to keep in mind that formation of exudates requires a competent immune system in the host, as a consequence meningeal enhancement is often less pronounced or even missing in elderly patients

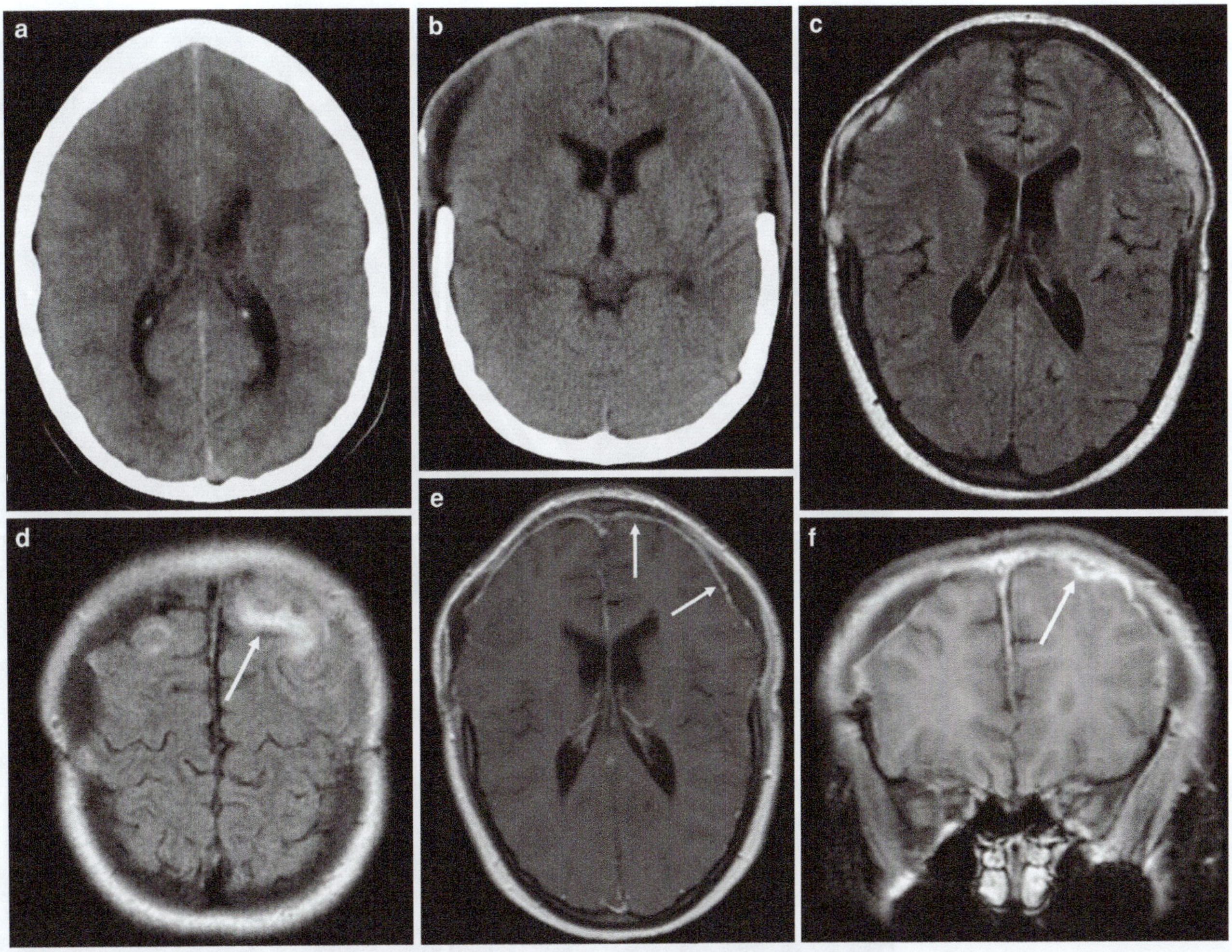

Fig. 4 Pneumococcal meningitis with complicating epidural empyema. A 14-year-old girl who presented initially with clouded consciousness and recurrent generalized seizures due to meningococcal meningitis. Indication for bifrontal hemicraniotomy was made due to pronounced general brain edema. **a** Axial CT before bifrontal hemicraniotomy. **b** Axial CT after bifrontal hemicraniotomy. **c, d** Axial FLAIR images after bifrontal hemicraniotomy. Pneumococcal meningitis with complicating epidural empyema. A 14-year-old girl who presented initially with clouded consciousness and recurrent generalized seizures due to meningococcal meningitis. Indication for bifrontal hemicraniotomy was made due to pronounced general brain edema. **e** Axial T1-weighted image after contrast administration after bifrontal hemicraniotomy. **f** Coronal T1-weighted image after contrast administration after bifrontal hemicraniotomy. Axial FLAIR images (**c, d**) show hyperintense signal in the epidural fluid collection within the bifrontal craniotomy defects and hyperintense changes of the frontal cortex (*arrow in* **d**). One month after the surgical intervention, the patient developed seizures again. Axial and coronal contrast-enhanced T1-weighted images (**e, f**) demonstrate bifrontal pachymeningeal enhancement, and additionally leptomeningeal and cortical enhancement of the adjacent frontal lobe (*arrows*), leading to the diagnosis of complicated bacterial meningitis with epidural empyema and beginning brain involvement

and individuals with immune deficiency (Srikanth et al. 2007).

Further imaging findings in TBM comprise hydrocephalus malresorptivus in approximately 50–80 % and infarcts due to secondary vasculitis in 30–40 % of TBM cases. Both ischemic and hemorrhagic infarcts are diagnosed best with DWI and T2*-sequences on MRI; however, studies comparing CT and MRI have shown that advantages of MRI are minimal in terms of hydrocephalus and basal enhancement (Garg 2010). Advantages of MRI are confirmed for patients with cranial nerve palsy: Imaging should always be performed in the axial and coronal plane using contrast-enhanced T1-weighted images with fat saturation to check for potential cranial nerve enhancement in the basal cisterns, the cavernous sinus, or the orbital cavities (see also "Neurotuberculosis").

4.3 Differential Diagnosis

Other causes of infectious and carcinomatous meningitis have to be considered for differential diagnosis. While TBM causes predominantly basilar meningeal enhancement,

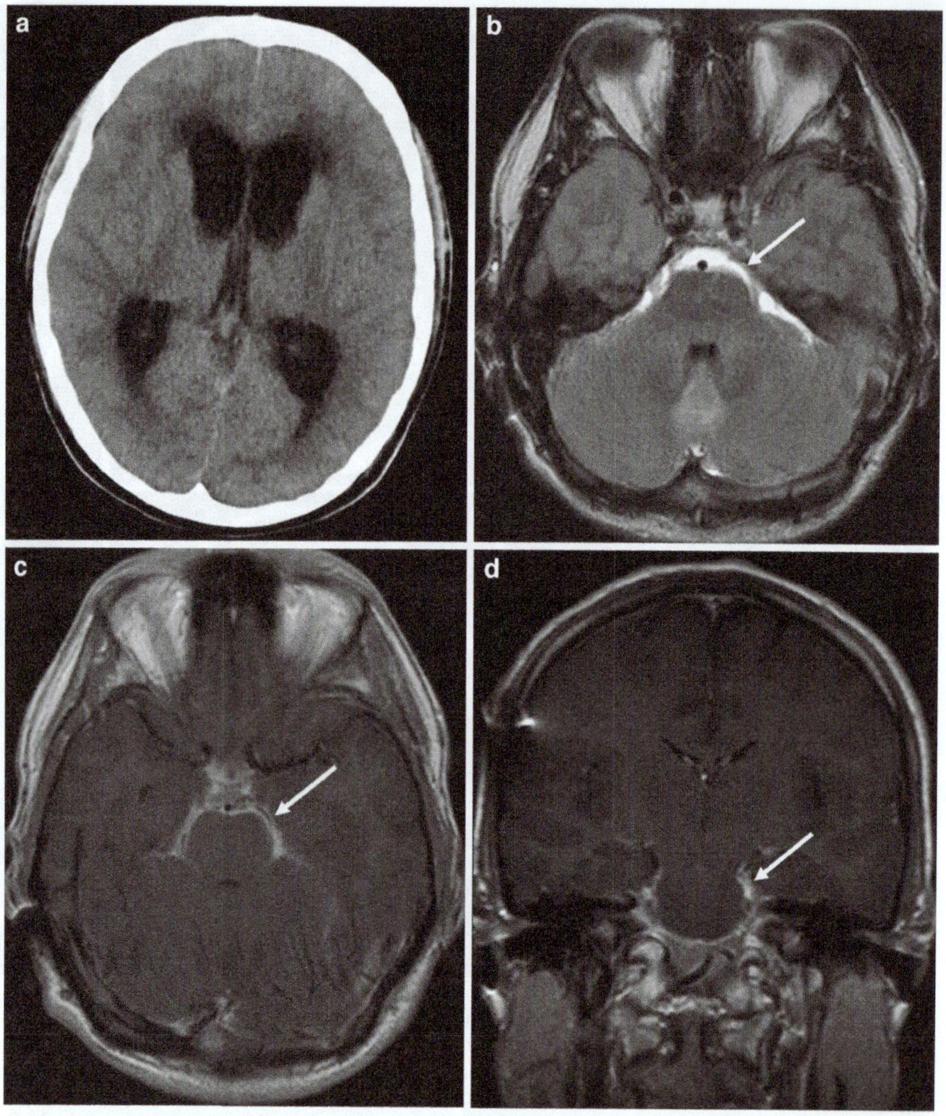

Fig. 5 Tuberculous meningitis. A 24-year-old patient, with a history of intravenous drug abuse, presented with headache and abducent nerve palsy. **a** Axial CT. **b** Axial T2-weighted image. **c** Axial T1-weighted image after contrast administration. **d** Coronal T1-weighted image after contrast administration. Initial CT (**a**) showed hydrocephalus. MRI revealed basal meningitis with hyperintense exudates in the prepontine and basal cisterns and thick, linear leptomeningeal enhancement (*arrow* in **b, c**) around the pons, the pedunculi cerebelli, and within the quadrigeminal cistern. Examination of the CSF confirmed tuberculous meningitis

bacterial meningitis affects more often the leptomeninges of the convexities. Furthermore, the combination of meningitis and parenchymal lesions suggests tuberculosis; however, some primary or metastatic tumors and some parasitic CNS infections (e.g., coccidiomycosis) may be indistinguishable from TBM.

5 Viral Meningitis

5.1 Epidemiology, Clinical Presentation, Therapy

Isolated inflammation of the meninges due to virus infection is rare. Most viruses cause encephalitis or meningoencephalitis (described in detail in Chap. 9). Virus predominantly affecting leptomeningeal structures and the underlying cortex are HSV type 1, the most common causative agent for viral meningoencephalitis, and the arbovirus, that causes tick-borne meningoencephalitis (TBME). Additionally, parainfectious meningitis is a common finding in many systemic viral infections and after antiviral vaccination. Initial symptoms of viral meningitis are lassitude, fever, headache, and an altered sensorium. Epileptic seizures, aphasia, hemiparesis, clouded consciousness, or psychotic symptoms indicate an advanced "encephalitic state" of viral CNS infection. Analysis of the CSF might reveal mild, mononuclear pleocytosis (< 300 cells/m^3), normal glucose and lactate, and normal or elevated protein. Specific treatment with antiviral chemotherapeutics (e.g., acyclovir, gancyclovir, foscarnet) is not always possible and depends on the causative agent which should be diagnosed with PCR.

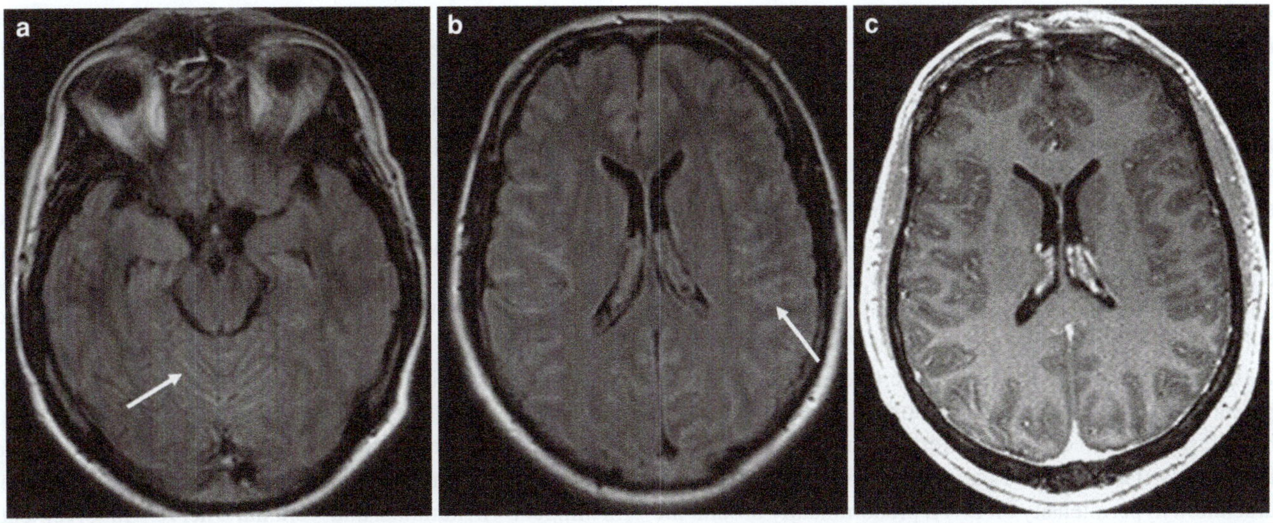

Fig. 6 Viral meningitis. A 36-year-old patient, who was admitted with fever, headache, and confused mental state. Lumbar puncture revealed moderate pleocytosis, normal glucose, and lactate. **a, b** Axial FLAIR images. **c** Axial T1-weighted image after contrast administration. Slightly hyperintense signal in the SAS of the sulci (*arrow* in **a, b**), suggestive of protein-rich inflammatory exudates due to viral infection. Pathological enhancement of the meninges is absent (**c**)

5.2 Imaging

In many cases and in early stages of viral meningitis, neuroimaging reveals no abnormalities or only unspecific changes such as focal or diffuse brain edema and swelling, or signal abnormalities in the SAS due to an increased protein content of the CSF (Fig. 6). In the later stage of HSV-1-meningoencephalitis, leptomeningeal, and cortico-medullary enhancement of the affected lobe may be visible; however, these changes follow the more specific changes of the disease with hyperintensity on T2-weighted and FLAIR images in limbic structures. Although patients with TBME develop meningitis in over 70 %, the majority of MRI scans are normal. Pathological findings indicating the presence of encephalitis comprise hyperintensities on T2-weighted images in the thalami, brain stem, caudate nucleus, or the cerebellum.

5.3 Differential Diagnosis

In cases of isolated viral meningitis, other infectious and neoplastic diseases, especially bacterial meningitis, have to be excluded. The diagnosis is made by testing of the CSF. In case of HSV meningoencephalitis, differential diagnosis includes paraneoplastic (limbic) encephalitis, ischemia, infiltrating neoplasm, other encephalitides (e.g., neuro-syphilis), and status epilepticus.

6 Fungal Meningitis

6.1 Epidemiology, Clinical Presentation, Therapy

Fungal infections of the CNS are most frequent in immunocompromised patients with AIDS, long-lasting diabetes mellitus, or after organ or bone marrow transplantation. Fungal hyphae (e.g., *Candida albicans*) primarily affect the meningeal microcirculation, whereas infections with *Cryptococcus neoformans, Aspergillus fumigatus*, or *Aspergillus flavus* involve predominantly larger cerebral vessels, leading to encephalitis, brain abscess, or vasculitis. The most common fungal infection of the CNS is cryptococcal meningoencephalitis, followed by aspergillosis and candidiasis. Cryptococcal meningoencephalitis manifests weeks after asymptomatic lung infection with clinical symptoms of basal meningitis, cranial nerve palsy, and hydrocephalus. The diagnosis is made through direct confirmation of the fungus in the CSF. Even under intensified treatment with amphotericin B and 5-flucytosine, mortality of cryptococcal meningoencephalitis is high; treatment is successful in only 30–50 % of cases.

Aspergillus may reach the CNS via hematogenous spread or through direct invasion from sinunasal aspergillosis. The infection manifests predominantly with solitary or multiple brain abscess or granulomata, less often with meningitis or ventriculitis. Mortality of CNS infection with *Aspergillus* is extremely high.

6.2 Imaging

Cryptococcal meningoencephalitis typically manifests with diffuse meningeal enhancement and ventriculitis beside characteristic cystic, punctuate lesions in the basal ganglia due to cryptococcal invasion of the perivascular spaces, the "soap-bubble lesions" (Kastrup et al. 2005; Hähnel et al. 2005). Hydrocephalus is found more often in immunocompetent patients as arachnoid reactions with exudates in the basal cisterns often do not manifest in immunocompromised individuals. Generally, fungal meningitis may cause subarachnoid hyperintensity on DWI, predominantly around the frontal lobe (Kawaguchi et al. 2012).

Imaging features of Aspergillus meningeal infection comprise pachymeningeal enhancement nearby the affected nasal sinus or the orbit; typically, bony structures are involved in the inflammatory process. More than 50 % of the patients develop hemorrhagic infarctions due to vasculitis of the perforating arteries of the basal ganglia. Parenchymal aspergillosis may appear as edematous and hemorrhagic lesions or solid, ring-like enhancing "tumoral" lesions with low signal intensity on T2-weighted images, which may be due to paramagnetic elements such as manganese and iron as well as blood-breakdown products. As laboratory findings of fungal infection do not always confirm the causative pathogen, knowledge of neuroradiological appearance of aspergillosis is helpful for early diagnosis (see also "Fungal infections").

6.3 Differential Diagnosis

Other infectious and neoplastic diseases, especially bacterial meningitis and TBM, have to be excluded. Fungal meningitis often causes a thicker and lumpier meningeal enhancement than bacterial or viral meningitis. In case of pachymeningeal enhancement and involvement of the skull base, neoplasms arising from the nasopharynx of the sinus have to be ruled out.

7 Neurosyphilis

7.1 Epidemiology, Clinical Presentation, Therapy

Syphilis is a curable sexually transmitted disease caused by the spirochete *Treponema pallidum*. The use of penicillin has reduced the incidence of syphilis during the past century; however, the trend has reversed since the 1980s due to the exchange of sex for drugs, unprotected sex, and the number of people with multiple sexual partners. The incidence of syphilis in industrialized countries is approximately 2–4/100,000 persons. The central nervous system may be involved at any stage of the infection in about 5–10 % of untreated patients; it is most common in patients with HIV infections. Neurosyphilis (Neurolues) is classified into four syndromes: syphilitic meningitis; meningovascular syphilis; as well as parenchymatous and gummatous neurosyphilis, these latter ones ending in general paresis and tabes dorsalis.

Syphilitic meningitis occurs usually in the second stage of the disease within the first 2 years after infection. It is thought to be the consequence of direct meningeal inflammation due to small-vessel arteritis. Patients present with headache, meningeal irritation, and cranial nerve involvement, especially the optic nerve, facial nerve, and the vestibulocochlear nerve.Meningovascular syphilis is assigned to the tertiary or late stage of syphilis. After prodromal symptoms that may last for weeks to months, focal deficits with unilateral numbness, paresthesias, hemiparesis, headache, vertigo, or psychiatric abnormalities are identifiable. These symptoms are caused directly by the inflammation of the meninges and the parenchyma or secondarily by infarctions and (aneurysm associated) bleedings due to vasculitis. The first-choice treatment for all manifestations of syphilis, including neurolues, is penicillin.

7.2 Imaging

There is only little systematic data about neuroradiological findings in neurosyphilis. Approximately one-third of the patients have normal findings (Brightbill et al. 1995). The majority of cases presents with non-specific white matter lesions or cerebral infarctions, less often with cerebral gummata. Syphilitic meningitis is a rare finding: The leptomeninges may present with thick and lumpy enhancement; predominantly the basal cisterns and the prepontine SAS are affected. In case of cranial nerve palsy, the involved nerve shows swelling and increased enhancement. Vasculitis is a common finding in MRA or DSA. Typical features include stenosis and interruption of large and medium-large arteries, and vasculitic aneurysms (see also "Neurolues").

7.3 Differential Diagnosis

In case of isolated syphilitic meningitis, other granulomatous diseases, especially tuberculosis, have to be excluded. The diagnosis is made by serological testing of the CSF and blood.

8 Neurosarcoidosis

8.1 Epidemiology, Clinical Presentation, Therapy

Sarcoidosis is a multisystem inflammatory disease characterized by non-caseating epithelioid-cell granulomas. Women are affected more frequently than men, and the onset of the disease is in the third and fourth decade. The CNS is involved in approximately 10 % of cases. In up to 50 % of cases, neurosarcoidosis is asymptomatic or self-limiting, and the remainder develop a chronic relapsing–remitting course of the disease. Typically, patients present with cranial nerve palsy, most often the facial nerve or the abducens nerve is affected. Further symptoms comprise meningeal irritation, signs of increased intracranial pressure, seizures, and hypothalamic or pituary gland dysfunction (e.g., diabetes insipidus). A specific treatment is not known, but corticosteroids are useful in most patients.

8.2 Imaging

Plain radiography and native CT may reveal osteolytic skull lesions. Contrast-enhanced CT and MRI will show a wide spectrum of leptomeningeal enhancement, especially of the basal SAS, and cranial nerve involvement; therefore, imaging of neurosarcoidosis should always include contrast-enhanced T1-weighted images with a slice thickness of 1–2 mm. Typically, neurosarcoid infiltration affects the infundibulum, chiasma, and hypothalamus. The granulomatous changes of the pachymeninges and in the SAS show focal or diffuse low signal intensity on T2-weighted images and isointense on T1-weighted images. More than 50 % of the patients present with periventricular hyperintense lesions on FLAIR and T2-weighted images, representing perivascular infiltrates in the Virchow–Robin spaces and vasogenic edema due to vasculitis of the small arteries. Diffusion-weighted imaging helps to distinguish acute cytotoxic edema from neurosarcoid-induced vasogenic edema (see also "Cerebral vasculitis" and "Granulomatous disease").

8.3 Differential Diagnosis

Known as the "great mimicker," differential diagnosis of neurosarcoidosis should include all types of meningitis, as well as neoplastic infiltration of the dura or the meninges (e.g., meningioma). The diagnosis is made by analysis of the chest X-ray, laboratory findings, and the CSF. In unclear cases, biopsy has to be considered for validation of the diagnosis.

References

Brightbill TC, Ihmeidan IH, Post MJD, Berger JR, Katz DA (1995) Neurosyphillis in HIV-positive and HIV-negative patients: neuroimaging findings. Am J Neuroradiol 16:703–711

Chang KH, Han MH, Roh JK, Kim IO, Han MC, Kim CW (1990) Gd-DTPA-enhanced MR imaging of the brain in patients with meningitis: comparison with CT. Am J Neuroradiol 11(1):69–76

Garg RK (2010) Tuberculous meningitis. Acta Neurol Scand 122(2):75–90

Hähnel S, Storch-Hagenlocher B, Kress B, Stippich C, Sartor K, Forsting M, Seitz A, Jansen O (2005) Infectious diseases of brain parenchyma in adults: imaging and differential diagnosis aspects. Rofo 177(10):1349–1365

Kamra P, Azad R, Prasad KN, Jha S, Pradhan S, Gupta RK (2004) Infectious meningitis: prospective evaluation with magnetization transfer MRI. Br J Radiol 77(917):387–394

Kastrup O, Wanke I, Maschke M (2005) Neuroimaging of infections. NeuroRx 2(2):324–332

Smirniotopoulos JG, Murphy FM, Rushing EJ, Rees JH, Schroeder JW (2007) Patterns of contrast enhancement in the brain and meninges. Radiographics 27(2):525–551

Kawaguchi T, Sakurai K, Hara M, Muto M, Nakagawa M, Tohyama J, Oguri T, Mitake S, Maeda M, Matsukawa N, Ojika K, Shibamoto Y (2012). Clinico-radiological features of subarachnoid hyperintensity on diffusion-weighted images in patients with meningitis. Clin Radiol 67(4):306-312. Epub 2011 Dec 20. PMID: 22192625 [PubMed–in process]

Srikanth SG, Taly AB, Nagarajan K, Jayakumar PN, Patil S (2007) Clinicoradiological features of tuberculous meningitis in patients over 50 years of age. J Neurol Neurosurg Psychiatry 78(5): 536–538

Van de Beek D, de Gans J, Spanjaard L, Weisfelt M, Reitsma JB, Vermeulen M (2004) Clinical features and prognostic factors in adults with bacterial meningitis. N Engl J Med 351(18):1849–1859

Weisfelt M, Hoogman M, van de Beek D, de Gans J, Dreschler WA, Schmand BA (2006) Dexamethasone and long-term outcome in adults with bacterial meningitis. Ann Neurol 60(4):456–468

Part III

Specific Topics

Granulomatous Diseases

Bodo Kress

Contents

Abstract

Granulomatous diseases of the central nervous system include a variety of different syndromes which are defined by focal inflammation containing fused and non-fused granulomas. Depending on the disease, different anatomical structures are affected. In many cases, MRI shows characteristic pattern of lesions and allows a specific diagnosis or a very specific differential diagnosis.

1 Tolosa–Hunt Syndrome

1.1 Epidemiology, Clinical Presentation, Therapy

Tolosa–Hunt syndrome (THS) was first published by Eduardo Tolosa in 1954. The syndrome was described by William Edward Hunt in 1996. The cause of THS is unknown. The THS is characterized by a chronic granulomatous inflammation of the apex of the orbit. Often, the cavernous sinus and the cranial nerves are also affected. The clinical symptoms are characteristic with unilateral orbital or facial pain combined with diplopia. The THS mostly occurs in adults. In histological samples non-specific granulomatous tissue is found. Therapy of choice in THS consists of the application of steroids.

In 1988 the International Society of Headache proposed the following diagnostic criteria:

1. One or more episodes of unilateral orbital pain over a period of approximately 8 weeks associated (at least 2 weeks).
2. Association with cranial nerve palsies affecting the third cranial nerve (oculomotor nerve), fourth cranial nerve (trochlear nerve), and sixth cranial nerve (abducens nerve) in the temporal context with pain with a maximum time difference of 2 weeks.
3. Improvement of pain after steroid administration in 72 h at most.
4. Exclusion of other cranial causes using MRI.

B. Kress (✉)
Department of Neuroradiology,
Central Institute of Radiology and Neuroradiology,
Steinbacher Hohl 2–26, 60488 Frankfurt, Germany
e-mail: kress.bodo@khnw.de

S. Hähnel (ed.), *Inflammatory Diseases of the Brain*, Medical Radiology. Diagnostic Imaging,
DOI: 10.1007/174_2012_625, © Springer-Verlag Berlin Heidelberg 2012
Published Online: 22 May 2012

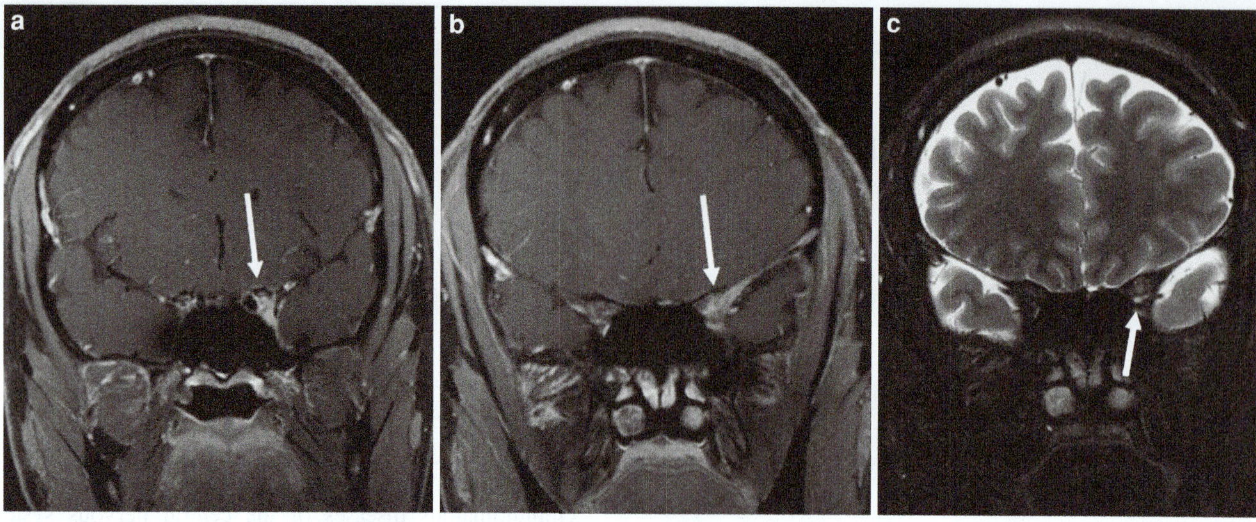

Fig. 1 Tolosa-Hunt syndrome . Patient with left-sided orbital pain and paresis of the left oculomotoric nerve. **a**, **b** Coronal T1-weighted image with suppression of the signal of fat (fat saturation) after contrast administration. **c** Coronal T2-weighted image with suppression of the signal of fat (fat saturation). On the left side the affected cavernous sinus is widened and reveals strong contrast enhancement (**a**, *arrow*). Pathological enhancement is evident also in the fat of orbital apex and the meninges (**b**, *arrow*). The paretic oculom\toric nerve in the left orbit has a high signal as a sign of damage (**c**, *arrow*)

1.2 Imaging

In some patients the enlargement of the cavernous sinus may be detectable even on CT. The imaging method of choice, however, is MRI. Coronal slices are most important. The slice package should cover the dorsal part of the ocular bulb, the cavernous sinus, and the pons (for detailed protocol recommendations see "Neurolues"). For planning the MR scan it is important to consider that the trochlear nerve arises from the back of the brain stem below the quadrigemine plate.

Lesions from THS are isointense relative to muscle on T1-weighted images and isointense to fat on T2-weighted images without fat saturation. On the affected side the cavernous sinus is enlarged, and the signal on non-enhanced T1-weighted sequences without fat saturation is intermediate; therefore, it is essential that the imaging protocol include also non-enhanced T1-weighted sequences without fat saturation: The hyperintense signal of normal fat of the pterygopalatine fossa, and of the orbital apex, are characteristic markers of non-affection. After contrast administration, the inflammatory tissue in the involved structures (cavernous sinus, orbital apex, pterygopalatine fossa) strongly enhances. The contrast enhancement typically does not involve the brain; meninges may sometimes reveal enhancement (Fig. 1).

1.3 Differential Diagnosis

The most important differential diagnosis is meningioma. The diagnosis can be confirmed by knowledge about the typical clinical and MR appearance of THS with slow clinical onset, combination of orbital or facial pain, and nerve palsies; however, sometimes the differential diagnosis may be difficult. In these cases follow-up MRI examinations after therapy are mandatory. Further differential diagnoses are sarcoid and lymphoma, both having different clinical courses with absent pain and a high and early recurrence rate after steroid therapy. Lymphoma, neurosarcoid, and meningioma are typically hypointense on T2-weighted images without fat saturation; however, pituitary adenomas, metastases, and rarely even meningiomas are isointense to fat on T2-weighted images without fat saturation.

2 Lymphocytic Hypophysitis

2.1 Epidemiology, Clinical Presentation, Therapy

Lymphocytic hypophysitis (LYH) is a rare autoimmune disease in which the pituitary gland is infiltrated by lymphocytes, plasma cells, and macrophages. The function of the pituitary gland is impaired. The LYH should be remembered in pregnant women and women of childbearing age with hyperprolactinemia, headache, visual field restrictions, and interference by one or more pituitary hormones with secondary disturbance of success organs, especially when the disease is combined with other autoimmune or endocrine disorders. Children, older women, and men are less commonly affected. Headaches, visual field restrictions, and infrequently diplopia, are caused by extrasellar enlargement of the pituitary gland with compression of the chiasma and

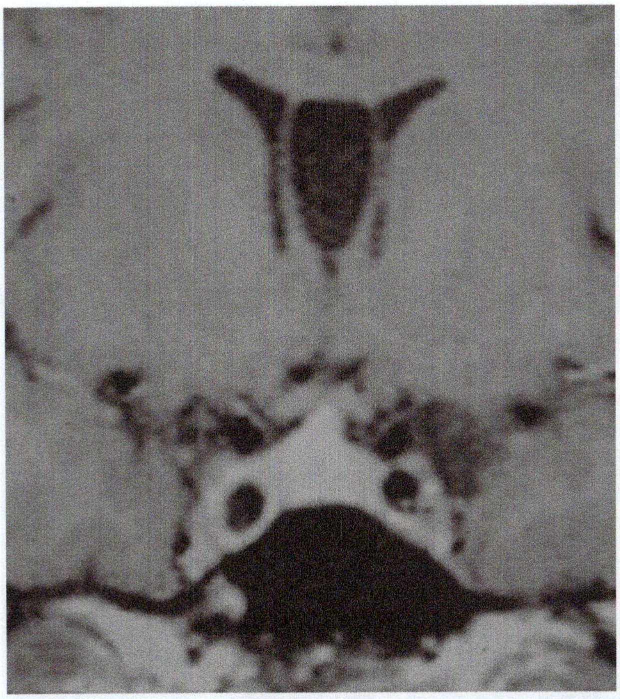

Fig. 2 Lymphocytic hypophysitis. Coronal T1-weighted image after contrast administration. Enlargement of the pituitary gland and stalk

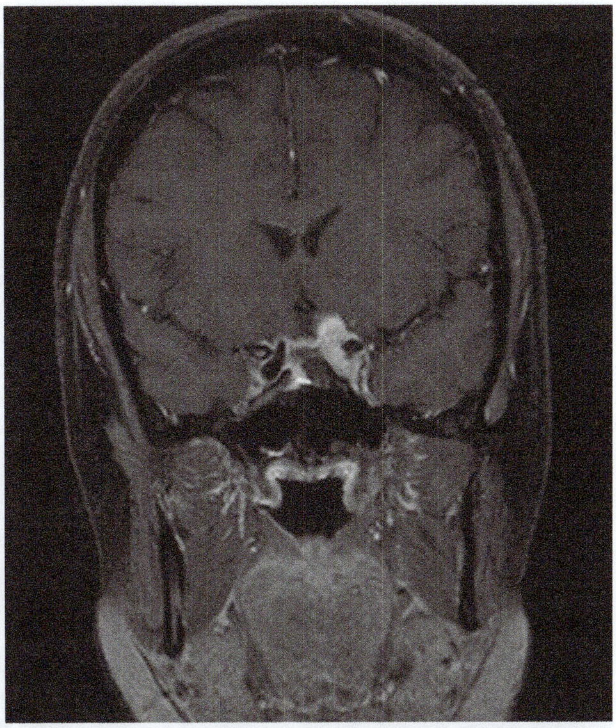

Fig. 3 Lymphocytic hypophysitis. Coronal T1-weighted image with suppression of the signal of fat (fat saturation) after contrast administration. Widened cavernous sinus on the *left* side. The granulomatous tissue does not respect the border of the cavernous sinus and spreads above to compress the enthorhinal cortex. Note that there is absent flow void in the distal left carotid artery

invasion of the cavernous sinus. Among the isolated endocrine deficits of the pituitary gland, ACTH deficit is the initial and most common deficit. A secondary adrenal insufficiency may occur with a high mortality. In some cases mass effect and infiltration of other structures are the main symptom of the disease.

Histopathological findings from pituitary biopsy reveal dense infiltrates of B- and T-lymphocytes, plasma cells with lymphoid aggregates surrounding atrophic acini of pituitary cells. Immunohistochemical analysis shows numerous mast cells randomly distributed and also localized in the vicinity of capillaries, suggesting a possible influence on capillary permeability and angiogenesis, thus favoring the inflammatory and immunological aggression against pituitary cells. Granulomas are absent. Antibodies against pituitary cells were found in many patients who suffered from LYH. The pathogenetic importance of these antibodies is unclear. Since possible spontaneous remission can occur, a careful follow-up is required in subclinical patients without important adrenal insufficiency or symptomatic extrasellar expansion. Therapy consists of endocrine replacement, neurosurgical decompression, and corticosteroids.

2.2 Imaging

The imaging method of choice is MRI. Coronal slices should be preferred. The slices should cover the dorsal part of the ocular bulb and the entire cavernous sinus (for detailed protocol recommendations see "Neurolues"). The pituitary gland and the cavernous sinus are enlarged on the affected side. Mostly, the infundibulum (pituitary stalk) and the adjacent meninges are also involved. The cavernous sinus contains substrate having hypointense signal on T2-weighted and non-enhanced T1-weighted images with homogeneous contrast enhancement. In addition, in some cases the internal carotid artery is involved and sometimes occluded by the tissue inflammation. Then the occluded artery enhances strongly (Figs. 2, 3, 4). New publications indicate that hypointense lesions in T2-weighted images around the pituitary gland and in the cavernous sinus might be pattern which might be characteristic for lymhocytic hypophysitis (Fig.5).

2.3 Differential Diagnosis

In contrast to pituitary adenomas, in LYH the sella is typically not enlarged. Another important differential diagnosis of LYH is THS, the latter neither affecting the pituitary gland nor the carotid artery. Moreover, in THS the symptoms improve within 72 h under steroid treatment, and hormone disorders are absent. Another important differential diagnosis is meningioma of the sphenoid wing and

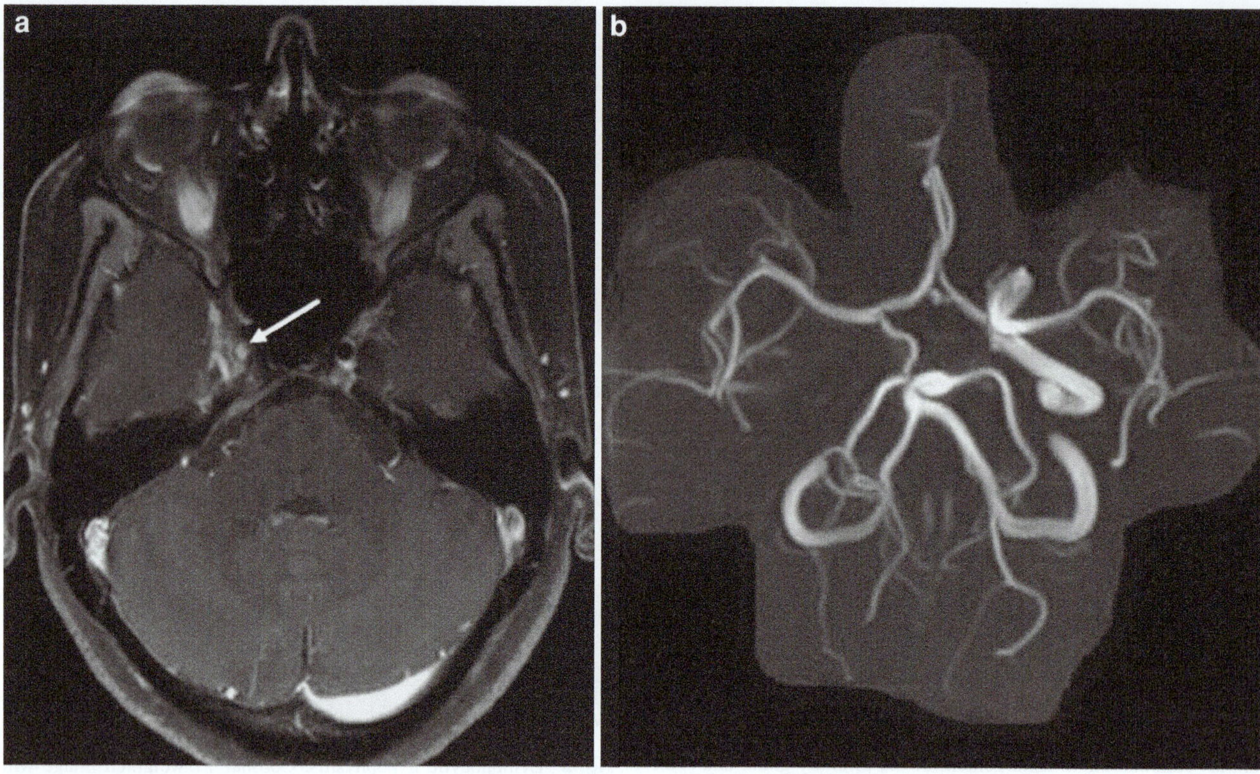

Fig. 4 Lymphocytic hypophysitis. **a** Axial T1-weighted image with suppression of the signal of fat (fat saturation) after contrast administration. **b** MIP of an arterial TOF MRA. There is a remarkable enhancement in the sphenoidal part of the right ICA (**a**, *arrow*) and in the right cavernous sinus. The enhancement is caused by granulomatous tissue which infiltrates the lumen of the right ICA (**a**). MRA confirms absent flow in the right ICA due to vessel occlusion (**b**)

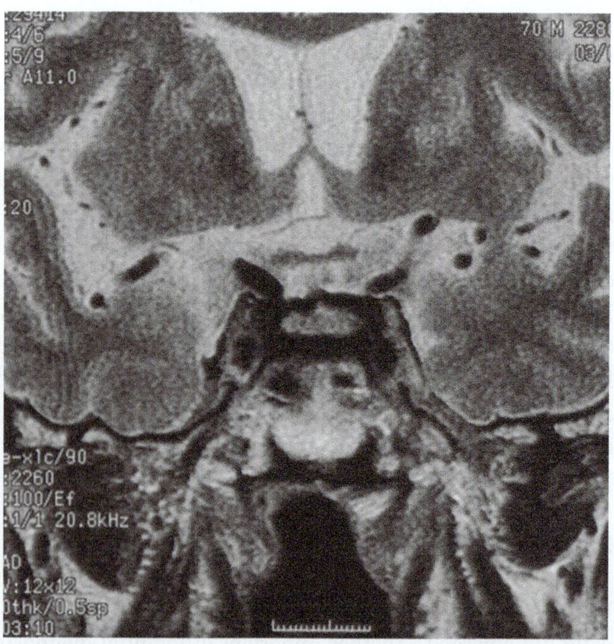

Fig. 5 Lymphocytic hypophysitis. Coronal T2w image. Enlarged pituitary gland is surrounded by a dark rim. Copyright permission granted by AJNR, image courtesy to Nakata et al. (2010)

meningioma of the tuberculum sellae, both accompanied by no hormonal disorders. Nevertheless, the differential diagnosis of LYH is difficult, because the MR signal of meningioma has a similar pattern as LYH. Meningioma does not diminish in size under high-dose steroid treatment. Other differential diagnoses are lymphoma and sarcoidosis. In many cases only biopsy can confirm the definitive diagnosis.

3 Neurosarcoidosis

3.1 Epidemiology, Clinical Presentation, Therapy

Sarcoidosis is a granulomatous disease with close topographic relationship to the vascular system. Typically, the systemic disease affects the lungs, in addition to the purely mediastinal lesions (lymphoma, stage I), and especially the pulmonary affection is typical. About 10 % of the cases affect the central nervous system, and in rare cases, the CNS is the sole place of disease. In stage I there might be an incidental finding on chest X-ray. Especially in stages IIb and III a

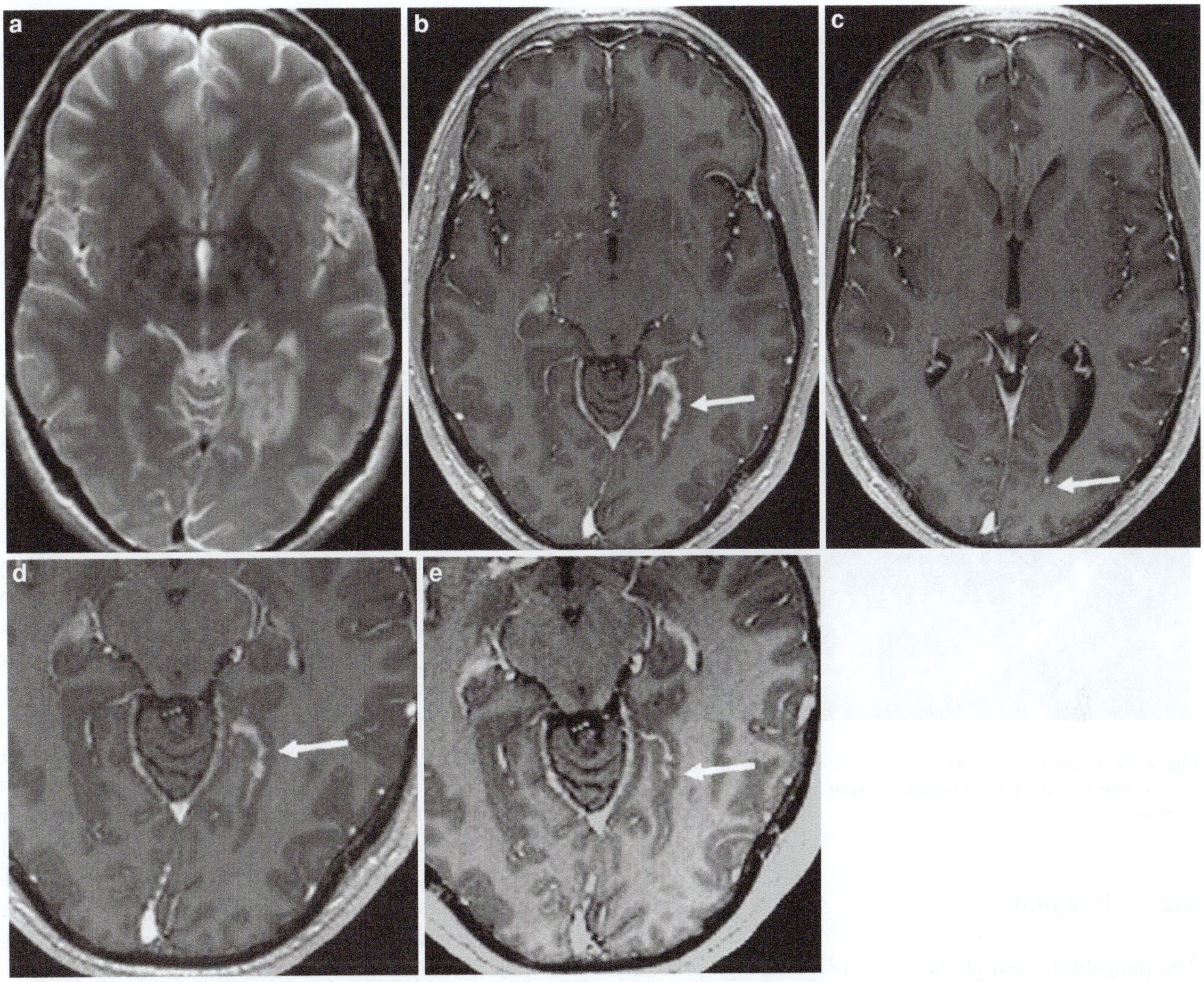

Fig. 6 Neurosarcoidosis before and under steroid treatment. **a**, **b** Initial examination. **d** Follow-up after 2 months. **e** Follow-up after 11 months. **a** Axial T2-weighted image. **b** Axial T1-weighted image after contrast administration. Sarcoid granulomas can lead to pearl-string thickening of the meninges, which may sometimes be difficult to differentiate from meningioma. In this case, the leptomeninges of the parietooccipital sulcus (**b**, *arrow*) and the ependyma of the occipital horn of the left lateral ventricle (**c**, *arrow*) are involved. Edema of the adjacent brain parenchyma (**a**) is evident. The granulomas diminished in size under steroid treatment (*arrows* in **d**, **e**). Neurosarcoidosis before and under steroid treatment. **c** Initial examination. **d** Follow-up after 2 months. **e** Follow-up after 11 months. **a** Axial T2-weighted image. **c–e** Axial T1-weighted image after contrast administration. Sarcoid granulomas can lead to pearl-string thickening of the meninges, which may sometimes be difficult to differentiate from meningioma. In this case, the leptomeninges of the parietooccipital sulcus (**b**, *arrow*) and the ependyma of the occipital horn of the left lateral ventricle (**c**, *arrow*) are involved. Edema of the adjacent brain parenchyma (**a**) is evident. The granulomas diminished in size under steroid treatment (*arrows* in **d**, **e**)

decrease in vital capacity and general symptoms happens as well as B symptoms with fever, night sweats, and weight loss. The symptoms of central nervous system affection are not specific enough. They range from simple headaches of visual impairment to neurological symptoms such as focal paresis and sensitivity disorders. The affection of the pituitary infundibulum can lead to disruption of hormone transport by, for example, the impact of diabetes insipidus. The drug of choice is an immunosuppressive medication with steroids and/or cytostatics. Despite aggressive therapy, often the disease turns into a chronic form. Non-caseating granulomas are typically macroscopic, showing giant cell nuclei histologically. Although there is no clear classification of the CNS affection, usually three different forms of affection are differentiated:

1. In the leptomeningeal form mainly the meninges are affected with inflammation and thickening. Sometimes neoplastic meningeal disease may be mimicked.
2. The most common form is the parenchymal form with affection of brain tissue, typically adjacent to the perivascular spaces. Also, affection of cranial nerves may occur.
3. In the vasculitic form primarily the vessel wall is involved.

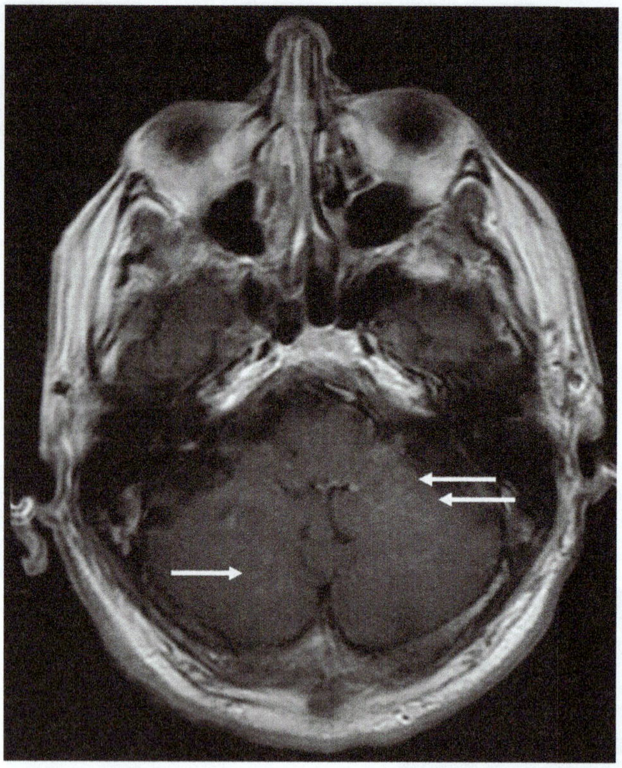

Fig. 7 Neurosarcoidosis. Axial T1-weighted image after contrast administration. Pathological enhancement of basal perivascular spaces (*arrows*)

3.2 Imaging

The imaging method of choice is MRI. Although primarily bigger, tumor-like lesions can be seen on CT; for the correct diagnosis; however, the high soft tissue contrast of MRT is indispensable (for detailed protocol recommendations see "Neurolues"). Both FLAIR and PD-weighted images are recommended for the detection of lesions adjacent to CSF. Magnetic resonance angiography is useful if the vasculitic form is suspected. To evaluate the leptomeningeal form, the coronal T1-weighted images with fat saturation should be performed additionally to standard non-fat-saturated images. In the case of cranial nerve affection, a T1-weighted 3D data set (e.g., T13D VIBE) contrast enhanced with a slice thickness below 1 mm should be performed. Subsequently, the multiplanar reconstruction of the cranial-nerve course is mandatory.

3.2.1 Leptomeningeal Form

Leptomeninges, and less commonly pachymeninges, are thickened and enhanced strongly and homogeneously. The thickening of the meninges can be so massive that the surrounding brain parenchyma is compressed with the consequence of edema (Fig. 6) and neurological symptoms due to the mass effect. Meningeal granulomas may even reach extracranial compartments by infiltration along the foramina of the skull base. The extension through the skull base is seen best on coronal T1-weighted images before and after contrast administration, if possible using fat saturation after contrast administration.

3.2.2 Parenchymal Form

The parenchymal form is the most common form of neurosarcoidosis with affection of the brain parenchyma adjacent to the perivascular spaces. The contrast enhancement in the brain is typically evident at the basal parts of the basal ganglia, in the crus cerebri, in the pons, and occipitoparietally (Fig. 7). As is true for other granulomatous diseases, the signal of granulomas on T2-weighted images is mostly iso- to hypointense.

Rarely, an expansion of the perivascular spaces may happen. Another typical location of sarcoid is the pituitary infundibulum (Fig. 8) with thickening and contrast enhancement. Typically, the lesion can be differentiated easily from the otherwise inconspicuous pituitary gland. If the neurohypophysis is infiltrated, the normal hyperintense granules of the neurohypophysis may appear dislocated on noncontrast T1-weighted images. These hyperintense granules are then usually seen above the sarcoid lesion in the pituitary infundibulum or in the hypothalamus (Fig. 9). Cranial nerves may also be affected. On T1-weighted high-resolution images the cranial nerves show pearl-string-like enhancing granulomas. The contrast enhancement can outlast clinical complaints by several months.

3.2.3 Vasculitic Form

This form is marked by vascular affection. In a benign course only slight irregularities of small arterial vessels are evident. If the major vessels of the circle of Willis are affected, the consequence may be hemodynamically relevant vasculitic stenoses and cerebral ischemia.

3.3 Differential Diagnosis

Neurosarcoidosis can mimic a variety of diseases. Bacterial or tuberculous meningitis, meningioma, and carcinomatous or lymphomatous meningiosis are the most important differential diagnoses of leptomeningeal sarcoidosis. Meningitis may be difficult to differentiate, especially in cases of unspecific CSF findings (see also Chap. 2). Parenchymal metastasis and primary intracerebral lymphoma are the most important differential diagnoses of the parenchymal

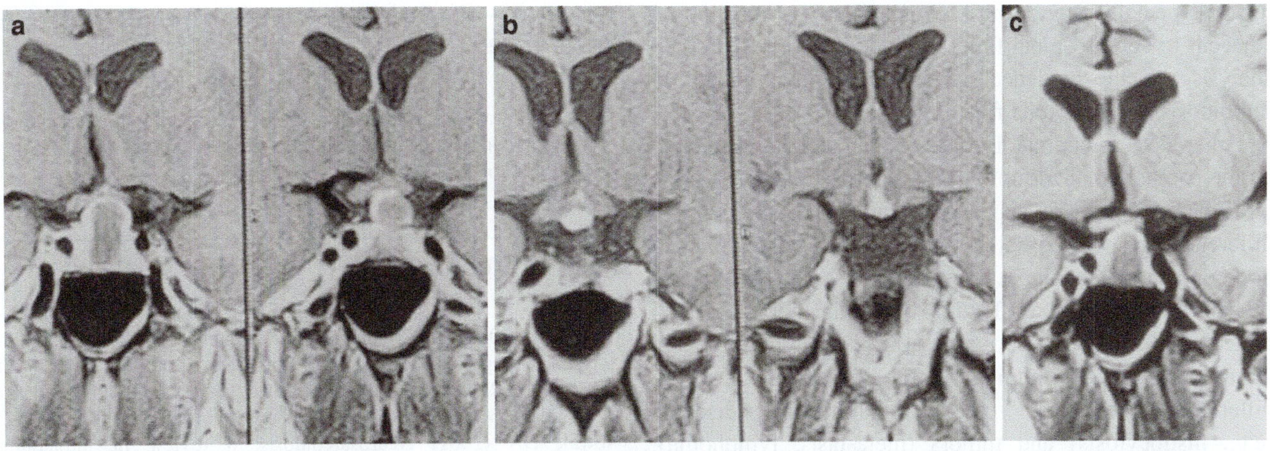

Fig. 8 Neurosarcoidosis with involvement of the pituitary stalk before, under, and after breaking off steroid treatment. **a–c** Coronal T1-weighted images after contrast administration. Enlargement of the pituitary stalk with ring enhancement at the initial examination (**a**). Under steroid treatment 2 months later the mass diminished in size (**b**). After breaking off treatment the mass relapsed (**c**)

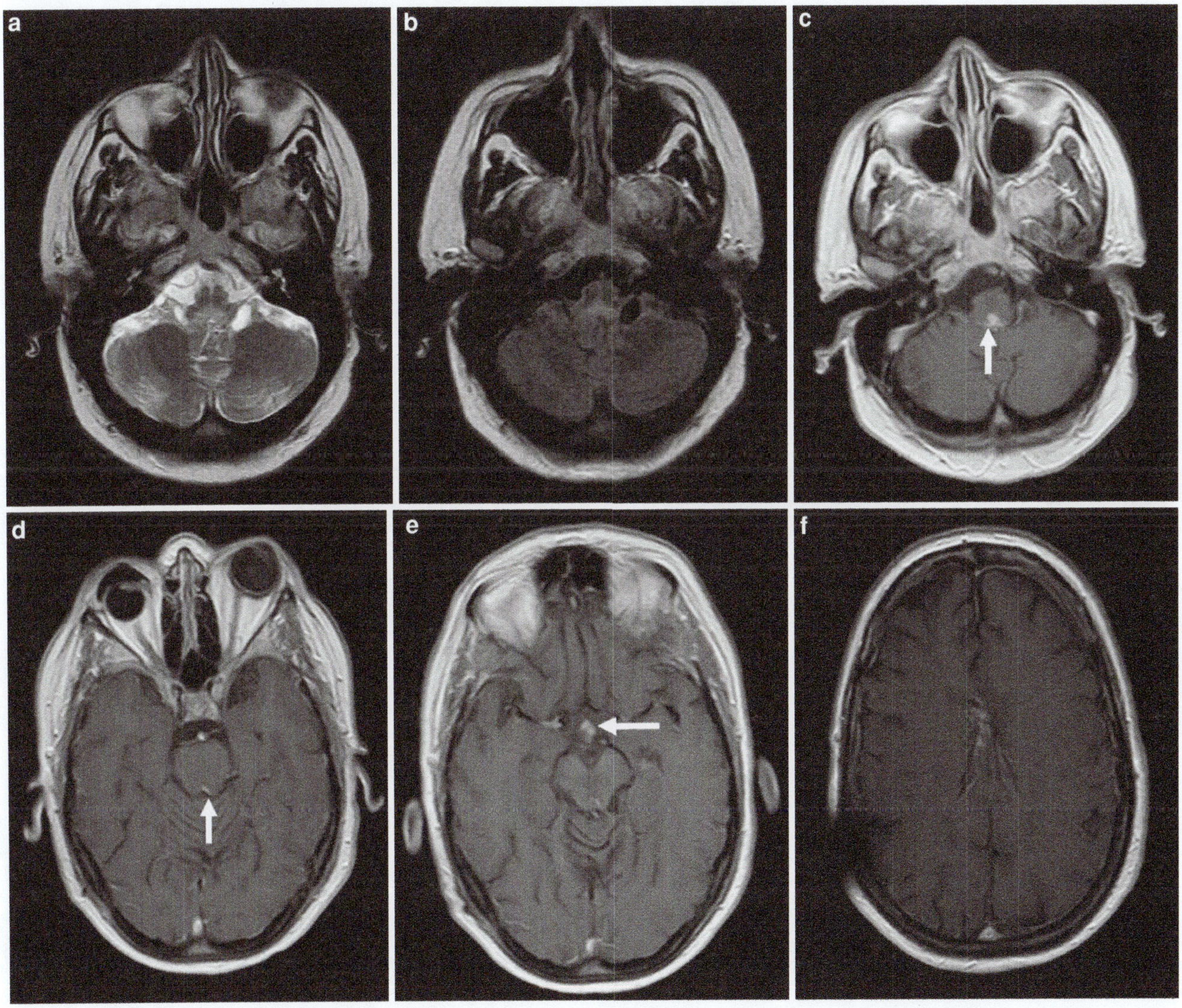

Fig. 9 Typical manifestations of neurosarcoidosis. **a** Axial T2-weighted image. **b** Axial FLAIR image. **c, d** Axial T1-weighted image after contrast administration. Enhancing granulomatous tissue in the fourth ventricle (**c**, *arrow*) and the adjacent parenchyma of the medulla oblongata with high signal in the medulla on T2-weighted images (**a**) and FLAIR images (**b**). Enhancing granulomatous tissue in the wall of the aqueductus cerebri (**d**, *arrow*), the hypothalamus and pituitary stalk (**e**, *arrow*), and the ependyma of the right lateral ventricle (**f**)

form. Especially angiocentric lymphomas are also found adjacent to cerebrospinal fluid and blood vessels. The CSF analysis and the evidence of pulmonary involvement in sarcoidosis are essentials for differentiation.

Other CNS inflammatory diseases can also be mimicked by the parenchymal form: multiple sclerosis plaques have a typical periventricular appearance and are often found in different stages with visualization of contrast-enhancing and non-contrast-enhancing lesions at the same time point. In neuroborreliosis the affection of cranial nerves is also typical, but usually the perivascular spaces are not affected. Granulomas of the pituitary infundibulum have to be differentiated against other inflammatory diseases (e.g., histiocytosis) and tumors (metastasis, lymphoma). Other forms of CNS vasculitis have to be included in the differential diagnosis of the vasculitic form of neurosarcoidosis (see also Chap. 2).

References

Nakata Y, Sato N, Masumoto T et al (2010) Parasellar T2 dark sign on MR imaging in patients with lymphocytic hypophysitis. Am J Neuroradiol 31:1944–1950

Further Reading

Carkirer S (2003) MRI findings in the patients with the presumptive clinical diagnosis of Tolosa-Hunt syndrome. Eur Radiol 13(1):17–28

de Bellis A, Ruocco G, Battaglia M et al (2008) Immunological and clinical aspects of lymphocytic hypophysitis. Clin Sci 114:413–421

Nowak DA (2001) Neurosarcoidosis: a review of intracranial manifestation. J Neurol 248:363–372

Shah R, Robertson GH, Cure JK (2009) Correlation of MR imaging findings and clinical manifestations in neurosarcoidosis. Am J Neuroradiol 30:953–961

Neuro-Infectious Disorders of Childhood

Birgit Ertl-Wagner and Angelika Seitz

Contents

B. Ertl-Wagner (✉)
Institute of Clinical Radiology,
Ludwig Maximilians University Munich,
Grosshadern Campus, Marchioninistrasse 15,
81377 Munich, Germany
e-mail: birgit.ertl-wagner@med.uni-muenchen.de

A. Seitz
Department of Neuroradiology,
Kopfklinik, University of Heidelberg,
Im Neuenheimer Feld 400, 69120 Heidelberg, Germany

Abstract

Children can be affected by the same or similar neuro-infectious disorders as adults. However, there are some neuro-infections that significantly differ between children and adults and/or between children of different age ranges in regard to the imaging pattern, the infectious agent and/or the route of infection. These include neuro-infectious diseases acquired in utero, neonatally, or during childhood and adolescence. Classic *congenital*, i.e., in utero acquired, are summarized in the so-called TORCH group, which stand for *TO*xoplasmosis, *R*ubella, *C*ytomegalovirus (CMV), and *H*erpes simplex virus (HSV) type II. These congenital infections have a characteristic imaging appearance that significantly differs from infections acquired later in life. Other congenital infections include lymphocytic choriomeningitis (LCM), syphilis, and HIV. *Viral infections* of the brain that preferentially affect children or those have a characteristic imaging appearance in childhood are the Rasmussen encephalitis, Subacute Sclerosing Panencephalitis (SSPE) as a complication of measles, the Reye syndrome, and varicella zoster encephalitis. Herpes simplex virus type 1 infections of the brain, tick-born encephalitis, and progressive multifocal leukoencephalitis (PML) may also have a somewhat different appearance, when occurring in childhood. In *bacterial encephalitis*, it is important to differentiate early and late cerebritis and abscess formation. Mycoplasma encephalitis tends to occur more often in children than in adults. *Fungal infections* of the brain usually only manifest themselves in the immunosuppressed child. They include candida and cryptococcal infections and coccidioidosis. Cysticercosis is a comparatively common *parasitic infection* of the brain that occurs both in children and in adults. Neuro-infectious diseases in childhood can have a variety of causes, including bacterial, viral, fungal and parasitic organisms. In addition to the type of infectious agent, pediatric neuro-infections are typically classified

S. Hähnel (ed.), *Inflammatory Diseases of the Brain*, Medical Radiology. Diagnostic Imaging,
DOI: 10.1007/174_2012_637, © Springer-Verlag Berlin Heidelberg 2012
Published Online: 09 June 2012

according to the age, at which infection occurred: congenital infections, i.e., in utero infections of the brain during embryonic and fetal development neonatal infections, i.e., infections that were either acquired perinatally or in the directly postnatal period infections that were acquired during the further course of childhood and adolescence.

1 Congenital and Neonatal Infections of the Brain

Congenital infections of the brain are caused by an infection of the developing brain in utero. The embryonic and fetal brain reacts differently to infectious agents than the neonatal brain or the brain of the older child. In addition, the extent and pattern of damage is also determined by the time of infection in regard to the gestational age (Table 1) (Barkovich 2005).

The congenital/neonatal infections of the brain are also called TORCH infections. This is an acronym that stands for:

- *To*xoplasmosis,
- *R*ubella,
- *C*ytomegalovirus, and
- *H*erpes simplex virus

Infections of the TORCH group are sometimes also referred to as (S)TORCH infections or TORCH-S infections, in which S stands for congenital syphilis. Other classifications use the "O" in TORCH as an abbreviation for "Other infectious agents" (instead of using it as the second letter of Toxoplasmosis)—these other infectious agents typically include Syphilis and HIV, but may also include Coxsackie virus, Varicella Zoster Virus, and Parvovirus B19.

Congenital toxoplasmosis of the brain is caused by *Toxoplasma gondii*. Mothers-to-be are commonly infected by feline excrements or by raw or undercooked meat. In the United States, more than one-fifth of the population is seropositive for *T. gondii*. If an acute infection occurs during pregnancy, the risk for a congenital infection is considered to range between 20 and 50 %. The incidence of congenital *T. gondii* infections is estimated to be between 1:3000 and 1:5000 live births. Affected children usually suffer from developmental delays and epilepsy. Hydrocephalus can be caused by a secondary aqueductal stenosis. A chorioretinitis is a common finding as well. However, affected children are often clinically inapparent at birth and the diagnosis is often only made several months later.

Congenital toxoplasmosis typically leads to calcifications of the periventricular regions and the gray matter of the cortex and the basal ganglia. The MR imaging protocol in children with a suspected TORCH infection should therefore always include T2*-weighted sequences or SWI sequences. The lateral ventricles are commonly dilated and microcephaly can be present. The later the infection occurs in the course of pregnancy, the less pronounced the changes usually are.

Congenital rubella infection is an infection by a Toga virus that has become very rare in the Western world due to immunization programs and screenings of the immune status in early pregnancy. Again, the severity of the infection depends on the time the infection occurs—the most severe infections with a high rate of miscarriage arise in the first trimester of pregnancy. In severe cases, microcephaly and a dilatation of the lateral ventricles are usually present. Calcifications in the periventricular region, in the cortex and in the basal ganglia are a common finding as well, as are periventricular cysts. In addition to the cerebral involvement, children often suffer from cataracts with leukocoria and from cardiac abnormalities; they may also present with a petechial rash.

Congenital cytomegalovirus (*CMV*) *infection* is a common congenital infection—it is considered to be more than 10 times more common than congenital toxoplasmosis. There are estimates that about 1 % of newborns are affected. However, only about 10 % of infected newborns have signs of the disease and only about half of these demonstrate an involvement of the brain. Affected children commonly have a developmental delay, microcephaly, and inner ear deafness. At birth, hepatosplenomegaly and a petechial rash may be present.

The extent and pattern of cerebral affection again depends on the time of infection. In severe cases there may be a pronounced dilatation of the lateral ventricles, lissencephaly, and cerebellar hypoplasia. In later infections, polymicogyria and white matter abnormalities with patchy areas of hyperintensity in T2-weighted images are a common finding (Fig. 1). Calcifications are typically periventricular. When a CMV infection occurs close to term, areas of white matter glioses and periventricular calcifications are a common finding, while disorders of cortical development are typically absent (van der Knaap et al. 2004).

The patchy and sometimes confluent white matter signal alterations that occur in congenital CMV infections can resemble the imaging appearance of leukodystrophies (Fig. 1).

In our experience, patchy white matter signal alterations are the most common MR imaging finding in children with congenital CMV infections; these may or may not be accompanied by disorders of cortical development such as polymicrogyria. In our setting, the most common presenting symptom in children with such a rather mild MR imaging manifestations of a congenital CMV infection is inner ear deafness. These children commonly present for an

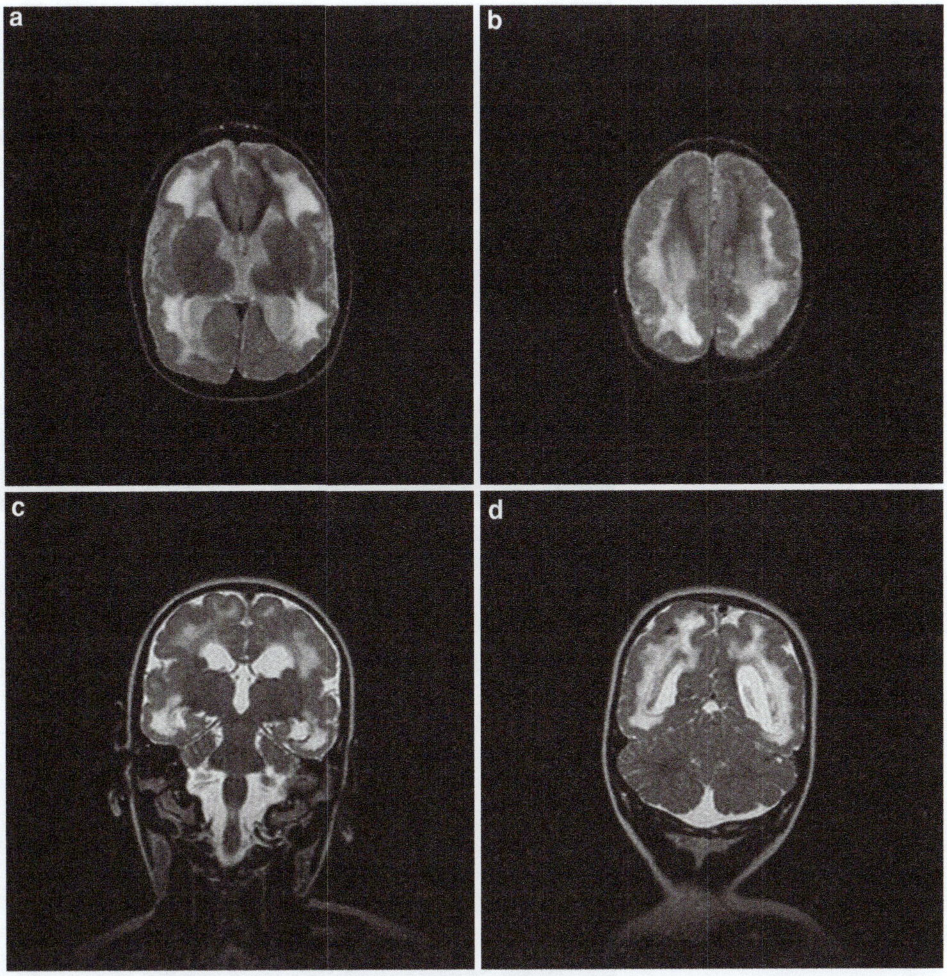

Fig. 1 Congenital CMV infection in a 3-year old boy. Axial (**a**, **b**) and coronal (**c**, **d**) T2-weighted sequences demonstrate pronounced confluent signal alterations in the *white matter* as well as polymicrogyria and microcephaly

MR imaging work-up prior to cochlear implantation and patchy white matter alterations are often the most salient MR imaging finding to suggest congenital CMV infection (Fig. 2, Table 2).

Herpes simplex virus (*HSV*) *encephalitis* in newborns is usually a neonatal infection that is caused by HSV type II. HSV type II is the genital subtype of HSV and is usually transmitted to the neonate during a vaginal delivery. Transplacental infections are possible, but less common. Congenital/neonatal HSV II encephalitis significantly differs from a later acquired HSV type I infection.

Children with HSV encephalitis that was acquired during delivery are usually severely affected and become symptomatic within the first 1–2 weeks of life with somnolence and seizures. In the rather rare instances, in which there was a transplacental infection of HSV type II, microcephaly, and parenchymal destructions of the brain are usually already present at birth.

Early in the course of the disease there are commonly patchy areas of increased signal intensity in T2-weighted sequences and decreased signal intensity in T1-weighted sequences with a concomitant diffusion restriction (Fig. 3). These are usually rapidly progressive. A patchy, relatively mild parenchymal contrast enhancement is usually present. Areas of hemorrhage are often observed in the further course. Cerebral atrophy and cystic encephalomalacia typically ensue (Fig. 3).

Congenital lymphocytic choriomeningitis (*LCM*) is caused by an adenovirus that is transmitted by rodents. Congenital infections in the second and third trimester can resemble congenital CMV infections and toxoplasmosis, while infections in the first trimester cause spontaneous abortions (Wright et al. 1997).

In addition to causing a chorioretinitis, LCM commonly leads to a necrotizing ependymitis, which eventually results in aqueductal stenosis and hydrocephalus. If hydrocephalus is absent, microcephaly may be present. The affected child may therefore have a macrocephalus or a microcephalus. Calcifications may be present, especially in a periventricular location. In addition, polymicrogyria may be found. Overall, LCM may closely resemble a congenital CMV infection.

Congenital syphilis has become a rare disease. Screening programs are typically conducted in the first trimester of pregnancy. The transmission usually occurs perinatally.

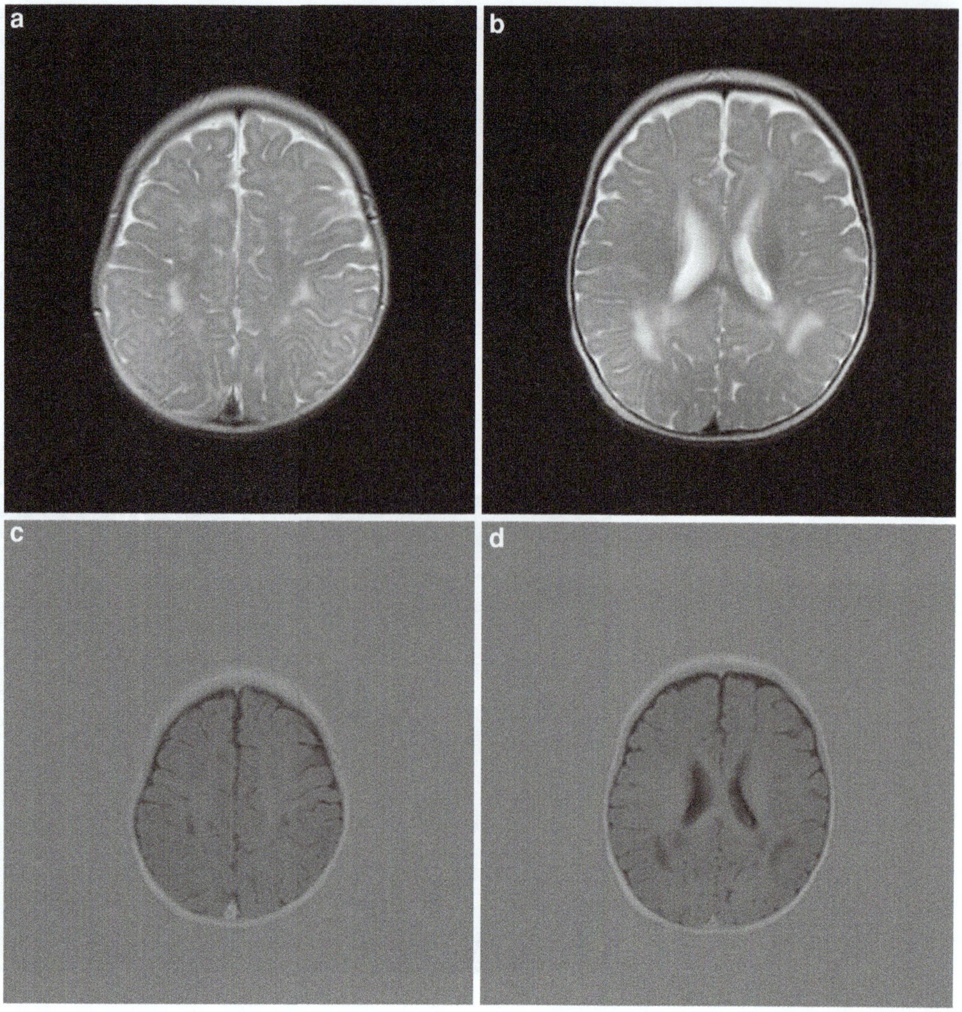

Fig. 2 Congenital CMV infection in a 6-month old boy, who presents for MR imaging prior to cochlear implant surgery. Axial T2-weighted (**a**, **b**) and T1-weighted IR (**c**, **d**) sequences demonstrate patchy signal alterations in the *white matter* in the absence of overt cortical malformations

Affected children tend to become symptomatic later than children with HSV II encephalitis. Symptoms are sometimes not noted until the children are 2–3 years old. Epilepsy and inner ear deafness are common symptoms.

MR imaging typically demonstrates inflammatory changes of the meninges that commonly extend into the perivascular spaces. There is a pronounced enhancement of the meninges—especially the basal meninges—after the administration of intravenous contrast medium, which may extend into the brain parenchyma. Cerebral ischemias can ensue.

While the incidence of *congenital HIV infections* is decreasing in the Western world, the global incidence still is rising. When the mother is untreated, there is an about 30 % chance of transmission to the child. However, in a treated mother undergoing a Cesarian section, this risk of transmission is reduced to 2 %. The infection is most commonly transmitted during a vaginal birth, but can also be acquired during the third trimester and during breast feeding.

Clinically, affected children usually become symptomatic during the first years of life.

A congenital HIV infection leads to a cerebral atrophy in most affected children. This cerebral atrophy is usually progressive in nature. A mineralizing microangiopathy leads to calcifications, especially in the basal ganglia. The basal ganglia may enhance prior to the calcium deposition. Subcortical calcifications may also be present.

In later stages, a fusiform vasculopathy may ensue that can be discerned in MR angiography. This vasculopathy can lead to cerebral ischemia.

In the further course of the disease, a PML may occur. PML is caused by an opportunistic infection with a papovavirus that leads to zones of demyelination by destructing oligodendrocytes.

Opportunistic infections with toxoplasmosis and primary cerebral lymphomas are somewhat less common in children with HIV infections than in adults.

There are several important *differential diagnoses* to the congenital TORCH infections to consider, which may closely mimic the imaging appearance of TORCH infections. These include the pseudo-TORCH syndrome, tuberous sclerosis, and neurocysticercosis.

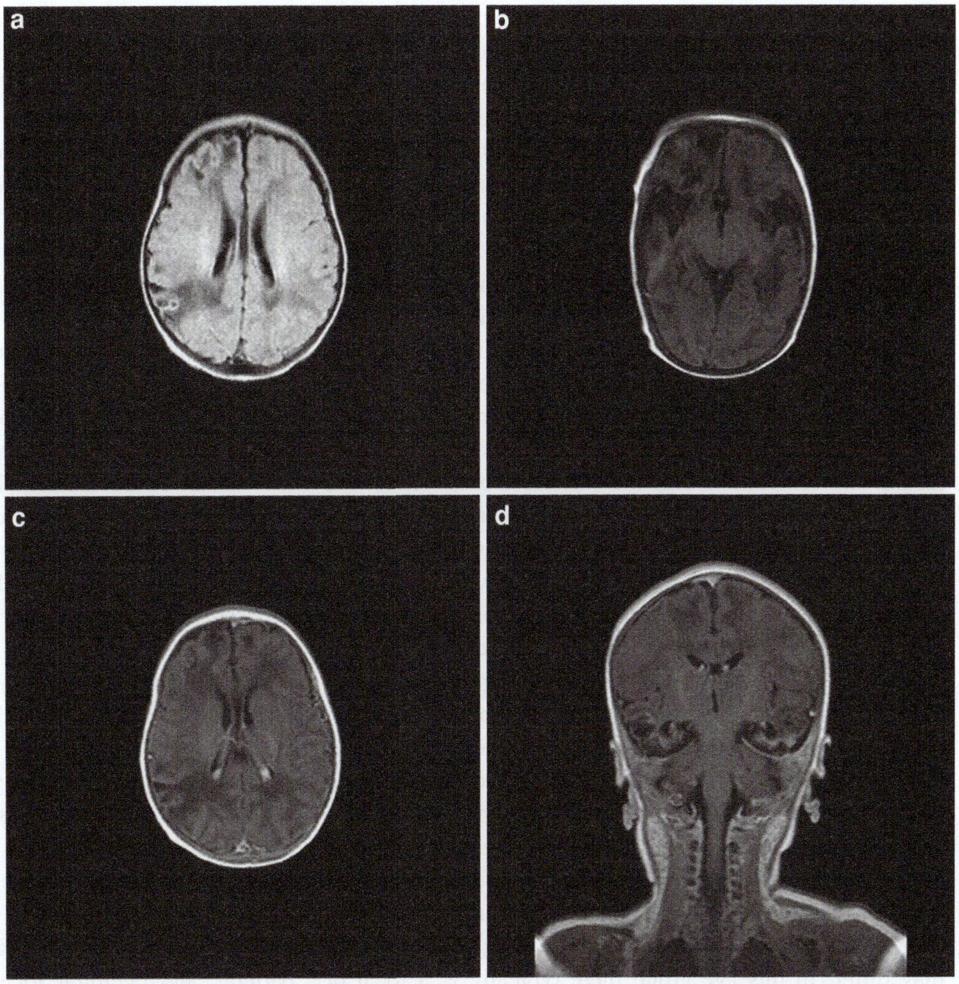

Fig. 3 Neonatal HSV type II encephalitis in a 3-week old girl. Axial FLAIR (**a**), axial unenhanced (**b**) and axial coronal contrast enhanced (**c, d**) T1-weighted sequences demonstrate areas of edema as well as areas of hemorrhage and atrophy

Pseudo-TORCH syndrome is also referred to as Aicardi-Goutières syndrome or Cree encephalitis. This syndrome has an autosomal recessive mode of inheritance. Hallmark features include basal ganglia and also periventricular calcifications, as well as a lymphocytosis of the cerebrospinal fluid, thereby closely resembling congenital infections of the TORCH type. In addition, a progressive leukodystrophy of the supratentorial and infratentorial white matter is present.

Neurocysticercosis is a rather common disorder worldwide leading to cerebral calcifications. Neurocysticercosis cysts most commonly affect the subarachnoid spaces over the convexities of the cerebral hemispheres, but may also be found in the basal cisterns, in the brain parenchyma and in the ventricles. Neurocysticercosis is caused by *Taenia solium*, the pork tapeworm. It can occur in any age and may resemble TORCH infections mostly because of the intracranial calcifications associated with both disorders.

Tuberous sclerosis—also referred to as the Bourneville–Pringle syndrome is a neurocutaneous syndrome. Hallmark features of cerebral imaging in patients with tuberous sclerosis include subependymal nodules and cortical/subcortical tubers. The subependymal nodules may calcify in the course of time and thereby resemble calcifications in TORCH infections. Moreover, cortical tubers may resemble cortical dysplasias in TORCH infections, such as in congenital CMV infections.

2 Neuropediatric Viral Infections and Disorders of Unresolved Etiology

HSV encephalitis in older children is almost always caused by HSV type I—as opposed to HSV type II infections in neonates. Affected children initially commonly suffer from flu-like symptoms. These are followed by increasing fever and altered levels of consciousness. Seizures, nausea, and vomiting, and pareses may also occur. Initial symptoms can be largely unspecific in children with mostly behavioral changes. About one-third of all HSV type I encephalitis cases occur in the pediatric age group—as symptoms in this age group tend to be less specific than in adults, HSV encephalitis is rather commonly an important differential diagnosis to consider. HSV encephalitis typically represents a reactivation of the virus in immunocompetent patients.

Whenever HSV encephalitis is suspected, intravenous acyclovir needs to be started immediately, as mortality rates are very high without treatment. The definite diagnosis is usually established by polymerase chain reaction (PCR) of the cerebrospinal fluid.

MR imaging is the imaging method of choice in suspected HSV encephalitis, as the sensitivity of CT is very limited, especially in early stages. Preferentially, MR imaging should include high resolution FLAIR sequences of the temporal lobe and thin-slice diffusion-weighted sequences.

HSV type I has an affinity for the limbic system. Therefore, the medial temporal lobes, the inferior frontal lobes, the insular/peri-insular regions, and the cingulated gyri are preferentially affected. An asymmetric involvement is common. Very rarely, the midbrain and pons may be affected.

There is an early restriction of diffusion in diffusion-weighted sequences that may precede the changes in T2-weighted and FLAIR sequences. Hemorrhage may ensue in the affected regions, which leads to "blooming" foci of signal hypointensity in T2*- weighted and SWI sequences. Enhancement of the affected gyri usually does not occur until about 1 week after the start of the symptoms; it preferentially affects the cortical ribbon. Generally, the MR imaging appearance of an HSV type I infection in older children and adolescents is similar to that in adults. However, in infants and young children the imaging appearance may differ. In this age group there typically is a focal or multifocal vascular distribution that may affect any lobe (Leonard et al. 2000).

Differential diagnoses to consider include limbic encephalitis, cortical edema secondary to an epileptic seizure or status epilepticus, ischemic changes, and neoplasm.

Rasmussen encephalitis is a rare disease also called chronic focal encephalitis. The definite pathogenesis of Rasmussen encephalitis has not been elucidated yet. It may be caused by an autoimmune mechanism, by a viral infection, or by an immune-mediated response triggered by a viral infection (Bien et al. 2005).

Symptoms are commonly preceded by an inflammatory episode. The onset is usually in childhood, especially in the preschool and school years. In the early stages of the disease, seizures usually occur with a comparatively low frequency and a mild hemiparesis is noted. In later stages there is an increase in seizure frequency and a progressive hemiparesis with cerebral atrophy. In the late stage of the disease there is permanent hemiparesis. Cognitive decline is also a common symptom. Generally, the prognosis of Rasmussen encephalitis is poor and seizures are largely refractory to antiepileptic medication. Hemispherectomy is a potential treatment option.

In early stages of the disease, there is usually a swelling of the gyri with a mild hyperintensity of the cortex and the underlying gray matter in T2-weighted and FLAIR sequences with a preferential affection of the frontal and parietal lobes. These hyperintense areas increase over time. In the further course of the disease, progressive atrophy ensues that eventually involves the entire hemisphere (Fig. 4). Contrast medium enhancement is usually absent; rarely, a mild degree of cortical or leptomeningeal enhancement may be observed.

MR spectroscopy may show a decrease in N-acetyl aspartate (NAA) and choline and an increase in myoinositol and glutamine/glutamate. PET usually shows a hypometabolism and hypoperfusion of the affected hemisphere, already early in the course of the disease. A transient increase in metabolism can be due to recent seizure activity.

Differential diagnoses to consider include the Sturge-Weber syndrome, cerebral infarctions, and mitochondrial encephalopathies such as MELAS.

Progressive multifocal leukoencephalitis is a disease that is encountered in patients with a deficiency of cellular immunity—most commonly in patients with AIDS or those under immunosuppressive therapy. It can occur in children and in adults and is caused the JC polyomavirus.

In MRI, there are patchy, often confluent white matter lesions with an increased signal intensity in T2-weighted and FLAIR sequences and a decreased signal intensity in T1-weighted images. These correspond to areas of demyelination. There is a typical involvement of the subcortical U-fibers with a preferential involvement of the frontal, parietal, and occipital lobes. The involvement is usually bilateral, albeit asymmetric. Generally, there is neither a mass effect nor a contrast enhancement. In late stages of the disease, cystic changes may ensue. Differential diagnoses to consider include HIV encephalitis, acute disseminating encephalomyelitis (ADEM), and CMV infection.

Varicella zoster encephalitis is caused by the varicella zoster virus—the same virus that causes chicken pox and—if reactivated—shingles. A Varicella zoster encephalitis is comparatively rare occurring in less than 0.1 % of chicken pox cases. Affected children most commonly present with cerebellar symptoms such as ataxia or dysarthria.

On MR imaging there is usually a diffuse cerebellar edema with swelling of the cerebellum and a diffuse signal hyperintensity on T2-weighted and FLAIR images. Additional signal abnormalities may occur in the basal ganglia and at the gray matter- white matter junction. Very rarely, a late-onset complication of a varicella zoster infection may occur, usually one to 4 months after an episode of chicken pox. Affected children usually present with hemiplegia due to an ischemia of the basal ganglia or infarctions of the cerebral cortex. MR angiography reveals a pronounced narrowing of the distal internal carotid artery, and the proximal middle, and anterior cerebral arteries (Ciccone et al. 2010).

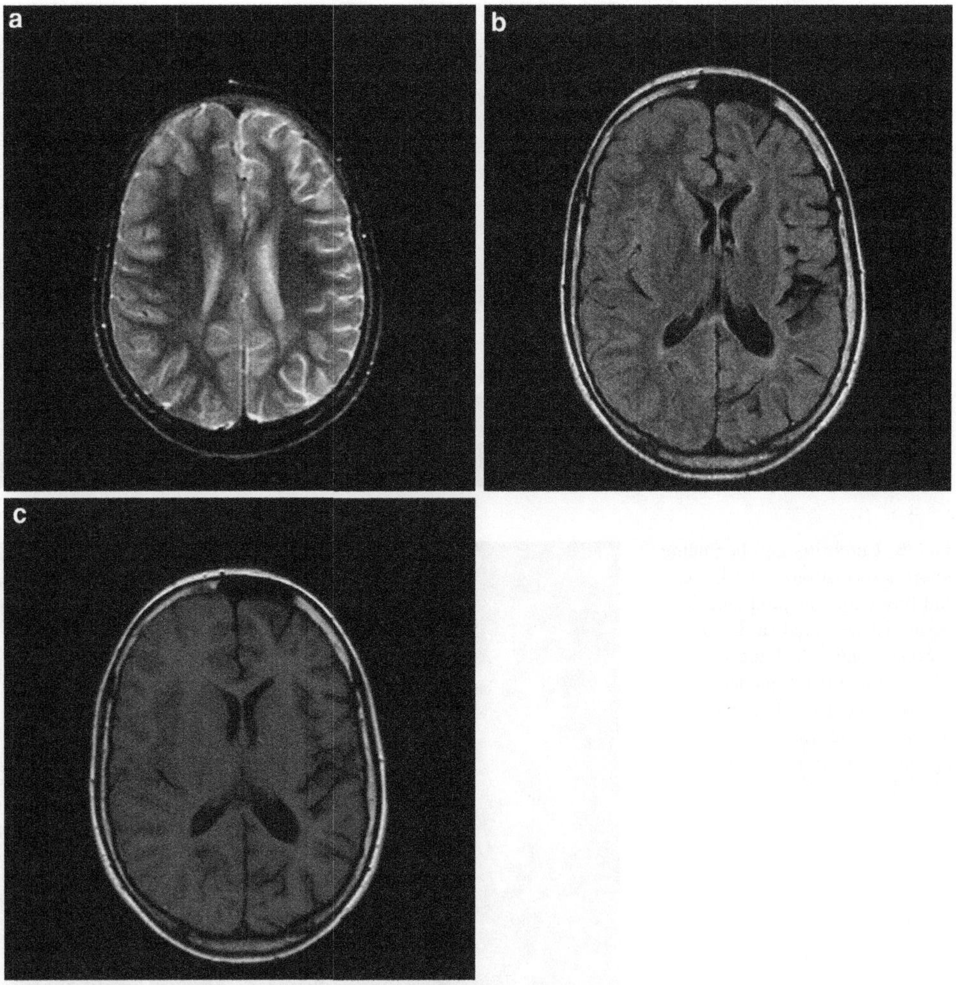

Fig. 4 Rasmussen encephalitis in an 11-year old boy. Axial T2-weighted (**a**), axial FLAIR (**b**), and axial T1-weighted (**c**) sequences demonstrate a hemiatrophy of the *left* hemisphere

Due to immunization programs, *measles infections* have become a comparatively rare disease. However, recent outbreaks have occurred in many countries usually caused by parents not immunizing their children. The measles virus can affect the brain in different ways: as an acute postinfectious encephalitis, as a progressive infectious encephalitis and as a SSPE.

Acute postinfectious encephalitis usually manifests itself within 1–2 weeks from the onset of the measles rash. The mechanism is considered to most likely be autoimmune. Affected children suffer from somnolence, headaches, and seizures.

On MR imaging there is a predominant affection of the basal ganglia, especially the caudate nucleus and the putamen, the thalami and the cerebral cortex with edema being present in the affected regions in the acute stage. Later, atrophy may ensue.

In progressive infectious encephalitis, symptoms usually appear around 3–6 months after the initial measles infection with seizures and somnolence. Symptoms are progressive in nature.

Subacute sclerosing panencephalitis, also referred to as Dawson encephalitis, is considered to be a late complication of an infection with measles. This type of encephalitis is progressive in nature and eventually fatal, usually in the course of 1–3 years. Affected children usually present with a progressive mental deterioration, behavioral alterations, and pareses.

MR imaging may be normal in the initial stages of the disease. In the further course, areas of increased signal intensity are usually noted in the cortex und subcortical white matter in T2-weighted and FLAIR sequences (Fig. 5). The parietal and temporal lobes are most commonly affected and the corpus callosum may be involved as well. Eventually, these signal alterations spread throughout the brain and severe atrophy ensues.

MR spectroscopy usually reveals an increase in cholin and myoinositol and a decrease in NAA. These MR spectroscopic changes may become apparent prior to the signal alterations on structural MR imaging. Generally, the degree

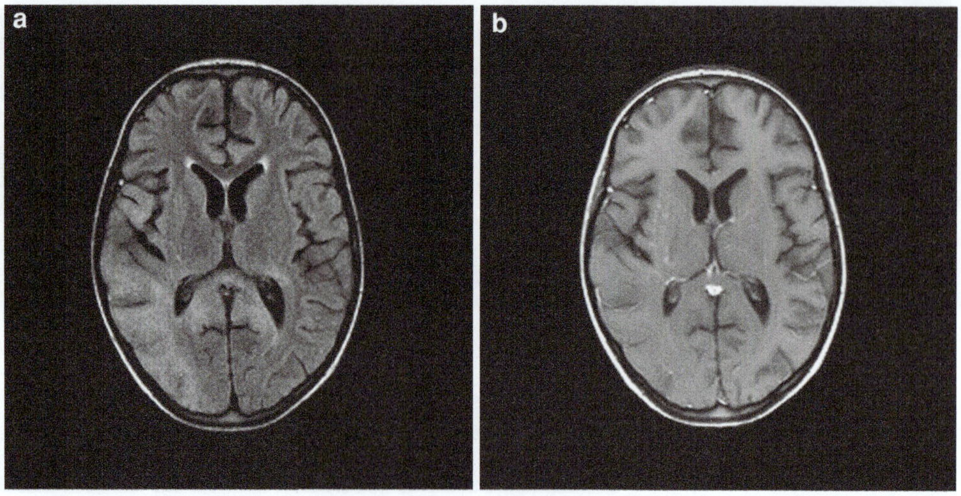

Fig. 5 Subacute Sclerosing Panencephalitis in a 9-year old girl. Axial FLAIR (**a**) and contrast-enhanced T1-weighted (**b**) sequences demonstrate swelling and signal alterations in the cortical and subcortical regions

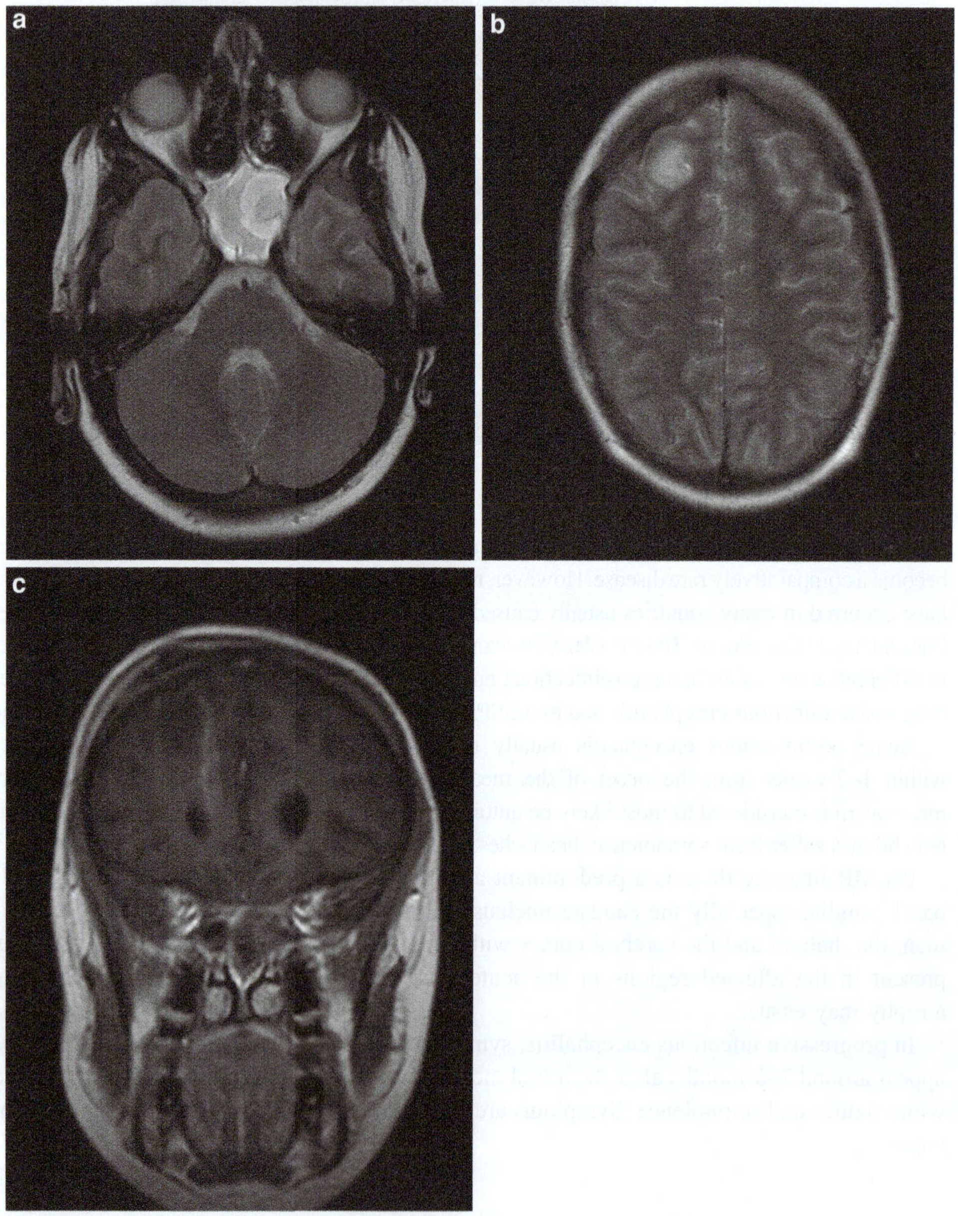

Fig. 6 Cerebritis and beginning abscess formation in a 14-year old boy with sphenoid sinusitis. Axial T2-weighted (**a**, **b**) and coronal contrast-enhanced T1-weighted (**c**) sequences demonstrate a focal signal alteration and a contrast-enhancement in the right frontal lobe

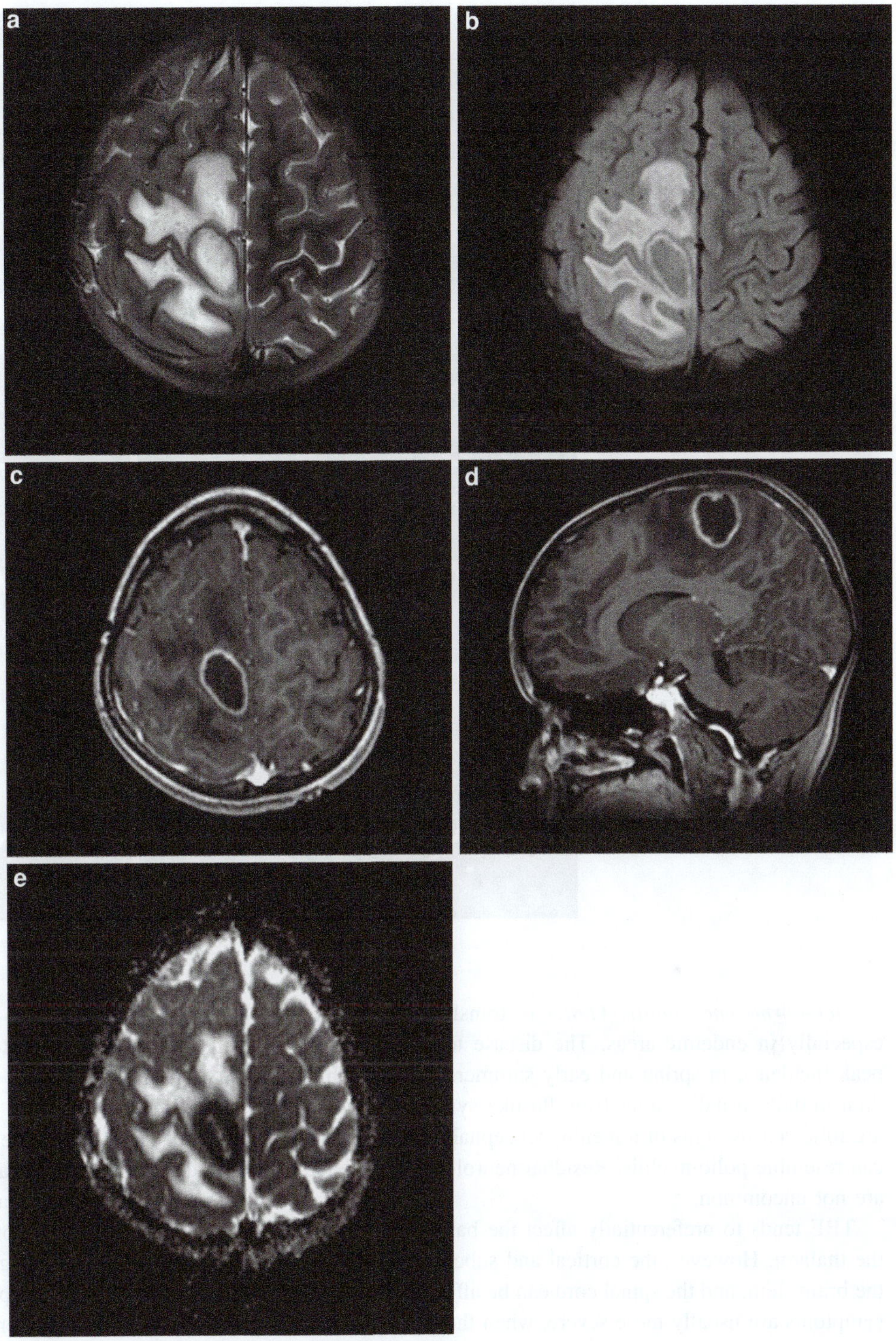

Fig. 7 Cerebral abscess in a 6-year old boy with a chronic tooth infection. Axial T2-weighted (**a**), and FLAIR (**b**), sequences as well as contrast-enhanced axial (**c**), and sagittal (**d**) T1-weighted sequences demonstrate a smooth-walled lesion with a contrast-enhancing rim and perifocal edema. The ADC map (**e**) shows a concomitant diffusion restriction

of involvement on MR imaging correlates only poorly with the clinical progression.

Differential diagnoses to consider include ADEM, HIV encephalitis, and progressive multifocal encephalitis.

Reye syndrome is an encephalopathy with a rather high mortality rate that tends to develop shortly after viral infections. An interaction between viral infections and toxins, such as salicylates, has been discussed even though the mechanism has not been fully elucidated yet. The incidence has been declining over the past years, though.

Symptoms usually present acutely with headaches, reduced consciousness, and seizures. Affected children often also suffer from acute hepatic failure with steatosis.

On MR imaging, there are usually signs of cerebral edema with swelling and signal hyperintensities of the cerebral hemispheres on T2-weighetd and FLAIR sequences.

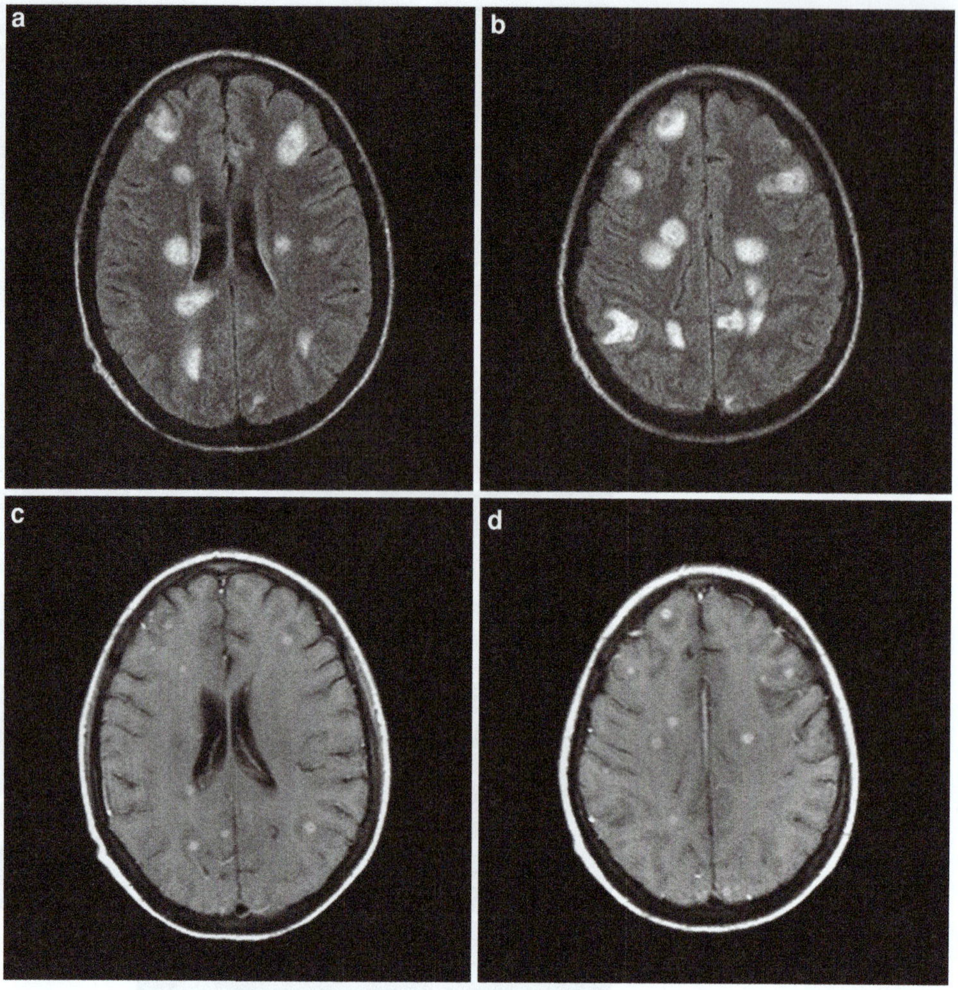

Fig. 8 Systemic nocardiosis in a 16-year old immunosuppressed boy. Axial FLAIR sequences (**a**, **b**), and contrast-enhanced T1-weighted sequences (**c**, **d**) show multiple foci of signal alterations with enhancement and perifocal edema

Tick-borne encephalitis (*TBE*) is transferred by ticks especially in endemic areas. The disease tends to have a peak incidence in spring and early summer. Affected children initially usually suffer from flu-like symptoms, which are followed by signs of a meningoencephalitis. Symptoms can resemble poliomyelitis. Residual neurological sequelae are not uncommon.

TBE tends to preferentially affect the basal ganglia and the thalami. However, the cortical and subcortical regions, the brain stem, and the spinal cord can be affected as well—symptoms are usually more severe, when the spinal cord is involved. MR imaging can be completely normal as well, though.

There are a multiple other causes of viral encephalitis, including various enterovirus infections and influenza infections. Not uncommonly, however, the cause of the encephalitis remains enigmatic.

3 Bacterial Infections of the Brain in Childhood

A *bacterial cerebritis* is the first stage of a bacterial infection of the brain, which can progress to form a cerebral abscess. A cerebritis can arise from an infection of the adjacent structures, e.g., from a mastoiditis or an infection of the paranasal sinuses (Fig. 6) (De Muri and Wald 2011). It can, however, also be spread via a hematogenic route, e.g., in sepsis or in a bacterial endocarditis. Children with cardiopulmonary malformations are more prone to suffer from cerebritis or cerebal abscesses. Sometimes, a cerebritis can also be caused by a direct inoculation of bacteria either by a penetrating wound or by an operation.

In a cerebritis, surgical interventions are usually not necessary—the mainstay of therapy is an antibiotic treatment.

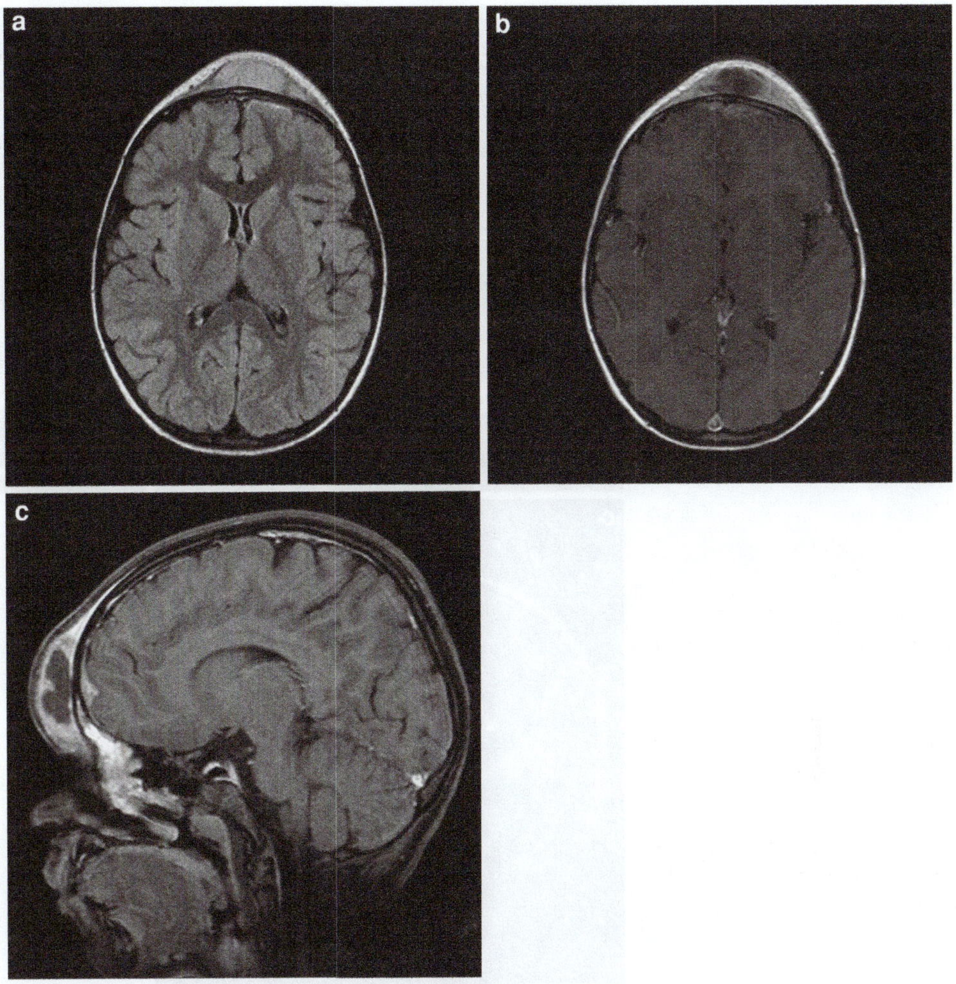

Fig. 9 Meningitis in a 3-year old girl with sinusitis and a subcutaneous abscess. Axial FLAIR (**a**), and axial (**b**), and sagittal (**c**) contrast-enhanced T1-weighted sequences demonstrate a thickening and an increased enhancement of the frontal meninges, as well as a pronounced subcutaneous abscess formation

On CT, there is usually an area of diffuse hypodensity, which correspond to a signal hyperintensity on T2-weighted and FLAIR sequences and a hypointensity on T1-weighted images (Fig. 6). There can be a patchy enhancement in the affected region. It is important to perform a follow-up examination in order to ascertain improvement and not to miss an abscess formation.

An *abscess formation* follows a bacterial cerebritis if the infection is not properly treated or does not respond to treatment. Abscess formations in neonates and babies are commonly found in a periventricular region and can be rather large, while abscesses in older children tend to occur in the basal ganglia or in subcortical regions.

On CT, a cerebral abscess presents as an area of focal hypodensity with an enhancing rim. There is usually a marked perifocal edema. On MR imaging, the center of the abscess is usually hyperintense on T2-weighted and hypointense on T1-weighted sequences. The abscess rim demonstrates a pronounced enhancement after the administration of contrast media (Fig. 7). The inner portion of this rim usually has a smooth border. In contrast to brain neoplasms, the enhancing rim of an abscess is usually comparatively thin. The perifocal edema presents with an increased signal intensity on T2-weighted and FLAIR sequences.

The differential diagnosis between a cerebral neoplasm and an abscess can often be difficult on conventional sequences alone, though. A helpful distinction can be the different diffusivity of these lesions. In contrast to cerebral neoplasms, the center of an abscess usually shows a markedly restricted diffusivity with a decreased ADC (Fig. 7) (Fanning et al. 2006). MR spectroscopy can also be a helpful adjunct to conventional MR imaging—there usually is an increased lactate peak and peaks of several amino acids including leucine, isoleucine, valine and alanine, and absent peaks of normal cerebral tissue.

It is always important to control cerebral abscesses to verify a complete remission.

Differential diagnoses for intracranial abscesses include cerebral neoplasm, demyelinating disorders such as ADEM or tumefactive demyelination, subacute parenchymal hemorrage, or subacute cerebral ischemia.

Mycoplasma pneumoniae is a potential cause of cerebral encephalitis. Mycoplasma encephalitis occurs more commonly in children than in adults. A central nervous system infection with mycoplasma pneumoniae can manifest itself

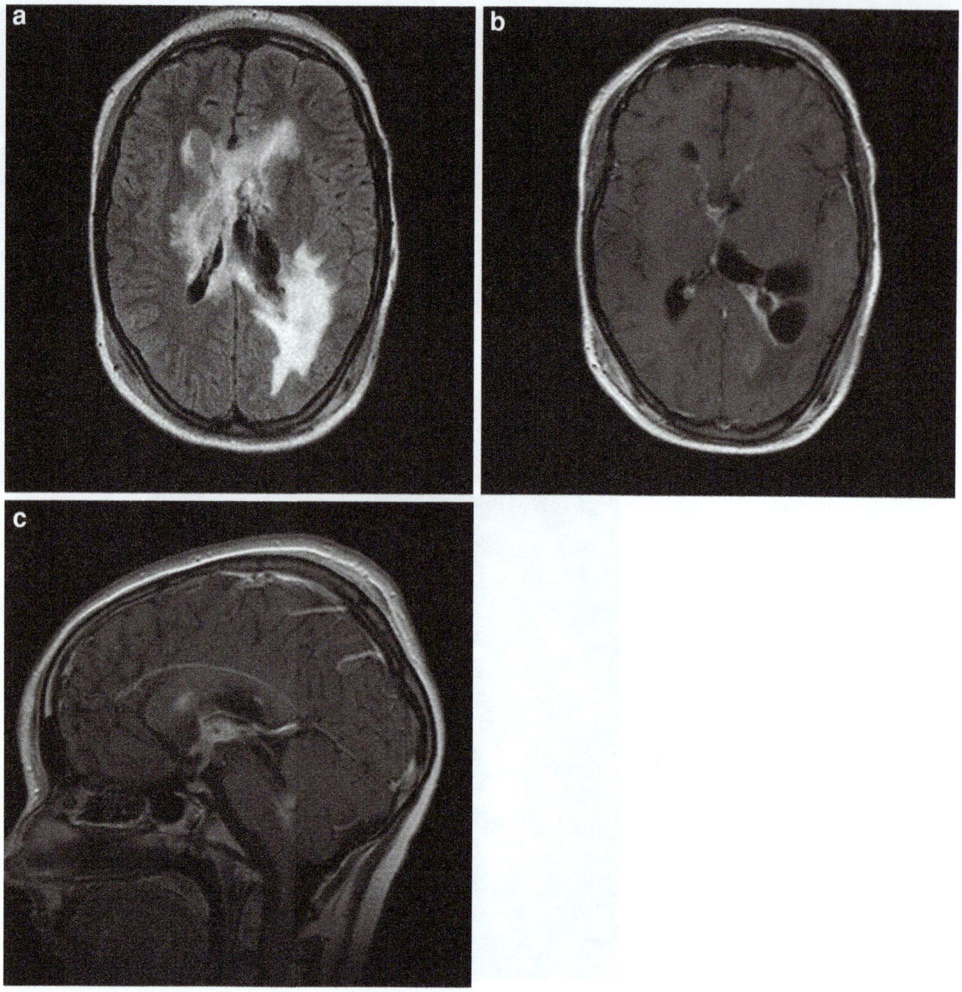

Fig. 10 Ventriculitis in a 14-year old boy with a status post sinogenic meningitis and abscess formation. Axial FLAIR (**a**), axial (**b**), and sagittal (**c**) contrast-enhanced T1-weighted sequences show pronounced periventricular signal alterations and cyst formations as well as an ependymal contrast enhancement

as encephalitis, meningitis, myelitis, polyradiculitis, and peripheral, and cranial neuropathy. However, encephalitis seems to be the most common presentation in children. A possible pattern of involvement is an acute striatal necrosis with high-intensity T2 signal in the caudate and putamen.

A *nocardiosis* only affects immunosuppressed patient. In systemic nocardiosis, there is a hematogeneous spread to various organ systems. In about one-third of cases, the central nervous system is affected as well. A cerebral nocardiosis usually leads to multiple brain abscesses with a ring-like enhancement and to a meningeal affection (Fig. 8).

4 Fungal and Parasitic Infections of the Brain in Childhood

Fungal infections of the brain are comparatively rare in children. They are usually opportunistic infections in an immunocompromised child.

A *candida* meningitis and cerebritis can occur in immunocompromised neonates or in children who have been treated with steroid or antibiotics for a long time. A secondary vasculitis can arise. On MR imaging, candida infections tend to resemble tuberculous infections of the brain. The basal meninges are preferentially involved with a pronounced enhancement. There can be adjacent abscesses. These usually have a comparatively thick and irregular enhancing rim.

A *cryptococcal infection* also preferentially leads to an affection of the basal meninges, but may also cause a ventriculitis or a vasculitis. Hydrocephalus and pseudocysts of the basal ganglia can be a complication. An abscess formation is rare in cryptococcosis.

A *coccidioidomycosis*, also known as "Valley fever," is mostly observed in the South-Western United States. It is caused by the fungi *Coccidioides immitis* or *Coccidioides posadasii*. The infection is exceedingly rare in Europe. Again, there is a preferential affection of the basal meninges. Hydrocephalus is a common complication.

A *cerebral cysticercosis* is a relatively common infection worldwide. Due to increasing international travel and migration, infections are increasingly seen in the Western world as well. The infection is caused by the parasite *T. solium*, a porcine tapeworm.

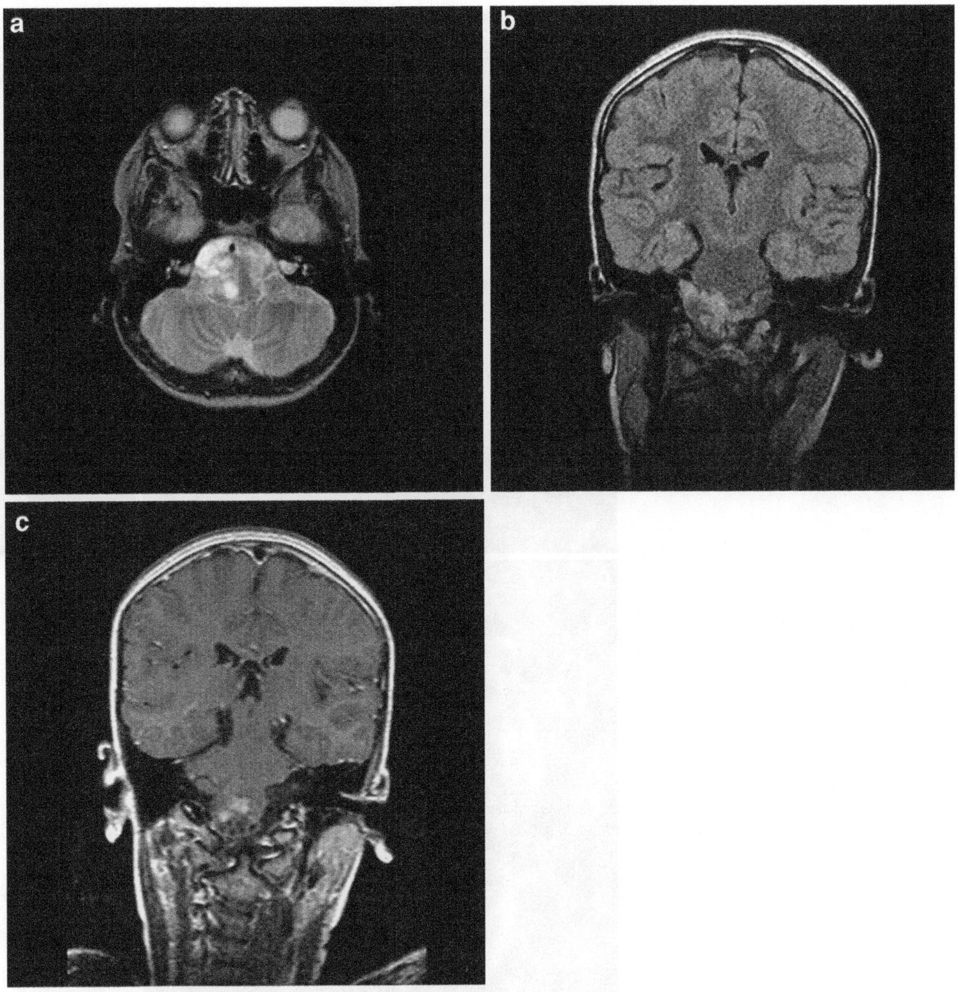

Fig. 11 Tuberculous meningitis and tuberculomas in an 8-year old boy who presented with a facial palsy. Axial T2-weighted (**a**) as well as coronal FLAIR (**b**) and contrast-enhanced T1-weighted sequences demonstrate contrast-enhancing lesions in the brainstem and in the basal meninges

Affected children often suffer from epileptic seizures. However, the clinical presentation can be quite variable. Headaches and difficulty concentrating can be common complaints as well.

There are different MR morphological presentations of cerebral cysticercosis. The most common finding is parenchymal cysticerci. These can occur anywhere in the brain—most commonly they are found in the gray matter, though. The content of the cyst can be solid or liquid. There can be an enhancement of the rim. Commonly, the cysts have a central dot.

Cysticerci can also occur in an intraventricular location—these can lead to an acute hydrocephalus.

A leptomeningeal cysticercal affection preferentially leads to an involvement of the basal meninges and may resemble a tuberculous meningitis. Calcifications may occur.

Racematous cysticerci have a grape-like appearance with septae. These cysts do not contain scolices anymore, but may increase in size over time.

5 Meningeal Infections of the Brain in Childhood

Meningitis is the most common intracranial infection in childhood. There are different modes of infection. A meningitis can be caused hematogeneously, by direct spread from an adjacent infection such as a mastoiditis or a paranasal sinusitis (Fig. 9), by a direct inoculation through a penetrating wound or an operation, by rupture of a subcortical abscess, or by spread from the choroid plexus.

Acute meningitis can be viral or bacterial. There are also chronic forms, e.g., tuberculous meningitis or granulomatous meningitis. Vaccination programs have markedly reduced the incidence of Hemophilus influenza meningitis in children.

The diagnosis is generally made by lumbar puncture with analysis of the cerebrospinal fluid. CT or MR imaging is usually only performed to rule out contraindications to a lumbar puncture or to diagnose complications.

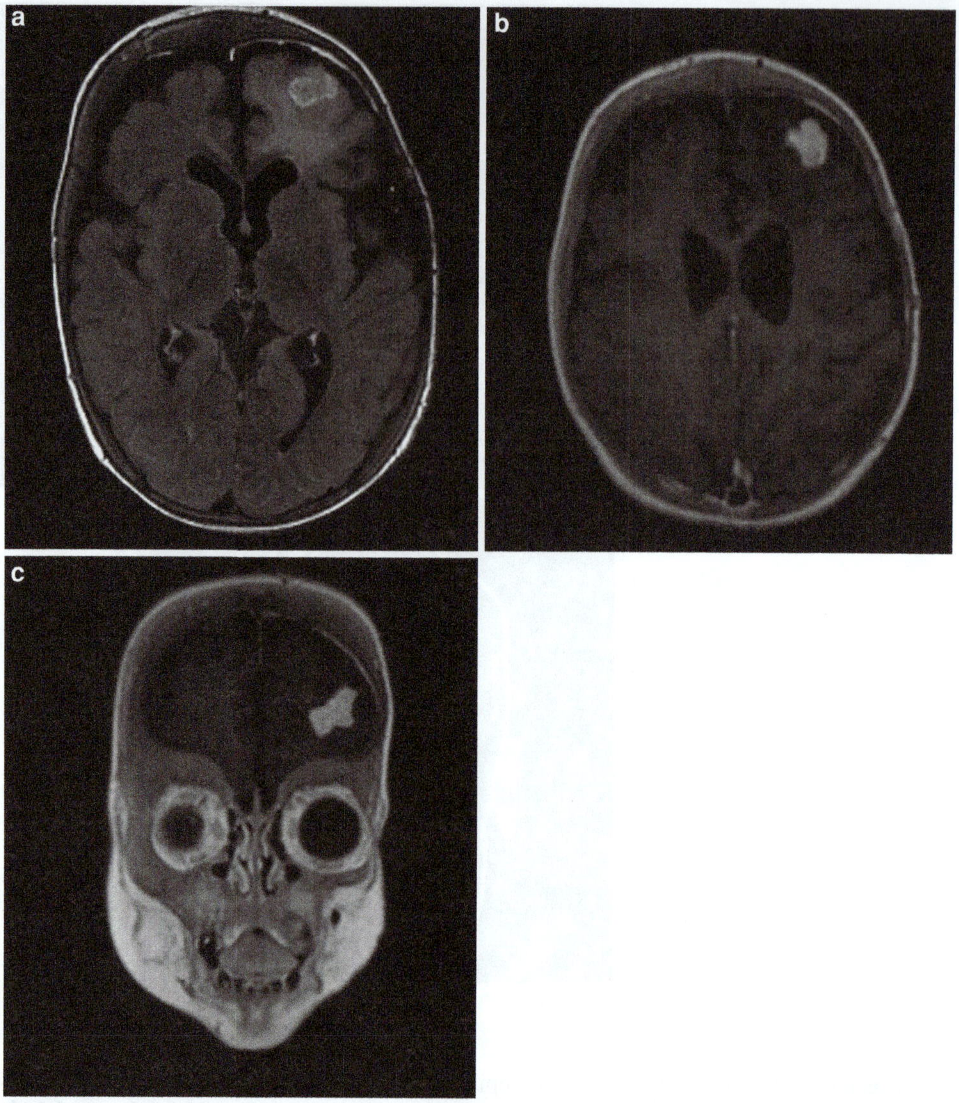

Fig. 12 Tuberculoma in a 2-year old boy with chronic tuberculous meningitis. Axial FLAIR (**a**), and axial (**b**), and coronal (**c**) contrast-enhanced T1-weighted sequences show a contrast-enhancing lesion of the *left* frontal lobe

The most common imaging sign of meningitis is usually a thickening and an increased enhancement of the meninges (Fig. 9). The most sensitive MR imaging sequence to detect leptomeningeal enhancement is a delayed contrast-enhanced FLAIR sequence. In addition, diffusion-weighted sequences should be performed to detect potential complications, such as cerebral ischemia, empyema, or abscess formation. However, MR or CT can be completely normal even in the presence of a pronounced meningitis.

Complications are generally more common in bacterial than in viral meningeal infections.

One of the most common complications of meningitis is hydrocephalus. This can be due to an occlusion of the passage of the cerebrospinal fluid (CSF) or to an impaired CSF absorption.

Meningitis can also affect the cerebral vessels and thereby cause a vasculitis. Subsequently, ischemic strokes can evolve with territorial or lacunar infarctions. A cerebral venous thrombosis including a cavernous sinus thrombosis can also occur.

When the meningitis involves the brain parenchyma, a cerebritis or an abscess formation may ensue.

Especially in newborn children, but also in older children, meningitis can lead to ventriculitis. This may lead to cyst formations and necroses of the periventricular white matter (Fig. 10).

In young children, bilateral subdural hygromas are a comparatively common complication of meningeal infections—they are especially common in Haemophilus influenzae meningitis. These hygromas are sterile effusions that eventually resolve.

If an empyema arises, the prognosis is generally worse. An empyema is a collection of pus that can lead to a compression of the adjacent brain parenchyma. It is usually unilateral. The signal intensity of the empyema is not completely isointense to CSF. It can be heterogeneous and

Table 1 Congenital and neonatal infections of the brain

Infection	Imaging characteristics
•Congenital toxoplasmosis	Calcifications of the periventricular white matter, basal ganglia and gray matter May cause hydrocephalus or microcephaly No malformations of cortical development
Congenital rubella infection	Very rare due to immunization programs Calcifications of the periventricular white matter, basal ganglia and gray matter Microcephaly and dilated lateral ventricles Delayed myelination and patchy signal alterations in T2-weighted images Cataracts and cardiac malformations
Congenital CMV infection	Most common congenital infection Calcifications especially of the periventricular white matter Malformations of cortical development such as polymicrogyria or lissencephaly Delayed myelination Patchy areas of white matter gliosis, can resemble a leukodystrophy; these may present in the absence of other abnormalities May cause cerebellar hypoplasia
Neonatal HSV II infection	Patchy to large confluent areas of hyperintensity on T2-weighted sequences Initially usually rapidly progressive Meningeal enhancement Cerebral atrophy and encephalomalacia Calcifications may occur
Congenital lymphocytic choriomeningitis (LCM)	Resembles congenital CMV and congenital toxoplasmosis Ependymitis with aqueductal stenosis and hydrocephalus May cause microcephaly or macrocephaly Periventricular calcifications Polymicrogyria
Congenital syphilis	Thickening and enhancement of the leptomeninges Extension into the perivascular spaces Cerebral infarctions may ensue
Congenital or neonatal HIV infection	If congenital, calcifications of basal ganglia and white matter Progressive atrophy Opportunistic infections, such as PML or toxoplasmosis, rarer in children than in adults Cerebral infarctions, and hemorrhages possible

Table 2 Viral infections of the brain in childhood

Infection	Imaging characteristics
HSV type I infection	About 30 % of infections occur in childhood Preferentially affects limbic system Hyperintense signal in T2 and FLAIR, restricted diffusion Thin-section FLAIR sequence of the temporal lobes recommended
Rasmussen encephalitis	Chronic focal encephalitis Early: swelling of gyri and cortical hyperintensity in T2 Later: progressive hemiatrophy
Varicella zoster encephalitis	Preferentially affects the cerebellum Diffuse cerebellar edema May also affect basal ganglia and gray—white matter junction
SSPE	Late complication of measles infection Hyperintense areas at the gray—white matter junction in T2- weighted sequences, progressive over time Later progressive atrophy
Reye syndrome	May be due to an interaction between viral infection and toxins (e.g. salicylates) Swelling, edema, and enhancement in the cerebral hemispheres
Tick-borne encephalitis	Preferential involvement of basal ganglia and thalami May also involve brain stem and spinal cord

septations may be present. An enhancement of the rim structures is usually noted.

A hyperintense signal in the subarachnoid spaces on FLAIR sequences must not always be due to meningitis—it is generally unspecific. Differential diagnoses for signal alterations in the subarachnoidal spaces on FLAIR sequences include ventilated patients with a high degree of oxygen, subarachnoid hemorrhage, vascular congestion due to parenchymal edema or retained gadolinium-based contrast medium in patients with end-stage renal disease. Most commonly, an increased or inhomogeneous signal may be simply due to artifacts.

Tuberculous meningitis is a comparatively common infection worldwide. The beginning is usually insidious. Tuberculous meningitis preferentially affects the basal meninges (Fig. 11). This commonly leads to a disorder of CSF circulation or to pareses of the cranial nerves.

MR imaging typically demonstrates a thickening and an increased enhancement of the basal meninges. A hydrocephalus is a common finding. Affection of the cerebral vessels can lead to ischemic strokes, which most commonly affect the basal ganglia.

In addition to causing meningitis, cerebral tuberculosis may also lead to tuberculomas of the brain parenchyma (Fig. 12). These are typically slightly hyperdense in CT and hyperintense on T1-weighted sequences with an enhancement after the administration of contrast media. In addition, they are characteristically hypointense on T2-weighted images. However, imaging characteristics can vary.

References

Barkovich AJ (2005) Infections of the nervous system. In: Barkovich AJ (ed) Pediatric neuroimaging. Lippincott Williams & Wilkins, Philadelphia, pp 801–868

Bien CG et al (2005) Pathogenesis, diagnosis and treatment of Rasmussen encephalitis: a European consensus statement. Brain 128:454–471

Ciccone S, Faggioli R, Calzolari F, Sartori S, Calderone M, Borgna-Pignatti C (2010) Stroke after varicella-zoster infection: report of a case and review of the literature. Pediatr Infect Dis J 29(9):864–867

DeMuri GP, Wald ER (2011) Complications of acute bacterial sinusitis in children. Pediatr Infect Dis J 30(8):701–702

Fanning NF et al (2006) Serial diffusion-weighted MRI correlates with clinical course and treatment response in children with intracranial pus collection. Pediatr Radiol 36:26–37

Leonard JR et al (2000) MR imaging of herpes simplex type I encephalitis in infants and young children: a separate pattern of findings. AJR Am J Roentgenol 174:1651–1655

Van der Knaap MS et al (2004) Pattern of white matter abnormalities at MR imaging: use of polymerase chain reaction testing of Guthrie cards to link pattern with congenital cytomegalovirus infection. Radiology 230:529–536

Wright R et al (1997) Congenital lymphocytic choriomeningitis virus syndrome: a disease that mimicks congenital toxoplasmosis or cytomegalovirus infection. Pediatrics 100:1–6

MR Imaging and Spectroscopic Specifics and Protocols

Axel Wetter

Contents

A. Wetter (✉)
Institute of Diagnostic and Interventional Radiology and Neuroradiology, University Hospital Essen, Hufelandstrasse 55, 45147 Essen, Germany
e-mail: wa2007@gmx.de

Abstract

Different protocols for MR imaging and spectroscopy are presented as well as special imaging features of inflammatory diseases of the cerebral parenchyma as described in this book. Advanced MR techniques such as DWI, PerfMRI, DTI, MT, as well as MRS, and their use in inflammatory diseases of the cerebral parenchyma are presented.

1 MR Fundamentals

1.1 DWI, DTI, PerfMRI

Diffusion-weightedimaging measures the molecular movement of water and thus allows characterization of the microstructure of tissues. For DWI strong magnetic field gradients are used in all three spatial levels before and after a refocusing pulse of 180°. The subsequent data acquisition is performed via an EPI sequence. The b-value is a sequence-specific factor that determines the sensitivity for the water diffusion. The SNR of the images decreases with increasing b-value, so that maximum b-values of 1.000 are normal at 1.5 T. A b-value of 0 complies with a T2-weighted image. On DWI T2 effects and diffusion effects are superimposed: Both restriction of diffusion and prolongation of T2 result in hyperintensity on DWI; therefore, hyperintensity on DWI is not unconditionally the result of diffusion restriction. By calculating the ADC, information about water diffusion without T2 superimposition is obtained. A decreased ADC shows reduced water diffusion, whereas an increased ADC is consistent with an elevated water diffusion. Cytotoxic edema typically reveals restricted diffusion, whereas vasogenous edema comes along with elevated diffusion. Examples of ADC changes in inflammatory diseases of the brain are listed in Table 1.

With DTI anatomically determined differences of water diffusion can be presented, for example, alongside fiber bundles

S. Hähnel (ed.), *Inflammatory Diseases of the Brain*, Medical Radiology. Diagnostic Imaging,
DOI: 10.1007/174_2012_667, © Springer-Verlag Berlin Heidelberg 2012
Published Online: 31 July 2012

Table 1 Examples of ADC changes of several inflammatory diseases of the brain as compared with normal values. *NAWM* normal-appearing white matter, *ADC* apparent diffusion coefficient, *ADEM* acute demyelinating encephalomyelitis, *SSPE* subacute sclerosing panencephalitis

	Parameter
Entity	ADC
Multiple sclerosis	
NAWM	↑
Chronic lesions with substantial tissue defects ("black holes")	↑↑
Acute MS lesions	↑
Very acute MS lesions	↓
ADEM	
NAWM	↔
Lupus, NAWM	↑
Bacterial infections	
Bacterial abscess (cavity)	↓↓↓
Tuberculoma	↔
Viral encephalitis	
Herpes simplex type 1 (early stage)	↓↓
SSPE, NAWM	↑
Fungal abscess (cavity)	↓↓
Neurocysticercosis	↑

of white matter. In isotropic diffusion, the ADC as a tissue-specific parameter is the same in all directions, while in anisotropic diffusion, it is greater in one direction than in the other one.

In contrast to cerebral gray matter, the cerebral white matter can be normally characterized by anisotropic diffusion, which is based on the course of the fiber bundles. Here the diffusion parallel to the direction of the fiber bundles is greater than vertical to this direction. If gradients are switched parallel to the preferred course of the fiber bundles, the direction of the diffusion results in a signal decrease along the gradients, while switching of the gradients vertically to the preferred direction of the diffusion has no influence on the signal intensity. If the measurements of different gradient directions are combined, a diffusion tensor can be described from the resulting varying signal decrease. For a complete description of the diffusion tensor, measurements have to be carried out in at least six gradient directions. For quantitative evaluation, ROI measurements of gray or white matter can be carried out and the parameters MD and FA can be calculated. The MD describes the extent of the average diffusion, while the FA is a measure for the direction-depending diffusion, taking values between 0 (complete isotropic diffusion) and 1 (diffusion in only one direction).

PerfMRI measures the microvascular blood flow in the brain tissue using susceptibility contrast of EPI sequences after administration of a paramagnetic contrast agent. A contrast bolus results in a signal decrease in the respective cerebral region by reducing the T2* relaxation time. The time course of this signal loss can be used to calculate a variety of hemodynamic parameters such as rrCBV, MTT, rrCBF, and TTP.

1.2 Magnetization Transfer Contrast

In comparison to free protons, protons bound to macromolecules are considerably limited in their mobility. Thus, the dephasation effects are emphasized with an extreme reduction of the T2 relaxation time. Thus, these bound protons normally cannot be demonstrated. Bound and free protons interact via a chemical exchange and dipol–dipol interactions and have a different resonance width, but the same mean resonance frequency. Via a high frequency pulse, which is placed outside the resonance of free water, the protons bound to macromolecules are saturated, while the free protons are not involved; however, magnetization transfer via the chemical compounds between bound and free protons also results in a loss of transverse magnetization and thus in a reduction of the T2 time of the free protons. In addition, the so-called cross relaxation also results in a reduction of the T1 time. For quantifying the changes of the magnetization transfer, MTR is used, which is calculated from the signal intensity before and after irradiation of the MT pulse.

1.3 Proton MR Spectroscopy

The chemical composition of tissues can be examined using proton MRS. Two acquisition techniques, the spin-echo and the stimulated-echo acquisition method (STEAM), are used. In contrast to the spin-echo technique, the STEAM technique allows shorter echo times; however, SNR of the STEAM technique is only half of the SNR of the spin-echo technique.

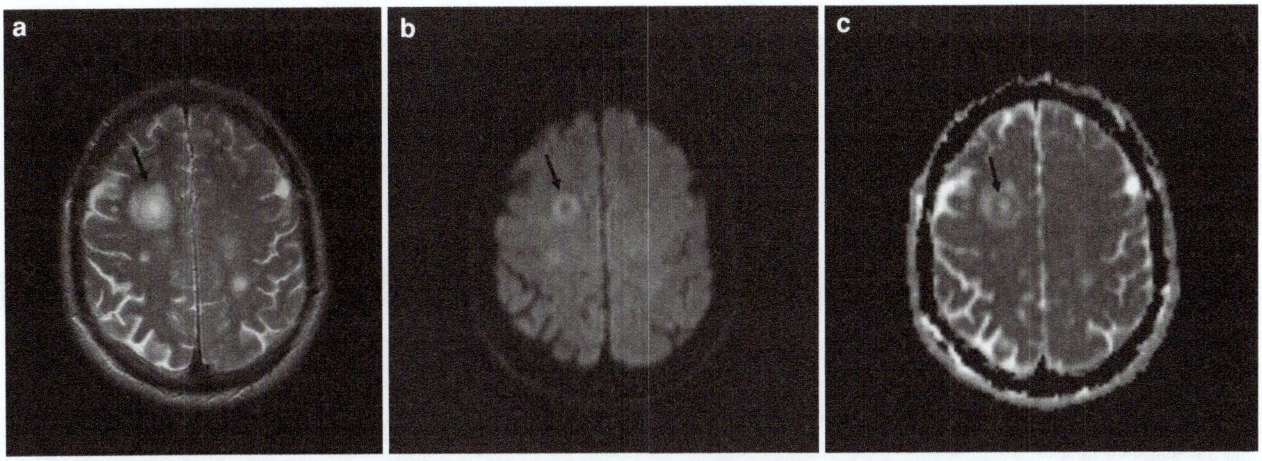

Fig. 1 **a–c** T2-weighted and Diffusion-weighted imaging of a very acute MS lesion. The T2-weighted image **a** shows a hyper-intense white matter lesion with a surrounding vasogenic edema (*arrow*). The DWI image **b** shows a hyper-intense rim which is hypo-intense in the corresponding ADC map **c** indicating a cytotoxic edema (*arrows*)

Table 2 Typical MRS features of several inflammatory diseases of the brain. *NAWM* normal-appearing white matter, *NAGM* normal-appearing grey matter, *ADEM* acute demyelinating encephalomyelitis, *SSPE* subacute sclerosing panencephalitis

	Metabolites						
Entity	tNAA	Choline	Creatine	Myoinositol	Lactate	Lipids	Amino acids
Multiple sclerosis							
NAWM	↓	(↓)		↑			
NAGM	↓	(↓)					
Black holes	↓↓	(↑)		(↑)			
Lesions, contrast enhancing	↓	↑	↑		(↑)		
Lesions, not contrast enhancing	↓	(↑)					
Chronic lesions	↓↓			↑			
ADEM	↓	↑	(↑)		(↑)		
Neuropsychiatric lupus	↓	↑		(↑)			
Bacterial infections							
Bacterial abscess					↑	↑	↑↑
Tuberculous abscess					↑	↑↑	
Viral encephalitis							
SSPE, early stage, NAWM		↑		↑			
SSPE, late stage, lesion	↓↓	↑		↑	↑	↑	
PML	↓ – ↓↓	↑	↑	↑	↑↑	↑↑	
Spongiforme encephalopathy, *"pulvinar sign"*	↓			↑			
Fungal abscess					↑	↑	(↑)
Toxoplasmosis						↑↑	

In addition to single-voxel spectroscopy, spectroscopic imaging (chemical-shift imaging) is increasingly used; thus, greater cerebral areas can be assessed and compared. Currently, using a 3-T scanner, it is possible to acquire a 2D chemical-shift imaging sequence in acceptable quality in not more than 8 min; thus, it can also be used in a clinical routine protocol.

In MRS, signal intensities are not applied depending on the frequency but instead on the chemical shift to a reference substance, the frequency of which is already known. The intervals of the resonances among each other and relative to the reference substance are specified as parts per million (ppm), a parameter which is independent of the field strength used.

Table 3 Brain MR imaging protocol recommended for MS. (Adapted from Simon et al. 2006)

	Sequence	Diagnostic scan for clinically isolated syndrome	MS baseline or follow-up scan	Comment
1	Three-plane (or other) scout	Recommended	Recommended	Set up axial sections through subcallosal line
2	Sagittal fast FLAIR	Recommended	Optional	Sagittal FLAIR sensitive to early MS pathology, such as in corpus callosum
3	Axial FSE PD- and T2-weighted images	Recommended	Recommended	TE_1 minimum (e.g. $\leq$ 30 ms); TE_2 (usually $\geq$ 80 ms); PD series sensitive to infratentorial lesions that may be missed by FLAIR series
4	Axial fast FLAIR images	Recommended	Recommended	Sensitive to white matter lesions and especially juxtacortical-cortical lesions
5	Axial pregadolinium T1-weighted images	Optional	Optional	Considered routine for most neuroimaging studies
6	3D T1-weighted sequence	Optional	Optional	Some centers use this for atrophy measures
7	Axial gadolinium-enhanced T1-weighted images	Recommended	Optional	Standard dose of 0.1 mmol/kg injected over 30 s; scan starting minimum 5 min after start of injection

Section thickness for sequences 3–6 is $\leq$3 mm with no intersection gaps, when feasible. Partition thickness for 3D sequence 6 is $\leq$1.5 mm. In-plane resolution is approximately 1 × 1 mm. The subcallosal line joins the undersurface of the front (rostrum) and back (splenium) of the corpus callosum.

The metabolites N-acetylaspartate and N-acetyl-aspartyl-glutamate (total NAA; tNAA), creatine and phosphocreatine (Cr), choline, glycerophosphocholine and phosphocholine (Cho), myoinositol (Mi), and glutamate/glutamine (Glx) can be detected at an echo time of 30 ms. If the echo time increases to 120 ms, only tNAA, Cr, and Cho can be evidenced. tNAA resonates at 2.02 ppm and serves as marker substance of neuronal integrity. Creatine resonates at 3.04 ppm and normally serves as reference signal for metabolic quantification. Myoinositol resonates at 3.56 ppm and is a marker of the glia cell proliferation. The choline signal at 3.22 ppm represents the choline pool of the brain. Choline is an integral part of the cellular membranes. In addition, lactate (Lac) and lipid resonances (Lip) can be evidenced. At an echo time of 135 ms lactate forms a characteristic doublet directing downward. At an echo time of 270 ms the doublet turns up again. Lactate serves as marker of the anaerobic glycolysis. At an echo time of 135 ms lipids (Lip) can often be defined between 0.9 and 1.3 ppm. A lipid peak can often be detected in tissue necroses. The most typical MRS features for the differentiation of several inflammations are listed in Table 2.

2 MR Imaging and Spectroscopic Aspects Regarding Particular Diseases

2.1 Multiple Sclerosis

Imaging recommendations are given in Table 3 (see also in Chapter Multiple Sclerosis and other Demyelinating Diseases). In patients with MS, the ADC value of the normal-appearing white matter has been shown to be increased as compared with normal values in several studies. Furthermore, the ADC value may also differ in patients with relapsing–remitting MS: during an episode it was shown to be higher than during remission. Recent studies have shown that there are also differences in the water diffusion between the different subgroups of MS. Hypointense lesions on T1-weighted images without contrast enhancement ("black holes") typically show the highest ADC value of all MS lesions, in comparison with isointense and contrast-enhancing lesions (Table 1). Very acute MS lesions might also show a restricted water diffusion due to a cytotoxic edema going along with a decreased ADC and a high DWI signal (Fig. 1). Anisotropy cards of normal-appearing white matter of patients with MS without specifying the subgroups mostly show a decreased FA in the normal-appearing white matter in contrast to the control group. Moreover, a decline of the FA of normal-appearing white matter was detected via the brain region adjacent to the MS plaques. The ADC of normal-appearing gray matter in patients with MS seems to correlate more with the clinical impairment than with the T2 lesion volume. Using PerfMRI interferences of the microvascular blood flow can be demonstrated in patients with MS. In this respect, the normal-appearing white matter of patients with MS shows lower values of the cerebral blood flow and cerebral blood volume in comparison with the control group. Among the MS subgroups, PPMS shows lower values of rrCBF and rrCBV than RRMS. Moreover, the hemodynamic parameters rrCBV and rrCBF of the normal-appearing white matter seem to correlate with the grade of clinical impairment.

Diffusion tensor measurements of the spinal cord document a reduced FA and an increased MD in patients with MS as compared with a control group. In this connection, it is interesting that the FA and MD values of the spinal cord do not correlate with the calculated values of the brain parenchyma.

The MTR is proportional to the amount of myelin; thus, the white matter has a higher MTR than the gray matter. If the MTR is decreased, demyelinization can be assumed. The MTR of normal-appearing white and gray matter of patients with CIS has been shown to be lower than that of control persons. Moreover, patients with CIS who develop a manifest MS in the course of disease show a lower MTR of the white matter than those who do not develop a manifest MS. The MS plaques show a lower MTR than normal-appearing white matter. The MTR of MS plaques also differs among each other, e.g., hypointense lesions show a lower MTR than isointense ones. The normal-appearing white matter directly adjacent to MS plaques shows lower MTR values than the more distant normal-appearing white matter. Changes of the MTR are more severe in patients with SPMS than in patients with RRMS. The MT measurements of the spinal cord demonstrate decreased MTRs in MS patients in comparison with the control group. Moreover, there seems to be a tendency toward lower MTRs in PPMS vs RRMS.

Regarding MTR and MD, there is no significant difference of the normal-appearing white matter between patients with ADEM and control persons.

The spectroscopic examination of normal-appearing white and gray matter provides further insight into patients with CIS and patients with confirmed diagnosis than standard imaging alone. The normal-appearing white matter in patients with CIS as well as in patients with manifested MS shows a reduced tNAA as a sign of axonal damage in comparison with control persons. An increase in myoinositole in the normal-appearing white matter can be evidenced in patients with confirmed MS as sign of a glial cell proliferation. By comparing the initial tNAA values of the normal-appearing white matter in patients with CIS, those patients who develop a manifest MS in the course of disease show a lower tNAA value; thus, the initial tNAA value of the normal-appearing white matter might have a prognostic value. In RRMS, an increased MI of the normal-appearing white matter correlates with the grade of clinical impairment. Already at an early stage of PPMS decreased tNAA values in the normal-appearing gray matter as well as decreased tNAA values and increased MI values of the normal-appearing white matter can be evidenced, which also positively correlate with the grade of clinical impairment. Furthermore, the T2 lesion volume can be correlated with the increase of MI of the normal-appearing white matter. The tNAA values of the normal-appearing gray matter of patients with secondary progressive course of MS are lower than those of patients with relapsing–remitting course; however, the tNAA values of the normal-appearing white matter do not differ between the two subgroups. At the initial stage, acute MS plaques often show an increased choline due to the myelin decomposition, which can revert to normal in the further course of the disease at remyelinization. Hypointense lesions on T1-weighted images ("black holes") show low tNAA values as a sign of axonal damage. T1 hypointense plaques with contrast enhancement show increased values for choline and creatine, as a sign of membrane decomposition or transformation, while these are normally missing in non-enhancing T1 hypointense lesions. All enhancing and non-enhancing lesions, however, have a decrease of the tNAA value in common.

Spectroscopically, a lactate peak can often be detected in ADEM; the choline/creatine ratio is not as highly increased as in MS. Spectroscopic measurements of the cervical spinal cord in MS patients show a reduced tNAA as well as an increased MI and choline value.

2.2 Vasculitis

In suspected cerebral vasculitis MR imaging is often performed as diagnosis by exclusion. As TOF-MR-angiography typically emphasizes the rate of stenoses of the intracranial vessels, it is a useful instrument to search for vasculitic changes. Is the MR imaging inconspicuous a cerebral vasculitis is unlikely; however, some studies have shown that despite inconspicuous MR imaging, typical conventional angiographic findings for cerebral vasculitis were present. Infarction, edema, hemorrhage, as well as disturbances of the BBB are typical findings in vasculitis; therefore, the MR imaging protocol is relatively extensive (Table 4). Contrast-enhanced T1-weighted images with fat saturation are very useful for the detection of vessel wall inflammation. Regarding detection of vasculitis-suspected lesions, the FLAIR sequence is more sensitive than standard T2 or PD sequences, without differing in the quality of imaging of infarction or edema.

In patients with cerebral involvement of lupus erythematosus perfusion measurements using SPECT demonstrate a global hypoperfusion of the brain, which mainly develops in the frontal and temporal lobes. In this connection PerfMRI provides a possible further modality for sensitive detection of cerebral hypoperfusion on a microvasular level; however, PerfMRI in cerebral vasculitis has thus far not been systematically examined. Both DWI and DTI of the normal-appearing white and gray matter demonstrate characteristic features in terms of an alleviated diffusion with ADC increase and reduced FA, which is regarded as loss of the tissue integrity probably due to partial demyelinization.

Table 4 Imaging protocol recommendations for various inflammatory diseases of the brain. *CE* contrast enhanced

Entity	MR sequence parameters					
Bacterial infections	Axial/T1/ 5 mm	Axial/PD, T2/ 5 mm	Axial/FLAIR/ 5 mm	Axial/DWI/ 5 mm	Axial/T1 CE/ 5 mm	Coronal/ T1 CE/ 5 mm	
Viral encephalitis	Axial/T1/ 5 mm	Axial/PD, T2/ 5 mm	Axial/FLAIR/ 5 mm	Axial/DWI/ 5 mm	Coronal/PD, T2/4 mm	Axial/T1 CE/ 5 mm	Coronal/T1 CE/ 5 mm
Spongiforme encephalopathies	Axial/T1/ 5 mm	Axial/PD, T2/ 5 mm	Axial/FLAIR/ 5 mm	Axial/DWI/ 5 mm	Axial/T1 CE/ 5 mm	Coronal/ T1 CE/ 5 mm	
Fungal infections	Axial/T1/ 5 mm	Axial/PD, T2/ 5 mm	Axial/FLAIR/ 5 mm	Axial/DWI/ 5 mm	TOF MRA, arterial flow	Axial/T1 CE/ 5 mm	Coronal/T1 CE/ 5 mm
Parasitic infections	Axial/T1/ 5 mm	Axial/PD, T2/ 5 mm	Axial/FLAIR/ 5 mm	Axial/DWI/ 5 mm	3D-CISS/T2/ 0.7 mm	Axial/T1 CE/ 5 mm	Coronal/T1 CE/ 5 mm
Inflammatory diseases of the meninges	Axial/T1/ 5 mm	Axial/PD, T2/ 5 mm	Axial/FLAIR/ 5 mm	Axial/DWI/ 5 mm	TOF MRA, arterial flow	Axial/T1 CE/ 5 mm	Coronal/T1 CE/ 5 mm
Vasculitis	Axial/T1/ 5 mm	Axial/PD, T2/ 5 mm	Axial/FLAIR/ 5 mm	Axial/DWI/ 5mm	TOF MRA, arterial flow	Axial/T1 CE/ 5 mm	Coronal/T1 CE with fat saturation/ 3 mm
Granulomatous diseases	Axial/T1/ 5 mm	Axial/PD, T2/ 5 mm	Axial/FLAIR/ 5 mm	Axial/DWI/ 5 mm	Axial/T1 CE/ 5 mm	Coronal/ T1 CE/ 5 mm	Coronal/T1 CE with fat saturation/ 3 mm
THS, LYH	Axial/ FLAIR/ 5 mm	Coronal/T1 CE without fat saturation/3 mm	Coronal/T2 with fat saturation/ 3 mm	Coronal/T1 CE with fat saturation/ 3 mm	Axial/T1 CE with fat saturation/ 3 mm	TOF MRA, arterial flow	
Detection of blood products	Axial/T2* or SWI/4– 5 mm						
Cranial nerve involvement	Axial/T1 CE/1– 2 mm						
Calcification	Computed tomography						

All MR sequence parameters are listed as: slice orientation/weighting/slice thickness. At 3 T, MPRAGE instead of conventional spin-echo sequences can be used.

For lupus-associated vasculitis of the brain distinctive metabolic features have been demonstrated in the normal-appearing white matter using MRS. Patients with lupus-associated vasculitis of the brain showed an increase in Cho/Cr ratio in contrast to the control group. Moreover, this increase in the Cho/Cr ratio correlated well with the number of lesions of the white matter and is possibly even predictive for the appearance of such lesions, as new lesions of the white matter preferentially develop in regions with metabolic disorders. At spectroscopy, the distinctive features correlate with hypoperfusion as detected in SPECT or PerfMRI of the respective cerebral areas. In more pronounced forms of cerebral lupus-associated vasculitis reductions of the tNAA values can be detected which show an axonal damage. So far, it has not been examined systematically whether these metabolic changes also appear in patients with primary cerebral vasculitis.

Due to the limited spatial resolution, MRA at 1.5 T has only a limited value for showing vasculitic changes of the small cerebral vessels. Due to the increase of SNR and T1 time, MRA at 3 T allows an improved vessel visualization as compared with 1.5 T. Using high-resolution 3D TOF MRA at 3 T, also segments of the cerebral arteries located at the periphery can be detected.

2.3 Bacterial Infections of Brain Parenchyma: Pyogenic Cerebritis and Brain Abscess

A recommendation for the MR protocol is given in Table 4. Due to the high cellularity and increased viscosity of pus, the liquid core (abscess cavity) of abscesses typically shows high signal in DWI and corresponding low ADC values. In pyogenic as well as tuberculous abscesses diffusion is restricted within the wall and in the core of the abscess. On the contrary, in the core of necrotic brain tumors and metastases diffusion is mostly unrestricted, resulting in lower signal on DWI and high ADC values (Fig. 6d, e in "Pyogenic Cerebritis and Brain Abscess"); thus, DWI may be helpful in differentiating abscesses from other cystic brain lesions, but diffusion restriction is not specific and in the single case does not allow differentiation of abscesses from other cystic brain lesions. In some types of fungal abscesses, the cavity may show a trend toward an elevated diffusion with an increased ADC value. In the capsule of abscesses the rrCBV is lower compared with other enhancing brain lesions such as high-grade gliomas and metastases (Fig. 6g in "Pyogenic Cerebritis and Brain Abscess").

Typical findings in the liquid core of untreated brain abscesses in proton MRS include elevated Lip, Lac, and cytosolic amino acids (Fig. 6f in "Pyogenic Cerebritis and Brain Abscess"). With an extended echo time of 130 ms the lactate inverts and can thus be differentiated more easily from the lipid peaks.

The amino acids valine, leucine, and isoleucine (common peak at 0.9 ppm) are the end products of the degradation of proteins by macrophages in the pus. Succinate (2.4 ppm) and acetate (1.92 ppm) are found in anaerobic, but not in aerobic, brain abscesses, and thus, different spectroscopic patterns were demonstrated depending on whether there were predominantly anaerobe- (in addition to cytosolic amino-acids evidence of alanine and acetate, facultative presence of succinate) or aerobe (lack of alanine, acetate, and succinate)-caused abscesses; however, due to partial volume and susceptibility effects, the value of proton MRS is restricted in small lesions, especially in the periphery or near the skull base. In contrast to brain abscesses, in necrotic cerebral tumors only the resonance of lactate can be detected. In tuberculous abscesses only lipids and lactate can be detected.

Cerebritis is the earliest form of manifestation of a pyogenic cerebral infection and shows restricted water diffusion even before a definite formation of abscess; therefore, it can lead to a mix-up with the diagnosis of acute ischemia. In contrast to a higher-grade glioma, there is no hyperperfusion in abscesses. Application of MT sequences results in significantly stronger enhancement of inflammatory brain lesions following contrast injection. In addition, MT can be used to characterize the composition of cystic brain lesions. The MT ratio has been shown to correlate with the viscosity, total protein concentration, and cell density. In the wall of pyogenic abscesses the MTR is found to be higher as compared with tuberculous abscesses.

2.4 Bacterial Infections of Brain Parenchyma: Neurolues

Because neurolues may involve cerebral vessels with the consequence of stenoses and aneurysms, MRA should be performed.

2.5 Neurotuberculosis

A recommendation for the MR protocol is given in Table 4. In contrast to tuberculous abscesses, tuberculomas are mostly hypo- or isointense on T2-weighted images and show several lipid resonances in MRS. In diffusion weighted imaging the appearance of tuberculomas is quite variable typically without restricted diffusion. In contrast to bacterial abscesses tuberculous abscesses do not normally show amino-acid resonances and are often characterized by lipid resonances and a lactate peak. The MTR of abscess capsules are more significantly decreased in tuberculous abscesses than in pyogenic abscesses.

2.6 Viral Encephalitis

A recommendation for the MR protocol is given in Table 4. Several studies have demonstrated that DWI has a great value for the early detection of the disease when conventional T2-weighted or FLAIR images are still normal.

Progressive multifocal leukencephalopathy (PML) lesions show a significantly decreased tNAA as well as a considerable increase in lipid and lactate resonances. The choline and creatine peaks are moderately increased. Some study groups have already shown that the increase in myoinositol as an inflammatory marker positively correlates with the survival rate in PML. In the early stage SSPE shows an increase in myoinositol and choline in normal-appearing white matter, while tNAA is still normal. In later stages, the tNAA value decreases and the lactate and lipid resonances can be evidenced in the lesions which are at this stage also visible on MR imaging.

At an early stage of SSPE DTI reveals an increase in the MD and a decrease of the FA of the normal-appearing white matter in normal T2-weighted imaging.

The MT imaging may show differences between PML and HIV encephalitis: the MTR is significantly decreased in PML lesions relative to HIV encephalitis. In both PML and

HIV encephalitis a decreased MTR of the normal-appearing white matter is evidenced relative to normals.

2.7 Spongiforme Encephalopathies

A recommendation for the MR protocol is given in Table 4. In contrast to standard T2-weighted sequences, both PD-weighted and FLAIR images are more sensitive for visualizing signal changes of the basal ganglia and thalamus. The pulvinar sign, a hyperintensity of the posterior thalamic nuclei on T2-weighting, can be documented best using FLAIR sequences or DWI. For imaging distinctive signal features in sporadic or variant Creutzfeld-Jacob disease DWI is best suited to detect abnormalities of the cortex and basal ganglia. Spectroscopic examinations of the pulvinar sign demonstrate an increase in myoinositol in the posterior thalamic nuclei.

2.8 Fungal Infections

A recommendation for the MR protocol is given in Table 4. In the cavity, fungal abscesses have a tendency toward a higher ADC value in comparison with pyogenic abscesses; however, previous studies have also described a similar behavior of fungal and bacterial abscesses in DWI, so that diffusion alone does not provide a safe differentiation between bacterial and fungal abscesses. Spectroscopically fungal abscesses can show lipid and lactate resonances as well as amino-acid resonances so that spectroscopy does not allow a safe differentiation from pyogenic abscesses, either. The invasive cerebral aspergillomycosis can provide a broad variance of findings, mainly cerebritis and abscesses, but also quite often infarct areas and bleedings, which can be pathogenetically explained by the angioinvasivity of the aspergilli.

2.9 Parasitic Infections

A recommendation for the MR protocol is given in Table 4. By comparing conventional MR sequences for diagnosis of neurocysticercosis, FLAIR is most sensitive for detecting the scolex, while contrast-enhanced T1-weighted images most sensitively document the lesion volume. Using DWI pyogenic and tuberculous abscesses of neurocysticercosis can be well differentiated, as vesicular and also degenerative forms of neuocysticercosis normally have significantly higher ADC values relative to brain abscess. Using 3D-CISS images intraventricular vesicular lesions of neurocysticercosis can be better detected as compared with conventional T2-weighted spin-echo images.

A new, possibly promising approach for the detection of cisternal neurocysticercosis are FLAIR images before and after ventilation of 100 % oxygen: Oxygen ventilation leads to a relative hyperintensity of CSF and subsequently to a better differentiation of vesicular lesions of neurocysticercosis; however, systematic studies are still missing on this technique. A smaller MRS study revealed higher succinate concentrations and lower acetate concentrations in degenerative cysticerci as compared with abscesses caused by anaerobes.

Cerebral toxoplasmosis in association with AIDS normally shows circular-enhanced lesions on T1-weighted sequences after administration of contrast agent in the deeper nuclear regions and at the cortico-medullary border. On T2-weighted and FLAIR sequences multiple lesions often stand out with a hypointense ring and variable signal in the center in comparison with gray matter; however, contrast enhancement can be missing in pronounced immune deficiency such as AIDS or after immunosuppression after organ transplantation. Diffusion-weighted imaging of cerebral toxoplasmosis has mainly been performed for differentiating toxoplasmotic lesions from other entities such as lymphomas; however, there are no clear distinctive imaging features. Although lesions of toxoplasmosis tend toward a higher ADC value than cerebral lymphoma manifestations, there is a considerable overlapping area of ADC, which does not guarantee a safe diagnosis in daily clinical practice. Also, spectroscopically the differentiation between lymphoma and toxoplasmosis is difficult: Spectroscopically, a huge lipid peak is characteristic for toxoplasmosis, whereas the remaining metabolites can hardly be evidenced. Lymphomas also show a high lipid peak, which is, however, often less pronounced in comparison with toxoplasmosis. Few data, however, suggest that the rrCBV in lesions of toxoplasmosis is significantly lower than that in active lymphoma lesions.

2.10 Meningitis

A recommendation for the MR protocol is given in Table 4. Some studies could evidence the advantages of contrast-enhanced FLAIR sequences over conventional contrast-enhanced T1-weighted spin-echo sequences in the diagnosis of inflammatory meningeal diseases. A further approach is the delayed enhancement, i.e., the delayed sequence acquisition after administering a paramagnetic contrast agent: The sensitivity for the detection of meningeal thickening in the case of inflammation is higher on delayed scans as compared with scans which are acquired without time delay.

Using DTI, an increased FA of the meninges and the adjacent brain parenchyma has been detected in purulent neonatal meningitis. The DTI changes normalized under effective treatment. Using SPECT imaging generalized and local disturbances of the cerebral blood flow, which are closely connected to the clinical status of the patient, can be detected in patients with bacterial and viral meningitis.

2.11 Granulomatous Diseases

A recommendation for the MR protocol is given in Table 4.

References

Simon JH, Li D, Traboulsee A, Coyle PK, Arnold DL, Barkhof F, Frank JA, Grossman R, Paty DW, Radue EW, Wolinsky JS (2006) Standardized MR imaging protocol for multiple sclerosis: consortium of MS centers consensus guidelines. Am J Neuroradiol 27(2):455–461

Further Reading

Balashov KE, Aung LL, Dhib-Jalbut S, Keller IA (2011) Acute multiple sclerosis lesion: conversion of restricted diffusion due to vasogenic edema. J Neuroimaging 21(2):202–204

Baysal T, Dogan M, Karlidag R, Ozisik HI, Baysal O, Bulut T, Sarac K (2005) Diffusion-weighted imaging in chronic Behçet patients with and without neurological findings. Neuroradiol 47(6):431–437

Demaerel P, Van Hecke P, Van Oostende S, Baert AL, Jaeken J, Declercq PE, Eggermont E, Plets C (1994) Bacterial metabolism shown by magnetic resonance spectroscopy. Lancet 344(8931):1234–1235

Desprechins B, Stadnik T, Koerts G et al (1999) Use of diffusion-weighted MR imaging in differential diagnosis between intracerebral necrotic tumors and cerebral abscesses [see comments]. Am J Neuroradiol 20:1252–1257

Garaci FG, Colangelo V, Ludovici A, Gaudiello F, Marziali S, Centonze D, Boffa L, Simonetti G, Floris R (2007) A diffusion longitudinal MR imaging study in normal-appearing white matter in untreated relapsing-remitting multiple sclerosis. Am J Neuroradiol 28(3):475–478

Gonen O, Moriarty DM, Li BS, Babb JS, He J, Listerud J, Jacobs D, Markowitz CE, Grossman RI (2002) Relapsing-remitting multiple sclerosis and whole-brain N-acetylaspartate measurement: evidence for different clinical cohorts initial observations. Radiology 225(1):261–268

Gupta RK, Vatsal DK, Husain N, Chawla S, Prasad KN, Roy R, Kumar R, Jha D, Husain M (2001) Differentiation of tuberculous from pyogenic brain abscesses with in vivo proton MR spectroscopy and magnetization transfer MR imaging. Am J Neuroradiol 22(8):1503–1509

Hakyemez B, Erdogan C, Bolca N, Yildirim N, Gokalp G, Parlak M (2006) Evaluation of different cerebral mass lesions by perfusion-weighted MR imaging. J Magn Reson Imaging 24(4):817–824

Luthra G, Parihar A, Nath K, Jaiswal S, Prasad KN, Husain N, Husain M, Singh S, Behari S, Gupta RK (2007) Comparative evaluation of fungal, tubercular, and pyogenic brain abscesses with conventional and diffusion MR imaging and proton MR spectroscopy. Am J Neuroradiol 28(7):1332–1338

Mishra AM, Reddy SJ, Husain M, Behari S, Husain N, Prasad KN, Kumar S, Gupta RK (2006) Comparison of the magnetization transfer ratio and fluid-attenuated inversion recovery imaging signal intensity in differentiation of various cystic intracranial mass lesions and its correlation with biological parameters. J Magn Reson Imaging 24(1):52–56

Runge VM, Wells JW, Kirsch JE (1995) Magnetization transfer and high-dose contrast in early brain infection on magnetic resonance. Invest Radiol 30(3):135–143

Tortorella C, Viti B, Bozzali M, Sormani MP, Rizzo G, Gilardi MF, Comi G, Filippi M (2000) A magnetization transfer histogram study of normal-appearing brain tissue in MS. Neurology 54(1):186–193

White ML, Hadley WL, Zhang Y, Dogar MA (2007) Analysis of central nervous system vasculitis with diffusion-weighted imaging and apparent diffusion coefficient mapping of the normal-appearing brain. Am J Neuroradiol 28(5):933–937

Zeidler M, Sellar RJ, Collie DA, Knight R, Stewart G, Macleod MA, Ironside JW, Cousens S, Colchester AC, Hadley DM, Will RG (2000) The pulvinar sign on magnetic resonance imaging in variant Creutzfeldt-Jakob disease. Lancet 355(9213):1412–1418

Acronyms

2D	Two-dimensional
3D	Three-dimensional
9HPT	Nine-hole peg test
ACA	Anterior cerebral artery
ACTH	Adrenocorticotropic hormone
aCL	Anticardiolipin antibody
ACR	American College of Rheumatology
ADC	Apparent diffusion coefficient
ADEM	Acute demyelinating encephalomyelitis
AHEM	Acute hemorrhagic encephalomyelitis
AICA	Anterior inferior cerebellar artery
AIDS	Acquired immunodeficiency syndrome
ANA	Antinuclear antibody
ANCA	Antineutrophil cytoplasmic antibody
ARDS	Adult respiratory distress syndrome
ASVD	Atherosclerotic vascular disease
BA	Basilar artery
BBB	Blood-brain barrier
BCG	Bacille Calmette-Guérin
BSE	Bovine spongiform encephalopathy
CADASIL	Cerebral autosomal-dominant arteriopathy with subcortical infarcts and leukoencephalopathy
CD	Cluster of differentiation (cell surface molecule present on leukocytes)
CGA	Giant cell (temporal) arteritis
Cho	Choline
CSI	Clinically isolated syndrome (in the context of multiple sclerosis)
CISS	Constructive interference in steady state
CJD	Creutzfeldt-Jakob disease
CMV	Cytomegalovirus
CNS	Central nervous system
cPACNS	childhood PACNS
Cr	Total creatine (creatine phosphocreatine)
CRP	C-reactive protein
CSF	Cerebrospinal fluid
CT	Computed tomography or computed tomogram
CTA	Computed tomographic angiography
DD	Differential diagnosis
DLB	Dementia with Lewy bodies
DNA	Deoxyribonucleic acid
ds	Double stranded
DSA	Digital subtraction angiography
DTI	Diffusion tensor imaging

S. Hähnel (ed.), *Inflammatory Diseases of the Brain*, Medical Radiology. Diagnostic Imaging,
DOI: 10.1007/978-3-642-30520-7, © Springer-Verlag Berlin Heidelberg 2013

DWI	Diffusion-weighted MR imaging
EBV	Epstein Barr virus
EDSS	Expanded Disability Status Scale
EEG	Electroencephalography or Electroencephalogram
ELISA	Enzyme-linked immunosorbent assay
ENT	Ear-nose-throat
EP	Evoked potentials
EPI	Echo-planar imaging
ESR	Erythrocyte sedimentation rate
FA	Fractionized anisotropy
FOG	Fluorodeoxyglucose
FLAIR	Fluid-attenuated inversion recovery
FSE	Fast spin echo
FTAabs test	Absorption fluorescent treponema antibody test
FTY720	Fingolimode
GA	Glatiramer acetate
GCA	Giant cell (temporal) arteritis
Gd-DTPA	Gadolinium diethylenetriaminopentaacetic acid
Glx	Glutamate/glutamine quotient
GRE	Gradient echo
HE	Hematoxylin-eosin
HLA	Human Leukocyte Antigen
HIV	Human immunodeficiency virus
HSV	Herpes simplex virus
HU	Hounsfield unit
ICA	Internal carotid artery
Ig	Immunoglobulin
IL	Interleukin
ILR	Interleukin Receptor
INF	Interferon
IR	Inversion recovery
i.v.	Intravenous
IVIG	Intravenous immunoglobulin G
LA	Lupus anticoagulant
Lac	Lactate
LCM	Lymphocytic choriomeningitis
Lip	Lipids
LYH	Lymphocytic hypophysitis
M	Methionine (in the context of sCJD subtypes)
MBP	Myelin basic protein
MCA	Middle cerebral artery
MD	Mean diffusity
Mi	Myoinositol
MIP	Maximum intensity projection
MPR	Multiplanar reconstruction
MPRAGE	Magnetization prepared rapid acquisition gradient echo
MR	Magnetic resonance
MRA	Magnetic resonance angiography
MRI	Magnetic resonance imaging
MRS	Magnetic resonance spectroscopy or spectrogram
MS	Multiple sclerosis
MSFC	Multiple sclerosis functional composite
MT	Magnetization transfer

MTR	Magnetization transfer ratio
MTT	Mean transit time
NAA	N-acetyl aspartate
NAWM	Normal-appearing white matter
NMO	Neuromyelitis optica
PACNS	Primary angiitis of the CNS
PAME	Primary amoebic meningoencephalitis
PAN	Panarteritis nodosa or polyarteritis nodosa
PCA	Posterior cerebral artery
Pcom	Posterior communicating artery
PCR	Polymerase chain reaction
PD	Proton density
PDGF	Platelet-derived growth factor
PDL	Progressive diffuse leukoencephalopathy
PE	Plasma exchange
PerfMRI	Perfusion MRI
PET	Positron emission tomography
PML	Progressive multifocal leukencephalopathy
ppm	Parts per million
PPMS	Primary progressive multiple sclerosis
PR	Progressive-relapsing (in the context of multiple sclerosis)
PRES	Posterior reversible encephalopathy syndrome
PrP	Prion protein
PSWCs	Periodic sharp and slow wave complexes
PVL	Periventricular leukomalacia
RNA	Ribonucleic acid
ROI	Region of interest
rMTT	Relative middle transit time of the contrast medium
rrCBF	Relative regional cerebral blood flow
rrCBV	Relative regional cerebral blood volume
SAH	Subarachnoid hemorrhage MPR
RRMS	Relapsing–remitting multiple sclerosis
SAII	Subarachnoid hcmorrhagc
SAS	Subarachnoid space
Sc	Scrapie
sCJD	Sporadic Creutzfeldt-Jakob disease
SDH	Subdural hematoma
SLE	Systemic lupus erythematosus
SNR	Signal-to-noise ratio
SPECT	Single photon emission computed tomography
SPMS	Secondary progressive multiple sclerosis
SSPE	Subacute sclerosing panencephalitis
STEAM	Stimulated echo acquisition method
Suc	Succinate
SWI	Susceptibility-weighted image
T	Tesla
TB	Tuberculosis
TBM	Tuberculous meningitis
TBME	Tick-borne meningoencephalitis
Thl	T-helper 1 cells
Th2	T-helper 2 cells
THS	Tolosa-Hunt syndrome
TIA	Transient ischemic attacks

tNAA	Total NAA
tNAA	Total N-acetyl aspartate
TOF	Time of flight
TPHA test	*Treponema pallidum* hemaglutination test
TTP	Time to peak
USPIO	Ultrasmall paramagnetic particles of iron oxide
V	Valine (in the context of sCJD subtypes)
VA	Vertebral artery
vCJD	Variant Creutzfeldt-Jakob disease
VIBE	Volumetric interpolated breath-hold examination
VZV	*Varicella zoster* virus
WBC	White blood cell

Index

S. Hähnel (ed.), *Inflammatory Diseases of the Brain*, Medical Radiology. Diagnostic Imaging,
DOI: 10.1007/978-3-642-30520-7, © Springer-Verlag Berlin Heidelberg 2013